Second Edition

The Scientific Basis of Orthopaedics

Second Edition

The Scientific Basis of Orthopaedics

Edited by

James A. Albright, M.D.
Professor and Chairman
Department of Orthopaedic Surgery
Louisiana State University School of Medicine
Shreveport, Louisiana

Richard A. Brand, M.D.
Professor of Orthopaedic Surgery and Biomedical Engineering
Department of Orthopaedic Surgery
The University of Iowa
Iowa City, Iowa

Appleton &Lange
Norwalk, Connecticut/Los Altos, California

0-8385-8504-3

87 88 89 90 91 / 10 9 8 7 6 5 4 3 2 1

Prentice-Hall of Australia, Pty. Ltd., Sydney
Prentice-Hall Canada, Inc.
Prentice-Hall Hispanoamericana, S.A., Mexico
Prentice-Hall of India Private Limited, New Delhi
Prentice-Hall International (UK) Limited, London
Prentice-Hall of Japan, Inc., Tokyo
Prentice-Hall of Southeast Asia (Pte.) Ltd., Singapore
Whitehall Books Ltd., Wellington, New Zealand
Editora Prentice-Hall do Brasil Ltda., Rio de Janeiro

Library of Congress Cataloging-in-Publication Data

The Scientific basis of orthopaedics.

 Includes bibliographies and index.
 1. Orthopedia. 2. Musculoskeletal system.
I. Albright, James A.   II. Brand, Richard A. [DNLM:
1. Orthopedics. WE 168 S416]
RD732.S36 1987   617'.3   86-32031
ISBN 0-8385-8504-3

Design: M. Chandler Martylewski

PRINTED IN THE UNITED STATES OF AMERICA

To our wives,
Merrilee and Daryl

Contents

Contributors

James A. Albright, M.D.
Professor and Chairman
Department of Orthopaedic Surgery
Louisiana State University School of Medicine
Shreveport, Louisiana

William F. Blair, M.D.
Associate Professor of Orthopaedic Surgery
Division of Hand Surgery
Department of Orthopaedic Surgery
The University of Iowa
Iowa City, Iowa

Richard A. Brand, M.D.
Professor of Orthopaedic Surgery and Biomedical
    Engineering
Department of Orthopaedic Surgery
The University of Iowa
Iowa City, Iowa

Joseph A. Buckwalter, M.D.
Professor of Orthopaedic Surgery
Department of Orthopaedic Surgery
The University of Iowa
Iowa City, Iowa

O. Donald Chrisman, M.D.
Clinical Professor of Orthopaedic Surgery
Department of Orthopaedics and Rehabilitation
Yale University School of Medicine
New Haven, Connecticut

Reginald R. Cooper, M.D.
Professor and Chairman
Department of Orthopaedic Surgery
The University of Iowa
Iowa City, Iowa

Charles A. DiSabatino, M.D.
Associate Clinical Professor of Medicine
Department of Medicine
Yale University School of Medicine
New Haven, Connecticut

Charles C. Edwards, M.D.
Associate Professor of Surgery
Division of Orthopaedic Surgery
University of Maryland School of Medicine
Baltimore, Maryland

Stanley M. Elmore, M.D.
Attending Orthopaedic Surgeon
Chippenham Hospital
Johnston-Willis Hospital
Richmond, Virginia

Gary E. Friedlaender, M.D.
Professor and Chairman
Department of Orthopaedics and Rehabilitation
Yale University School of Medicine
New Haven, Connecticut

H. M. Frost, M.D.
Orthopaedic Surgeon
Southern Colorado Clinic
Pueblo, Colorado

John P. Fulkerson, M.D.
Associate Professor of Orthopaedic Surgery
Division of Orthopaedic Surgery
University of Connecticut School of Medicine
Farmington, Connecticut

Dennis P. Grogan, M.D.
Assistant Chief of Staff
Shriners Hospitals for Crippled Children
Assistant Professor of Orthopaedic Surgery
University of South Florida College of Medicine
Tampa, Florida

Peter Jokl, M.D.
Associate Clinical Professor
Department of Orthopaedics and Rehabilitation
Yale University School of Medicine
New Haven, Connecticut

Preface to First Edition

This book is the outgrowth of a series of basic science seminars for orthopaedic residents which was initiated in the early 1960s. The thrust of the seminars has been directed toward the attainment of a sound background in the underlying mechanisms controlling the musculoskeletal system, with an attempt to maintain relevancy without sacrificing content. To this end, undue concentration on topics beyond the realm of orthopaedic surgery has in most cases been avoided. At the same time, it has been considered equally important to resist the natural inclination of clinicians to focus on specific disease states rather than mechanisms. This precludes the inclusion of clinical syndromes or pathologic entities except when helpful to illustrate a point, since such material represents the end result of determinative processes rather than the processes themselves.

The underlying assumption behind the seminars has been that learning is an active process requiring the direct participation of the student. A lecture, paper, or chapter, regardless of how well presented, can supplement, but not supplant, the personal efforts of the learner. The material presented here has been sifted from an enormous body of information over a period of time. The central concepts of each subject have been presented without trying to exhaust the subject. We have specifically not attempted a complete review of relevant literature. Rather, it is intended to expose the student to the prevailing concepts of musculoskeletal function or dysfunction. The text attempts to translate numerous technical details into a form which will be of practical value. Unproven theories and points of controversy have been deemphasized. References will allow the interested reader to investigate further the various areas.

The majority of topics selected for inclusion constitutes a nucleus of subjects essential to a comprehensive grasp of orthopaedic surgery. Other topics, such as inflammation and immunology, have achieved increasing recognition in recent years and can be expected to assume a more important role in the future.

We feel that emphasis on the normal structure and function of the musculoskeletal system and on the mechanisms of its response to abnormal conditions (disease or injury) is essential to good clinical practice. Only by transmitting an appreciation of present concepts can we produce physicians who will ask the appropriate questions and improve the quality of medical care in the future.

James A. Albright
Richard A. Brand

Acknowledgments

The unseen force behind this effort has been Dr. Wayne O. Southwick who, as Chief of the Yale Orthopaedic Residency, established the underlying tone for all levels of Department activity. His contagious enthusiasm and enlightened concepts of graduate education have catalyzed innate scholarly interests in ever increasing numbers of students and residents. The editors and many of the contributors to this book are former students of his, who were actively encouraged to expand to their maximum potential. He has accomplished this by relying on a rarely found ability to stir latent talents. Once awakened, the attraction toward productive activity has invariably served as its own stimulus, guaranteeing its continuation beyond the end of formal training. Perhaps most important has been his genuine concern for individuals, together with a maturity that allows the student to grow beyond his mentor. Without such an environment, this book, which will never adequately reflect its background, would have remained an abstraction.

Additionally, we would like to acknowledge the following individuals:

Subrata Saha for reviewing the manuscript for Chapter 7 on the physical properties of bone.

John P. Albright, Roland Baron, Z. A. Ráliš, and Subrata Saha for contributing original and previously unpublished photographs.

James A. Arnold, A. Ascenzi, Stig Backman, A. Boyde, Dennis Carter, A. Chamay, Jonathan Cohen, Donald H. Enlow, and Irving Redlar for contributing original negatives or prints which otherwise could not have been reproduced satisfactorily.

Ruth Nolan and Rose Britton for spending many hours in typing of manuscripts.

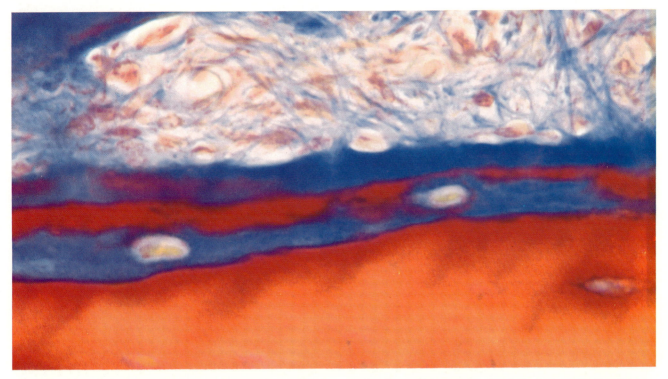

Figure 5–24. Ráliš' tetrachrome stain of a demineralized paraffin bone section. Bone which was mineralized prior to decalcification stains red and unmineralized osteoid stains blue. This section was taken from a patient with osteomalacia, so the osteoid, in contrast to normal osteoid tissue, is incompletely mineralized. This pathologic tissue, called "osteoid bone," is a mixture of patchy blue and red colors, sharply delineated against the normal mineralized red bone (about x 300). *(Contributed by Mr. Z. A. Ráliš.)*

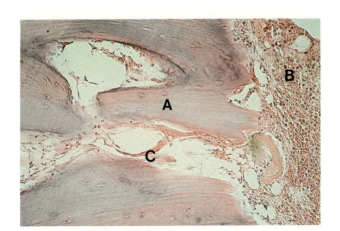

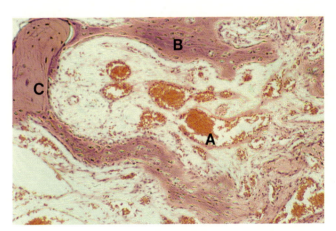

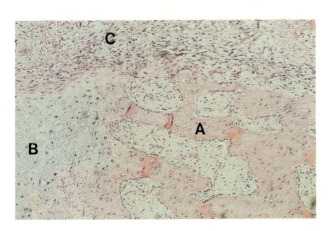

Figure 11–2. Top left: Inflammatory phase of fracture of human talus (3 days). Note dead bone (A) near fracture site, organizing hematoma containing inflammatory cells (B), and thrombosed blood vessel (C). **Top right:** Reparative phase of fracture of human ulna (19 days). Note abundant new capillaries (A) and new bone (B) laid down adjacent to old bone (C). **Bottom left:** Remodeling phase of fracture of human radius (48 days). Note mixture of new trabecular bone (A), cartilage (B), and periosteal fibroblastic tissue (C).

*Researchers have already cast much
darkness on the subject, and if they
continue their investigations, we shall
soon know nothing at all about it.*

Attributed to Mark Twain

Chapter 1

The Cells and Matrices of Skeletal Connective Tissues

Joseph A. Buckwalter and Reginald R. Cooper

If by some magic solution one could dissolve all the connective tissue of the body, all that would remain would be a mass of slimy epithelium, quivering muscle and frustrated nerve cells.

—Arcadi, 1952

SKELETAL CONNECTIVE TISSUES

Faced with learning matrix and cell biology, orthopaedists may respond that replacement or repair of cartilage, bone, ligament, or tendon requires technical skill and a sound sense of basic mechanics, not a knowledge of cells and matrices, and that these latter subjects are best left to the biologists. Failure to consider biologic phenomena, however, can lead to misinterpretation of diagnostic information, inappropriate surgical or medical interventions, and undesirable results of technically excellent and mechanically sound procedures. Equally important, future significant advances in the care of musculoskeletal problems will depend on increased knowledge of cell and matrix biology. Improved surgical techniques and applied bioengineering have changed the practice of orthopaedics through the development of microsurgery, internal fixation of the skeleton, replacement arthroplasty, arthroscopy, and new methods of correcting spinal deformity, but these advances have left the most fundamental questions unanswered. We still understand relatively little of the mechanisms of fracture and soft-tissue healing, the etiology of degenerative arthritis, the disturbances of growth and development of the skeleton, the underlying nature of congenital deformities such as clubfoot and congenital hip dislocation, and the cause of idiopathic scoliosis. Answers to these questions and ultimately improved treatment of musculoskeletal problems will come from increased understanding of the connective tissue cells and their matrices. In the words of Henry Mankin (1983), "future changes in Orthopaedics will be based in biology and more specifically in our ability to understand and alter its basic unit, the cell." To provide the basis for study of specific skeletal tissues and their properties, this chapter reviews the skeletal connective tissue cells and their matrices.

The term connective tissue (*Gewebe der Bindesubstanz*) comes from the work of the nineteenth-century histologists and pathologists. They were intrigued by the wide distribution of connective tissue and its role in binding the other tissues of the body together. Reichert, as reported by Virchow (1859), sought to prove that cartilage, periosteum, bone, tendons, and fascia formed a continuous mass, a basic tissue (*Gundgewebe*) or connective substance, extending throughout the body and that this tissue experiences certain specialized changes in different localities without altering its basic character. Before Virchow it was accepted that connective tissue consisted primarily of fibers, and many thought it was acellular. Reichert argued that folds in a homogenous substance produced the appearance of fibers, whereas Schwann felt that the fibers developed by splitting off from the cell body until only the nucleus remained. Virchow showed that direct splitting of cells into fibers did not occur and that intact cells existed in connective tissue. His histologic definition of connec-

tive tissue, "the greater part of the tissue is composed of intercellular substance, in which, at certain intervals cells lie embedded," remains unchanged.

The tissues of multicellular organisms depend on connective tissue for mechanical support; the lung, liver, kidney, and brain could not maintain their elaborate organization or the function of their parenchymal cells without a structural framework. Many forms of connective tissue are distributed throughout the body. Loose areolar connective tissue invests muscles, nerves, and vessel walls; dense irregular connective tissue forms the dermis, the fascia of muscles, the sclera of the eye, the coverings of the brain and spinal cord, and the capsules of glands and organs, and adipose tissue is found in the fat pads, subcutaneous tissues, and the bone marrow. A distinct group of connective tissues, the skeletal tissues, bone, cartilage, and dense fibrous tissue provide the remarkable strength and durability of the bony skeleton, the load-bearing and gliding surfaces of joints, and the fibrous tissue of ligament, joint capsule, and tendon that stabilizes joints and transmits muscle forces to bone. In skeletal connective tissues, densely packed collagen fibrils frequently form elaborate patterns specialized for their particular functions. Unlike the other tissues of the body, they lack a separate parenchymal component and they consist of relatively few cells in an abundant matrix.

Because the most obvious functions of skeletal connective tissue are mechanical, it is tempting to regard these tissues as homogeneous, inert, and passive, like plastic or metal. However, advances in connective tissue biology demonstrate that the skeletal connective tissues have elaborate molecular architecture that can change rapidly. Even in the mature skeleton these tissues remain metabolically active and responsive to hormonal, mechanical, electrical, and metabolic stimuli.

The skeletal connective tissues originate from a subdivision of embryonic mesenchyme. During embryonic development two morphologic and functional classes of tissues appear, epithelia and mesenchyme (Fig. 1–1). The term mesenchyme (Greek *mesos*, middle, and *enchyma*, infusion) was derived from the embryonic location of mesenchyme between the epithelial layers of endoderm and ectoderm. Epithelium may develop from endoderm, ectoderm, or mesoderm, but mesenchyme appears to develop only from mesoderm. Epithelia and mesenchyme are distinguished by the relationship of the cells to each other and the relationship of the cells to the matrix (Fig. 1–1). In epithelia the cells maintain close relationships with other cells, frequently linking themselves with specialized cell junctions and devoting a large portion of their cell membrane to contact with other cells. Basement membranes, a unique form of connective tissue matrix, frequently serve as a bed for epithelial cells and separate them from mesenchyme. In the mesenchyme that forms the skeletal tissues, the cells rarely establish contact with other cells and surround themselves with an extracellular matrix in which they migrate and proliferate. With development, undifferentiated mesenchymal cells can assume a variety of forms including blood, fat, and smooth muscle cells as well as the specialized connective tissue cells—fibroblasts, chondrocytes, osteoblasts, osteocytes,

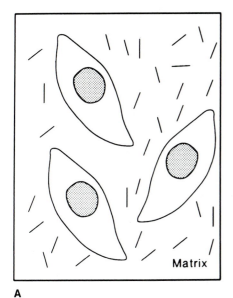

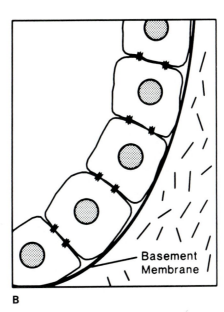

Figure 1-1. Diagrammatic representation of the differences between mesenchymal and epithelial tissues. **A.** Mesenchymal cells have little or no contact with other cells and are surrounded by an extracellular matrix. **B.** Epithelial cells establish and maintain close cell-to-cell contact and may rest on a basement membrane that separates them from mesenchymal tissue. Mesenchyme develops from the mesoderm; epithelium may arise from ectoderm, mesoderm, or endoderm.

and osteoclasts (Fig. 1–2). Cell differentiation creates a persistent, but not necessarily permanent, change in cell form and function. The differentiated form is stable in that it can persist through many generations of the cell. Since each somatic cell contains the entire genome, the complete set of genetic material, each cell can theoretically assume any form or function. During differentiation the genome remains constant, that is, no genetic information is lost, so cell differentiation requires that different cells express different parts of the genome. In any one cell only about 5 to 10 percent of the genes are active. These active genes can be grouped into "housekeeping" genes and "luxury" genes. Housekeeping genes maintain cells by directing synthesis of membranes, ribosomes, and mitochondria and must be active in all cells. Luxury genes are active in

differentiated cells and direct synthesis of the molecules that give the cells their special form and function (DeRobertis and DeRobertis, 1980). Various stimuli can activate specific luxury genes that induce cell differentiation, but once differentiation occurs, it persists even in the absence of the original stimulus. Even in the mature individual, some cells retain the ability to assume a different form. Fibroblasts and pericytes in particular have this ability and can develop into other types of cells given the appropriate stimuli (Fig. 1–2). Cell differentiation produces the variety of tissues necessary for the existence of complex organisms, but it also makes possible the survival of organisms following injury. Repair of injured tissue depends on the ability of cells to proliferate and maintain their special form, to differentiate into other specialized

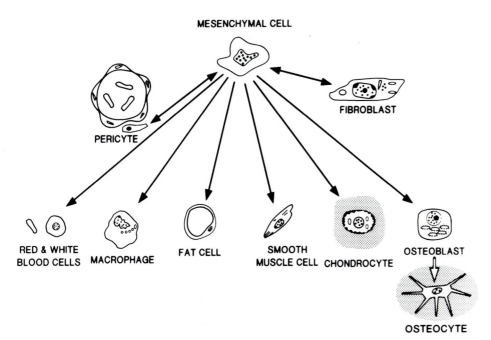

Figure 1-2. Diagrammatic representation of the differentiation of specialized connective tissue cells from undifferentiated mesenchymal cells. Even in mature skeletal tissue, pericytes, undifferentiated mesenchymal cells, and possibly fibroblasts retain the capacity to differentiate into other specialized connective tissue cells given an appropriate stimulus. Under certain circumstances other differentiated cells may dedifferentiate, migrate, and proliferate like the mesenchymal cells and then differentiate again.

forms or to dedifferentiate, and to regain their ability to migrate and proliferate rapidly and then differentiate into a specialized form again. For example, fracture healing usually depends on the differentiation of less-specialized cells into chondrocytes and osteoblasts. Even differentiated cells, however, may possess the capacity to assume another form and function.

The principle function of connective tissue cells is to produce and maintain the extracellular matrix. This matrix has made possible the organization and stability of multicellular organisms and thereby the evolution of complex forms of life. In particular, vertebrates benefit from the specialized matrices of the skeletal connective tissues, which give them unusual strength, mobility, and dexterity. All of the matrices have an elaborate structure consisting of complex macromolecules. These molecules may appear as the fibrils of collagen and elastin or as nonfibrillar matrix components including proteoglycans, structural glycoproteins, and the nonfibrillar collagens. Variations in the composition, properties, and arrangements of these macromolecules produce the different forms of the skeletal connective tissue matrices and reflect the function of the tissue. For example, the hyaline cartilage matrix, commonly subjected to compressive loads, has a high proteoglycan and water content and type II fibrillar collagen, whereas the tendon matrix, commonly subjected to tensile loads, has a lower proteoglycan and water content and type I fibrillar collagen.

The skeletal connective tissue matrices do not initially appear as cartilage, bone, or dense fibrous tissue. Like the mesenchymal cells, the mesenchymal matrix differentiates into distinct forms, and the differentiation of the matrix parallels the differentiation of the cells. In fact the development of specialized skeletal connective tissues requires simultaneous differentiation of cells and matrix and close interaction between them. During this process the matrix not only supports the cells mechanically, it also actively modifies cell behavior (Kosher and Church, 1975; Hay, 1981). Initially, mesenchymal matrix contains a large volume of water, and the macromolecular framework consists primarily of hyaluronate, a high molecular weight polysaccharide with sparse, loosely arranged collagen fibrils, usually type I. In this matrix the cells migrate freely and proliferate. Matrix differentiation begins with removal of much of the hyaluronate and loss of some water followed by the appearance of the definitive matrix macromolecules: a large concentration of type I collagen and tissue-specific proteoglycans and glycoproteins in bone and dense fibrous tissue or type II collagen, cartilage proteoglycans, and glycoproteins in hyaline cartilage.

THE CELL

The cell is the ultimate morphologic and functional unit of life. All living tissues consist of cells and cell products. Despite striking differences in form and function, cells share common biochemical composition and metabolic processes. Mechanical forces, electrical currents, nutritional and hormonal manipulations, drugs, and radiation change living tissues by acting through the cell or the cell matrix. With the ability to understand and direct cell function lies the potential for effective treatment of almost any disease or injury. The validity of these statements seems obvious, but their acceptance is surprisingly recent.

Cells have been studied for over 300 years; however, the past five decades have brought great changes in our concepts of the cell and the development of the science of cell and matrix biology. Robert Hooke in 1665, using lens systems considered crude by modern standards, examined the microscopic structure of cork and saw walls surrounding what appeared to be empty spaces. Because of their resemblance to clusters of small rooms, he labeled them cells, a misnomer in the etymologic sense (Latin *cella*, hollow space); nonetheless, the term cell has persisted. Van Leeuwenhoek in 1674, studying cells free in fluid, noted some internal structure (Dobele, 1960). In 1838 Schleiden, a botanist, and in 1839 Schwann, a zoologist, advanced the "cell theory" that all living beings consist of cells and cell products (DeRobertis and DeRobertis, 1980). Schwann believed that the intercellular matrix was the source of new cells. Rudolf Virchow in 1859 added the revolutionary concept that all cells necessarily derive from preexisting cells and that, rather than being the source of cells, the intercellular matrix is dependent on the cells, any given area of matrix being ruled over by a cell. From about the time of Virchow until 40 or 50 years ago, the view of the cell as simply a nucleated mass of more or less amorphous proteoplasm recurred with monotonous regularity from one textbook to the next. This perpetuated the mistaken concept that the cell constitutes a fixed structural building block in which complex chemical reactions of life occur. Two developments dramatically altered this concept and established the inseparability of cell structure and function:

1. Increased resolving power (i.e., the ability to separate two closely positioned points and see them as two instead of one) of instrumental analysis (x-ray diffraction, electron microscopy) allowed detailed examination of cells, cell organelles, and extracellular matrices.
2. Collapse of artificial barriers between previously separate disciplines (histology, histochemistry, electron microscopy, immunology, biochemistry, physiology, genetics, biophysics). The information generated by the combined efforts of researchers using techniques from all relevant fields provided an understanding of cell structure and function that would otherwise be impossible.

The current concept of the cell (Fig. 1–3) portrays these diverse self-regulating separate units as sharing certain common functions and structures. At a minimum cells reproduce, transform energy, and synthesize molecules. They must contain at least a cell membrane, genetic material, and the necessary machinery for protein synthesis. Within these broad limits cells vary greatly and acquire almost unlimited special structures and functions. All animal cells resemble each other, however, in possessing a

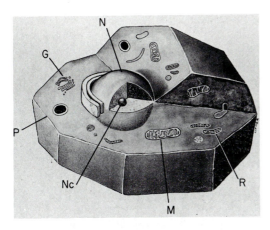

Figure 1-3. Diagrammatic representation of the cell showing the distinct structural and functional units (organelles): nucleus (N), nucleolus (NC), plasma membrane (P), mitochondria (M), rough-surfaced endoplasmic reticulum (R), and Golgi zone (G).

Structure

General

Size. Cell size varies over a broad range. The cells of some pleuropneumonialike organisms (PPLO) have a diameter of 0.1 μm, red blood cells have a diameter of 7.0 μm, and certain bird eggs may have a diameter of several centimeters. In humans, nerve and muscle cells may be as long as 1 ft. Cells of a specific type usually do not vary much in size. The size range of cells may depend upon physical requirements for cell metabolism. A unit smaller than 0.1 μm possibly prohibits the specialized structural parts necessary to maintain life. Conversely, larger distances might prevent the rapid diffusion of metabolites and nutrients necessary to maintain cellular metabolism.

Shape. Cell shape varies with cell function, external forces, cell wall structure, viscosity, and surface tension. The extracellular environment can alter cell shape, and these modifications may affect cell function. For example, Folkman and colleagues (1978, 1980) found that, for cultured cells, round cells stop making deoxyribonucleic acid (DNA), flatter cells have a high rate of DNA synthesis and proliferation, and taller cells require more growth factor to stimulate proliferation. Many intact cells assume a polyhedral form, but most animal cells are not rigid; they actively change their shape given the appropriate stimulus. Their ability to change their shape, however, may be limited by their extracellular matrix as in bone or cartilage. In fluids or in large masses, cells obey laws of minimal surface and often assume a round shape or become tetrakaidecahedrons (14-sided) (DeRobertis and DeRobertis, 1980).

Subcellular Components. Although structural segregation at the subcellular level provides a necessary, efficient, and effective functional division, the cell retains its identity as the unit of life by virtue of its ability to control and integrate the metabolic reactions of its organelles. Related enzymes involved in a given metabolic pathway cluster in membranes of the appropriate organelle, thus isolating specific reactions from each other. Organelles are not constant cell components. They differ in number and form from cell to cell and can differ in the same cell from one moment to the next depending on the needs and functions of the cell.

Membranes. In considering the essential parts common to all cells, logic dictates an initial review of biologic membranes. These sheetlike structures enclose the cell (plasma membrane) and the nucleus (nuclear membrane) and form most organelles. Without membranes cells could not exist, and even slight damage to the plasma membrane may cause cell malfunction or death. Equally serious consequences result from damage to the membranes of lysosomes and mitochondria. In addition to separating the cell from its environment, the plasma membrane acts as a receptor mechanism for the cell. Special receptor sites on

membrane-bound nucleus and distinct subcellular organelles (Brochet and Mirsky, 1961). To understand cell structure and function, we must examine these organelles and include a study of the composition, shape, aggregation states, and interrelationships of macromolecules. Study of cells, their organelles, and their molecules, however, is not sufficient. Recently we have learned that understanding cell form, size, migration, proliferation, metabolism, synthetic function, differentiation, and aging require full consideration of the extracellular matrix (Hay, 1981). Formerly the matrix was viewed as an inert, almost randomly arranged macromolecular framework created by the cells for their structural support. It is now clear that cells continuously interact with the matrix and that matrix composition and organization powerfully influence cell function. The cell membrane is intimately associated, structurally and functionally, with the matrix macromolecules so that, in a sense, drawing the boundary between cell and matrix at the membrane is artificial and promotes the misconception that connective tissue cells can be fully understood as units isolated from their matrix.

Because of distinct functional specializations, bone, cartilage, and dense fibrous tissue cells differ from each other and from other cells in shape, structure, and appearance; however, they are, first and foremost, cells. As such, they share the fundamental characteristics and metabolic processes common to all cells. An initial examination of cell composition, structure, and function provides the background for an analysis of specialized skeletal connective tissue cells to see how they represent adaptations of these common patterns.

Composition

Despite their diversity all cells consist of water, ions, and cellular macromolecules: proteins, carbohydrates, lipids, and nucleic acids. Water forms about 75 percent of most cells, protein 15 percent, lipid 2 to 3 percent, and carbohydrate 1 percent.

the plasma membrane interact with specific hormones and release internal messengers that influence cell function. The membrane also senses mechanical deformation and the ion fluxes produced by electrical fields and thereby makes possible the cellular response to these stimuli. Membranes consist largely of lipid and protein in varying ratios from 25 to 75 percent lipid. Lipid averages about 40 percent by weight (Siekevitz, 1970). Most animal cell membranes contain less than 1 percent carbohydrate. Particular configurations of lipids, proteins, and carbohydrates form the cell's antigenic markers and thus its immunologic identity. Membranes share several common properties. They are freely permeable to water and neutral lipophilic molecules, less permeable to polar (charged) molecules, and slightly permeable to polar ions. They maintain an electrical gradient, keeping the cell interior electrically negative relative to the exterior, and they have a high electrical resistance (Lehninger, 1975).

Because of common characteristics and composition that is lipid and protein, Danielli and Davson in 1935 postulated that all membranes share a common structure. They proposed that membranes consist of a bimolecular lipid layer sandwiched between two protein layers. By high-resolution electron microscopy, membranes frequently appear as two dense lines each about 1.5 nm thick separated by a 5.0 nm electron-lucent region. This electron microscopic image led Robertson (1959) to propose the "unit membrane hypothesis" along the lines of the Danielli–Davson model. This portrays membranes as a continuous bilayer of mixed polar lipids, with the nonpolar hydrocarbon chains projecting toward the midportion of the membrane and the polar ends outward, each surface of the lipid bilayer being covered by a monomolecular layer of protein, and perhaps some carbohydrate ionically linked to the lipid (Fig. 1–4). According to this model the electron-dense layers represent protein and the lucent middle layer, lipid. This would indeed maximize the interaction of the charged portion of the lipid molecule with water and minimize contact of the hydrophobic hydrocarbon chains with water (Fig. 1–5). Many doubt the universal validity of this model, and the electron microscopic image may be artifactual. In fact, much recent evi-

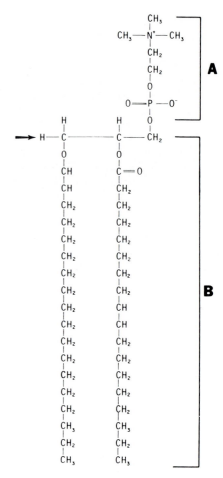

Figure 1-5. Structure of a phospholipid (phosphatidylcholine) showing the polar head **(A)** and nonpolar tails consisting of fatty acids esterified to glycerol (arrow).

dence supports a modification (Siekevitz, 1970; Lehninger, 1975) of the model. Lipids in membranes probably do form lipid bilayers. Various proteins seem, however, to occupy a variety of positions in relation to the lipids (Fig. 1–6). Some lie on the external surface only, some on the inter-

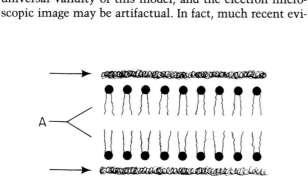

Figure 1-4. Diagrammatic representation of the unit membrane hypothesis, which suggests that all membranes consist of a bimolecular layer of lipids **(A)**, with the hydrophilic polar heads pointing toward the membrane surfaces and the hydrophobic nonpolar tails pointing toward each other. These are covered by a monolayer of protein (arrows) with attached carbohydrate. This model fits well with the typical trilaminar electron microscopic image of membranes.

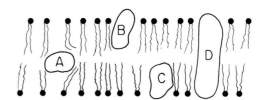

Figure 1-6. The modified unit membrane hypothesis, or fluid mosaic model, suggests that various proteins in membranes distribute themselves in **(A)**, on the external surface **(B)**, on the internal surface **(C)**, and across **(D)** the membrane. Molecules in membranes probably move with respect to each other, and the entire membrane also moves. Extracellular matrix molecules, especially glycoproteins, associate with specific membrane molecules.

nal surface, and some penetrate the thickness of the membrane. The most widely accepted model of membrane structure, the fluid mosaic model (DeRobertis and DeRobertis, 1980), accounts for these proteins. This model proposes that membrane lipids form a bilayer, but that the lipid and protein components arrange themselves in a mosaic pattern and that these components are not fixed. The fluidity of the membranes in this model implies that the lipids and proteins have considerable freedom of movement within the bilayer.

Membranes in different sites, mitochondrial membranes versus nuclear membranes, for example, differ slightly in composition and serve markedly different functions. They can do this and still retain similar structural features by varying the relative content and types of lipid and protein. More saturation of the lipid hydrocarbon chains provides more rigidity. Some unsaturation produces the fluidity necessary for membranes to function in transmitting metabolites. Many proteins in biologic membranes serve as highly specific enzymes for metabolic reactions. Variation in the protein content therefore provides diverse functional capabilities in different membranes.

Whatever the exact configuration of cell membranes, they contain literally thousands of vitally important enzymes, and most functions of cells occur on, in, or through membranes. They regulate ion and molecular transport, osmotic pressure, electrical potential, protein synthesis, energy transmission, phagocytosis, growth, cell division, and fluid transport.

Nucleus. The size and the ready absorption of basic dyes, resulting from the nucleic acid content, make the cell nucleus easily visible by light microscopy. Through its roles in cell replication and in directing protein synthesis the nucleus controls cell structure and activity. It can not function, however, without the appropriate cytoplasmic environment. Events in the cytoplasm help control the performance of the nucleus, and the cytoplasm along with the cytoplasmic organelles make possible the expression of the genetic material contained within the nucleus.

Nuclei differ in size and form in different classes of cells, but all cell nuclei share certain common features. The cell nucleus is surrounded by a double-layered nuclear membrane or nuclear envelope containing nuclear pores about 0.05 μm in diameter, some of which are covered with septa. The outer nuclear membrane is frequently studded with ribonucleoprotein (RNP) granules or ribosomes. The nucleus in the somatic cells of humans contains the diploid number of 46 chromosomes in which resides DNA. DNA acts as the repository of genetic information and directs cell activity. It does not exist in a free form, however, but rather as a complex with basic proteins called histones, nonhistone (more acidic) proteins, and RNA. This complex, called chromatin, condenses at the time of cell division to form chromosomes.

Nucleolus. Nucleoli may also be seen by light microscopy. They appear as dense granules within the nucleus and contain primarily protein and RNA with a small amount of DNA. Their size varies with the synthetic activity of the cell: they are large in synthetically active cells and smaller or absent in cells with limited or absent synthetic function. Nucleoli synthesize ribosomal RNA and assemble ribosomes. Ribosomes consist of roughly equal amounts of ribosomal RNA and protein. Genes in the nucleolus direct synthesis of most of the ribosomal RNA, and chromosomes outside of the nucleolus synthesize some ribosomal RNA. Ribosomal proteins are synthesized in the cytoplasm, migrate to the nucleolus, and combine with RNA to form ribosomes. The ribosomes then travel back into the cytoplasm to assume their function of protein synthesis.

Ribosomes. Ribosomes, complex cellular organelles consisting of 52 proteins and three RNA molecules (DeRobertis and DeRobertis, 1980), make possible protein synthesis. Ribosomes can only synthesize proteins at a limited rate. Cells thus differ in their number of ribosomes, usually in relation to their need for protein synthesis. For example, osteoblasts actively engaged in the synthesis of osteoid fill much of their cytoplasm with ribosomes. When the same cell becomes an osteocyte, the ribosomes almost disappear. Ribosomes may be membrane bound or free in the cytoplasm.

Rough-surfaced Endoplasmic Reticulum. This intracytoplasmic organelle, described by Claude et al. (1945) consists of membranes folded into stacks, tubules, vacuoles, and cisternae. The outer surface of these membranes is studded with ribosomes. The rough-surfaced endoplasmic reticulum concerns itself mainly with the production of protein for export from the cell or for transport to another site within the cell. Messenger RNA attaches to the ribosomes, transfer RNA matches amino acids to the genetic code of the messenger RNA, and the growing chain of amino acids passes into the lumen of the endoplasmic reticulum.

Polyribosomes. Free cytoplasmic ribosomes described by Palade (1955) or those collected into groups attached to molecules of mRNA (polyribosomes) exist in the cytoplasm without attachment to membranes or other structures. These free ribosomes and polysomes probably synthesize protein for intracellular use.

Smooth-surfaced Endoplasmic Reticulum. Smooth endoplasmic reticulum consists of membranes arranged primarily in tubular and vesicular forms and usually is associated with the Golgi complex. The most common function of the smooth endoplasmic reticulum is synthesis of lipids and sterols. The mechanisms of lipid production, in contrast to those for proteins, are poorly understood.

Golgi Apparatus. This organelle, usually located in a juxtanuclear position, consists of smooth-surfaced membranes folded into layers of tubules, vesicles, and vacuoles (Golgi, 1898). Usually the Golgi membranes take the form of flattened disk-shaped cisternae that have associated secretory vesicles on one side. Its functions remain incompletely elucidated. Among other activities, the Golgi zone concentrates and packages protein and lipids, links carbohydrates to protein (Godman and Lane, 1964), and secretes macromolecules from the cell. Many proteins are thus synthesized in the rough endoplasmic reticulum and transported to the Golgi membranes where carbohydrates are added. Virtually every macromolecule exits from the cell via the Golgi apparatus (Revel and Hay, 1963; DeRobertis and DeRobertis, 1980) (see Fig. 1–34).

Mitochondria. Mitochondria recover energy from nutrients that enter the cell and convert it into the high-energy phosphate bond of adenosine triphosphate (Lehninger, 1961, 1964). Mitochondria thus transduce chemical energy contained in foodstuffs into a form that the cell can use. Mitochondria contain DNA and ribosomes and are capable of protein synthesis. Mitochondria may be so numerous that they fill a large portion of the cell as in osteoclasts, or they may be rare as in chondrocytes. They can assume many forms including spheres, lamellae, and tubes. Their numbers may rapidly increase or decrease in response to the needs of the cell, and they can divide and unite within the cell. These 1- to 7-μm organelles consist of an outer membrane and an inner membrane (Lehninger, 1964). The inner membrane infolds into numerous cristae mitochondriales. This arrangement increases the surface area for metabolic reaction.

Centrioles. These organelles consist of cylinders 150 nm in diameter and 300 to 500 nm in length. Centrioles exist in pairs, each of which consists of nine sets of three tubules. They usually lie in a juxtanuclear position and function to organize microtubules during the formation of the mitotic spindle. They also serve as the attachment point for cilia in those cells that contain these structures.

Lysosomes. These single membrane-bound, 0.2- to 0.5-μm packets contain hydrolytic enzymes that become active in a mildly acidic environment (DeDuve, 1958, 1963). These enzymes include collagenase, acid phosphatase, cathepsins, sulfatase, and glycuronidase. They destroy worn-out cell parts and materials brought into the cell by phagocytosis. Excreted hydrolytic enzymes destroy extracellular components such as collagen and mucopolysaccharides.

Microfilaments. Cells have a cytoplasmic skeleton consisting of microfilaments and microtubules that gives them their form and mobility. Filaments 4 to 5 nm in diameter, more or less randomly arranged, pervade the cytoplasm of most cells and serve along with microtubules as a cytoskeleton. They appear to be the motile part of the cytoskeleton, providing a contractile system that allows the cell to move and change shape.

Microtubules. These tubules, 0.02 to 0.03 μm in diameter, occur in all cells. They form the centrioles and serve as part of the cytoskeleton determining the shape of the cell. Their role in determining cell shape may be especially important during differentiation. They are also associated with the transport of molecules, granules, and vesicles within the cell, with cell movement, and possibly in cellular sensory transduction.

Function

General Cell Functions. Despite obvious variations in form, location, differentiation, and response to stimuli, all cells share certain necessary functions. One can group the most important reactions in cells into three easily remembered functions that distinguish cells from inanimate objects (Lehninger, 1975).

1. Replication
2. Synthesis of biomolecules—nucleic acids, proteins, carbohydrates, lipids
3. Energy transformation—transducing the chemical energy in foodstuffs to synthesize molecules, replicate, and perform work

Fortunately, we now have methods to measure these functions, and these methods have been applied to skeletal connective tissue cells. By dealing with these three characteristics, we can see how skeletal connective tissue cells are specialized variations on the main theme of all cells.

Cell Replication. The hereditary determinants, or genes, which in the cells of higher organisms form part of the structure of chromosomes, ultimately control cell form and all cell activities. The chemical material of genes, DNA, contains encoded within it all genetic information. Although DNA was discovered in 1869 by Miescher (quoted by Lehninger, 1975), it was not implicated as having much, if any, genetic potential until 1943 when Avery et al. (1944) observed permanent and heritable changes in cell function by altering DNA.

DNA consists of two unbranched chains arranged in a double helix, a structure delineated by Watson and Crick in 1953 (Fig. 1–7). The backbone of the chain contains alternate molecules of a five-carbon sugar, deoxyribose (Fig. 1–8), connected by phosphate molecules that act as bridges between carbon number 3 and number 5 in adjacent sugar molecules. Bonded to either sugar moiety, one of four nitrogenous bases extends toward the opposite chain in the DNA molecule. These four bases consist of two purines (adenine and guanine) and two pyrimidines (thymidine and cytosine). The unit, consisting of sugar, phosphate, and one of the nitrogenous bases, is called a nucleotide. DNA may therefore be defined as a polynucleotide chain. The two

Figure 1-7. Scheme of DNA structure consisting of a double helix. The backbone of each strand consists of alternate sugar (S) (deoxyribose) and phosphate (P) groups. Strands are joined by hydrogen bonds between nitrogenous bases (A, T, C, G).

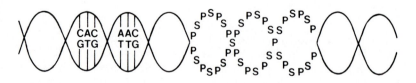

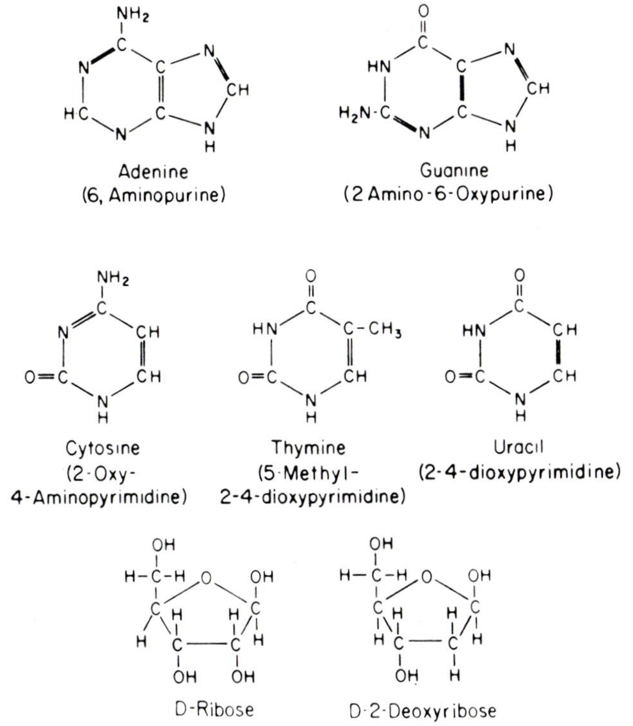

Adenine
(6, Aminopurine)

Guanine
(2 Amino-6-Oxypurine)

Cytosine
(2-Oxy-
4-Aminopyrimidine)

Thymine
(5-Methyl-
2-4-dioxypyrimidine)

Uracil
(2-4-dioxypyrimidine)

D-Ribose

D-2-Deoxyribose

Figure 1-8. Structural formulas of components of DNA and RNA. Deoxyribose is the sugar component of DNA, and ribose is the sugar component of RNA.

chains link with each other by joining the nitrogenous bases of one chain with those of the other chain through hydrogen bonds. Companion bases (those bases linked to each other) are never identical (i.e., adenine is never linked to adenine) but are always complementary (i.e., the same two bases are always linked to each other in the chain). Adenine always joins thymine and guanine always joins cytosine.

DNA, closely bound to proteins (histones and nonhistone proteins) and RNA, is divided among the chro-

mosomes in the nucleus. Chromosomes consist of chromatin, which contains about 30 percent DNA, 5 percent ribonucleic acid (RNA), 36 percent histones, and 28 percent nonhistone proteins (DeRobertis and DeRobertis, 1980). The full complement of genetic information for all cell activities and all characteristics is encoded in the DNA of every cell. This code depends upon the sequence of bases forming the nucleotide units. The preservation and expression of the information depends on three processes: (1) replication, the exact reproduction of DNA before cell division; (2) transcription, production of a copy (message) of a DNA segment (gene) concerned with coding for one polypeptide chain; (3) translation, changing the base sequence in the message into a polypeptide chain (protein), with an amino acid sequence corresponding exactly to that ordered by the genetic message as determined by the nitrogenous base sequence in the gene.

DNA must be faithfully reproduced each time a cell divides and must be transmitted exactly (with the bases in the sequence identical in the new DNA and in the original) to the daughter cells. Before the encoded information can be used, it must be transcribed in the nucleus in a manner that allows it to be transmitted to the cytoplasm. This encoded message must then be translated to be used during protein production.

Before cell division, DNA must be replicated with great fidelity so that one complete set of genetic instructions can be transmitted to each daughter cell. This replication takes place by an unwinding and splitting of the DNA strands (Fig. 1–9). In turn, the cell produces a new complementary DNA strand adjacent to each of the original strands, which serve as templates—a mechanism called semiconservative replication by Meselson and Stahl (1958). The base sequence in the original DNA molecule thereby becomes duplicated exactly. A complete set of genetic instructions can then be transmitted to each daughter cell. The term semiconservative replication denotes that half of the DNA received by each daughter cell originally resided in the mother cell nuclear DNA and the other half was formed just prior to cell mitosis. This proc-

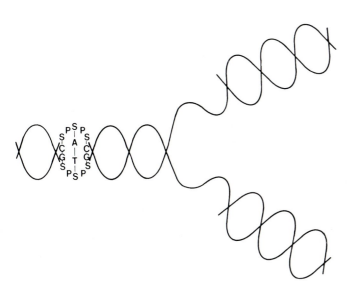

Figure 1-9. DNA replication involves an unwinding of the double helix. Each strand then serves as a template against which a new strand of DNA forms, with the nitrogenous base sequence exactly as it was in the original DNA molecule. In this way, genetic continuity is preserved and transmitted from one cell to another through countless generations. Transmission of the wrong sequence would constitute a genetic mutation. Flow of genetic information from one DNA molecule to a newly formed molecule by the template mechanism is called replication.

ess of replication requires an enzymatic mechanism, elucidated by Kornberg (1969), which ranks among the most remarkable known. The complex geometry, mechanics, and kinetics involved in unwinding the DNA helix, replicating it, and rewinding it maintains genetic continuity over billions of generations.

This replication of DNA before cell division provides an opportunity to find cells that are about to divide. Tritiated thymidine, a radioactive tracer, is incorporated into replicating DNA and labels these cells. The tracer subsequently goes with the DNA into cells derived from the originally labeled ones.

Synthesis of Biomolecules. Proteins constitute some of the most important biomolecules produced by cells. A protein contains one or more amino acid chains called polypeptides. Twenty common amino acids form nearly all proteins. An amino acid (Fig. 1–10A) is an organic acid whose alpha carbon contains an amino group, and one of its hydrogen atoms is substituted by one of several aliphatic or aromatic chains. This chain alone determines the differences between the 20 amino acids. A protein, or polypeptide chain, consists of amino acids joined by peptide linkages (Fig. 1–10B). A protein whose molecular weight exceeds 50,000 daltons usually contains more than one polypeptide chain.

A polypeptide chain or a protein can be viewed as a long word written in a language of 20 letters (the 20 amino acids). The number of amino acids in a polypeptide chain ranges from about 100 to 1800 (usually 100 to 300). The number and sequence of amino acids in the chain determine the primary structure of the protein. This primary structure makes each protein species unique. No two proteins or polypeptide chains contain exactly the same number and same sequence of amino acids. For this reason, there can be hundreds of thousands of different proteins in the human body. The primary structure in turn determines the way in which the polypeptide chain arranges itself in space, that is, how the chains loop and bond with themselves and to other chains. This native conformation (secondary and tertiary structure), specific for each protein, determines how the protein functions biologically. If the chains unfold (denature), biologic specificity ceases. Proteins have two major functions. They act as structural proteins comprising parts of a cell or the intercellular matrix, and they act as biologic regulators such as hormones or enzymes, which catalyze nearly all biologic reactions inside or outside the cell.

As noted, the genetic information to direct the production of a protein depends upon the base sequence in DNA. The central problem of genetics is how a four-letter alphabet (the base sequence in DNA) is transcribed, taken to the cytoplasm, and there translated into the 20-letter alphabet of amino acids in a polypeptide chain.

A specific segment of the DNA strand, called a gene or cistron, regulates the production of one polypeptide chain. Human cells contain about 1 million genes. The sequence of nucleotides in a gene bears a linear correspondence to the sequence of amino acids in the polypeptide chain of the specific protein for which the gene codes.

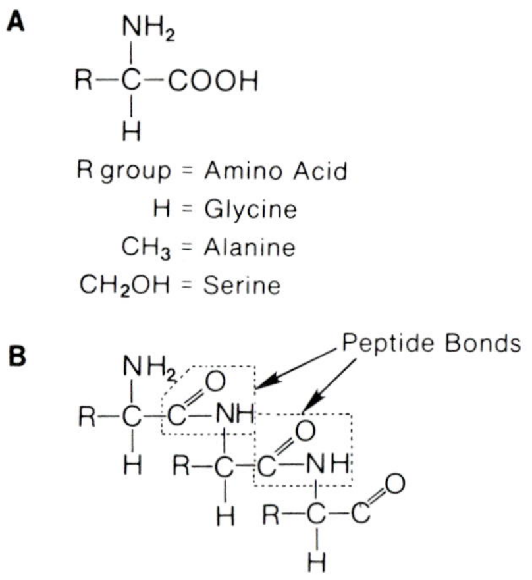

Figure 1–10. A. Chemical structure common to all alpha amino acids. **B.** Mechanism wherein amino acids join each other by peptide bonds to form polypeptide chains (proteins).

Each group of three nitrogenous bases (called a codon) along the DNA strand within the gene codes for one amino acid. Nirenberg and Mathali (1961) and Nirenberg and Leder (1964) performed fundamental research leading to the discovery of the code words (three-base sequences) for each of the 20 amino acids. During protein synthesis, to send a copy of the genetic message out of the nucleus, DNA again temporarily splits in the region of that gene containing the unique code for the specific protein. The DNA strand then serves as a template for the production of a copy of the code. This copy (Fig. 1–11), called messenger RNA (mRNA) by Jacob and Monod (1961), codes for a specific amino acid sequence needed to make a particular protein. Unlike DNA, mRNA contains ribose as its sugar instead of deoxyribose (see Fig. 1–8). Instead of thymidine, it contains a closely related nitrogenous base, uracil (see Fig. 1–8). In its other aspects, its structure resembles a single strand of a DNA molecule. The base sequence in mRNA is complementary to the base sequence in the DNA that acted as its template. Messenger RNA leaves the nucleus and moves to ribosomes in the cytoplasm, either those on the rough-surfaced endoplasmic reticulum, those remaining as free ribosomes, or those in polyribosomes (Fig. 1–12). Here, mRNA serves as a template for the sequential ordering of amino acids. Ribosomes bring together various components necessary for protein production: mRNA, transfer RNA, and amino acids. At the ribosomal site, mRNA acts as a template where amino acids assemble in the appropriate sequence and numbers to form a given polypeptide chain. Amino

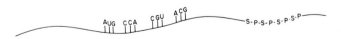

Figure 1–11. Diagram of mRNA made against the template in a region of DNA that codes for a specific polypeptide chain (gene). Transfer of genetic information from DNA to RNA is called transcription. In some RNA-containing viruses transcription may be reversed and information can flow from RNA to DNA, that is, RNA can be transcribed into DNA.

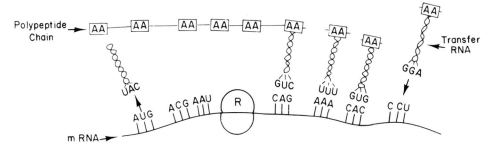

Figure 1-12. Messenger RNA (mRNA) moving along the ribosome in the cytoplasm where the genetic message in the codons (the three bases that signify one amino acid) is read. A transfer RNA specific for each amino acid carries the activated amino acid from the cell cytoplasm to insert it at the appropriate place in the growing polypeptide chain as directed by the codons on mRNA. Transfer RNA can recognize the appropriate codon for its amino acid, and therefore the amino acids in the polypeptide chain align in a linear sequence directed by mRNA. The transfer of genetic information from RNA to protein is called translation, or simply protein synthesis. This process cannot be reversed.

acids in the cytoplasm must first be activated by a specific enzyme and adenosine triphosphate. They then become attached to a specific transfer RNA, delineated by Zamecnik (1960), that brings the amino acid to the mRNA attached to ribosomes (ribonucleoprotein [RNP] granules). Transfer RNA has the ability to read the three-base genetic code on mRNA and insert its amino acid at the appropriate site in the growing polypeptide chain (Fig. 1-12). Amino acids then link by peptide bonds (see Fig. 1-10B). This process continues until the polypeptide chain terminates when all of the code on the mRNA has been used.

Obviously, any one cell uses only part of the total pool of genetic information available in nuclear DNA (the genome). Cell differentiation therefore depends upon the selection of a specific set of genes that controls the production of a specific set of proteins. A temporary activation of specified genes leads in turn to the temporary production of a certain protein. This is called cell modulation. If, on the other hand, certain genes become persistently activated, the result is cell differentiation. Determinants of which genes any cell uses seem to be factors that combine with regulator genes to turn on and off structural genes that code for various proteins. Much speculation has arisen, and much research has attempted to determine the exact nature of factors that influence regulator genes. These may include specific molecules, ions, pH changes, inductor substances, oxygen tension, piezoelectricity, or mechanical stress. In many instances, simple cell metabolites probably act on regulator genes through a negative feedback mechanism.

Radioactive tracers can be used to monitor metabolic processes in the cell and to follow protein exported from the cell. Histochemical techniques also determine the localization of enzymes used inside or outside the cell during the production of protein. Radioactive tracers (tritiated uridine) are incorporated into mRNA and thereby indirectly provide evidence of protein production.

Energy Transformation. Cells require a continual input of energy to perform the active transport of the ions and molecules necessary to sustain life, the synthesis of macro-

molecules, and specialized functions like cell movement, phagocytosis, and bone resorption. Most energy in human cells comes from the breakdown of glucose in a series of stages by one of several pathways that eventually transmit the stored energy to adenosine triphosphate (ATP) (Fig. 1-13). This convenient biomolecule stores energy in high-energy phosphate bonds. These serve as the universal cellular energy currency. The anaerobic glycolytic, or Embden-Meyerhof, pathway breaks down glucose from a six-carbon molecule into two three-carbon fragments, either pyruvate or lactate (Fig. 1-13A). The hexose monophosphate shunt serves as an alternate anaerobic pathway. After the process reaches this point, lactate may diffuse from the cell, go to the liver and be converted to glycogen, be converted to glycogen within the cell, or in the presence of oxygen, go back to pyruvate.

To metabolize pyruvate further and obtain the rest of the stored energy requires oxygen, an aerobic cycle (Fig. 1-13B). The first part of this, the familiar citric acid (or Krebs') cycle, is coupled to the cytochrome oxidase and electron transport system wherein energy-rich ATP is pro-

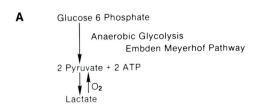

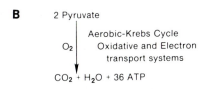

Figure 1-13. Pathways for energy production in cells. **A.** Anaerobic metabolism. **B.** Aerobic metabolism.

duced. These cycles can be studied by histochemical stains for enzymes used in the cycle or by using C-14–labeled glucose and tracing it into the by-products of each cycle. Bone, even in the presence of oxygen, metabolizes some of its glucose anaerobically. All bone cells have the enzymes necessary for anaerobic glycolysis. They all contain citric acid cycle and cytochrome oxidase enzymes in the mitochondria. Total enzyme activity is usually highest in osteoclasts, next highest in osteoblasts, and lowest in osteocytes (Fulmer, 1966).

Specialized Cell Functions. In addition to these three general functions common to all cell types, some cells perform highly specialized tasks. For example, nerve cells transmit electrical impulses, muscle cells contract, fat cells store large quantities of lipid, and red blood cells carry oxygen. In the skeletal tissues, cells also have specialized functions. Osteoblasts synthesize the organic matrix of bone and may help control the mineralization of osteoid, chondrocytes synthesize the cartilage matrix and may help control the mineralization of cartilage in growth plate, and osteoclasts resorb bone. Fibroblasts, chondrocytes, and osteoblasts not only have special abilities to synthesize large volumes of extracellular matrix macromolecules, they

probably also influence the organization of these macromolecules into the matrix.

SPECIALIZED CONNECTIVE TISSUE CELLS

The specialized cells of skeletal connective tissues are identified by their morphology, location, and function. They are usually classified as fibroblasts, chondrocytes, and bone cells. In bone, undifferentiated cells, osteoblasts, osteocytes, and osteoclasts can be identified.

Fibroblasts

Fibroblasts usually assume a spindle or flattened shape and have an unspecialized cell membrane, and in dense fibrous tissue they may have long cytoplasmic processes. They have a single nucleus, and when active, they contain a large volume of endoplasmic reticulum and prominent Golgi membranes. Less active fibroblasts tend to have more modest amounts of endoplasmic reticulum and Golgi membranes. In skeletal tissue, fibroblasts form the predominant cells of dense fibrous tissues: ligament, tendon, and joint capsules. In these tissues the cytoplasmic processes of fibroblasts extend for long distances as they weave

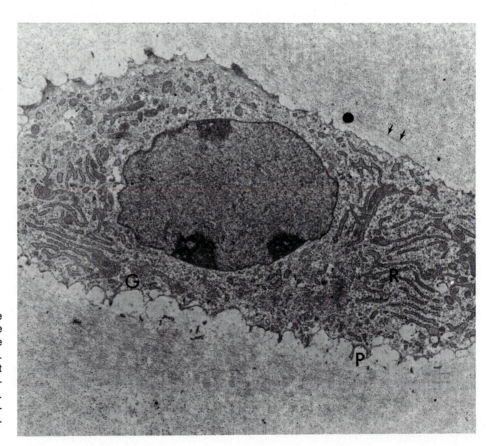

Figure 1-14. A chondrocyte whose nucleus contains three dense nucleoli. The cell surface has numerous cell processes (P). The cytoplasm contains abundant rough-surfaced endoplasmic reticulum (R) and Golgi vesicles (G). The matrix contains collagen fibrils (arrows). (Original magnification × 12,000.)

between the dense collagen bundles. Fibroblasts synthesize the matrix macromolecules of dense fibrous tissue including collagen, elastin, proteoglycan, and noncollagenous matrix proteins.

Chondrocytes

Cartilage cells lie in lacunae. Their size, shape, and ultrastructural features vary as a reflection of their function and metabolism. Chondrocytes tend to assume a spherical shape, or in the growth plate, a disk shape. The cell surface tends to be irregular because of relatively short cell processes. Active cells contain abundant rough-surfaced endoplasmic reticulum and prominent Golgi vesicles (Fig. 1–14). These contain precipitates of various sizes and shapes. At times, Golgi vacuoles merge with the plasma membrane and open onto the cell surface. Radioactive tracer studies demonstrate conclusively the role of chondrocytes in production of matrix collagen and protein polysaccha-

rides. Protein is produced in the rough-surfaced endoplasmic reticulum, moves to the Golgi zone where sugars and sulfates are added, and then exits from the cell (Godman and Lane, 1964; Revel and Hay, 1963).

Undifferentiated Cell of Bone

If tritiated thymidine is administered to an experimental animal and bone is examined within one hour, nearly all of the label remains in nuclei of undifferentiated mesenchymal cells (osteoprogenitor cells) adjacent to vessels and not yet directly applied to the surface of newly forming osteoid or bone. Only a few osteoblasts incorporate the tracers. With increasing time after the injection, the label is found, although to a lesser degree, in osteoblasts and osteoclasts. With further time, it permeates osteocytes. This indicates that cells in bone can arise from undifferentiated mesenchymal cells.

These cells lie close to vessel walls (Fig. 1–15). They

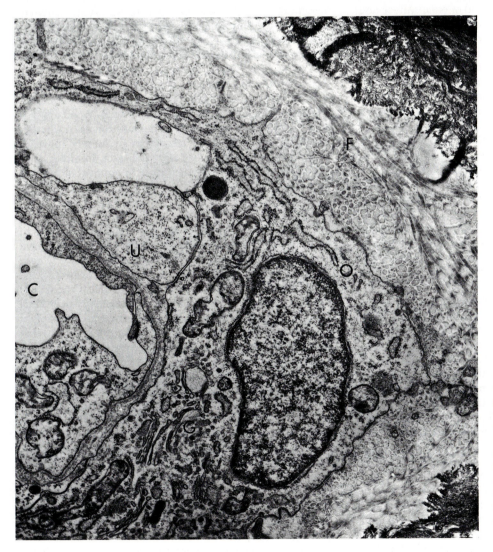

Figure 1–15. An undifferentiated cell (U) containing many cytoplasmic filaments lying adjacent to a bone capillary (C). The cell (O), probably a young osteoblast, contains a well-developed Golgi zone (G). Osteoid collagen fibrils (F) form layers and bone mineral deposits in this matrix, noted in the upper right corner. (Original magnification × 14,600.) *(Reprinted, by permission, from Cooper et al. 1966.)*

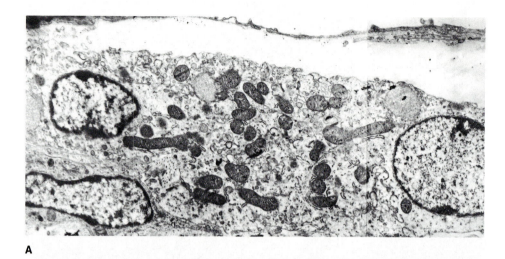

A

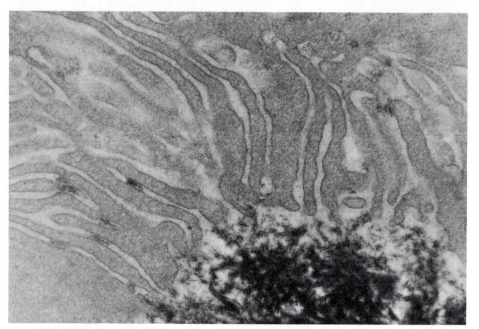

Figure 1-17. A. Cell body of multinucleated osteoclast containing numerous mitochondria with dense granules. Note the paucity of rough-surfaced endoplasmic reticulum. (Original magnification × 5700.) **B.** The brush border of an osteoclast consists of numerous cytoplasmic processes between which lie many bone crystals and collagen fibril fragments. (Original magnification × 15,000.) *(Reprinted, by permission, from Cooper et al.: 1966.)*

B

and at times contact processes from other osteocytes. Some specialized contact zones (tight junctions) have been found between bone cell processes (Cooper, et al. 1966). The osteocyte processes in canaliculi permeate the mineralized bone matrix. These processes, 0.08 to 0.10 μm in diameter, occupy about three fourths of the canalicular diameter. They contain dense granules and vesicles.

The extremely small bone matrix crystals (about 0.04 μm by 0.004 μm) have a surface area of about 100 m²/g, or a total of 100 acres in the adult human body (McLean and Urist, 1955). Most crystals lie deeply buried in bone, and cellular action would be necessary to tear them down and transfer the mineral into the extracellular fluid. This obviously could not account for the immediate exchange between serum calcium, extracellular fluid calcium, and bone. Haversian canals and lacunar walls form a large sur-

face area of bone crystals exposed to extracellular fluid. Canalicular walls with their small diameter constitute another vast surface area of about 3000 m² in the adult human body (Robinson, 1964). One cannot ignore the implication that such an interface between bone crystals and extracellular fluid by its very magnitude must have numerous physiologic functions. Osteocytes lie in an ideal position to monitor minute-to-minute, second-to-second calcium exchange between bone mineral and the extracellular fluid. This in turn leads to an exchange with serum calcium. This is of critical importance because the serum calcium–ion concentration is one of the most closely monitored concentrations in the human body because of its vital role in maintenance of cell functions that include cell membrane transport, muscle contraction, nerve irritability, and other processes that maintain life.

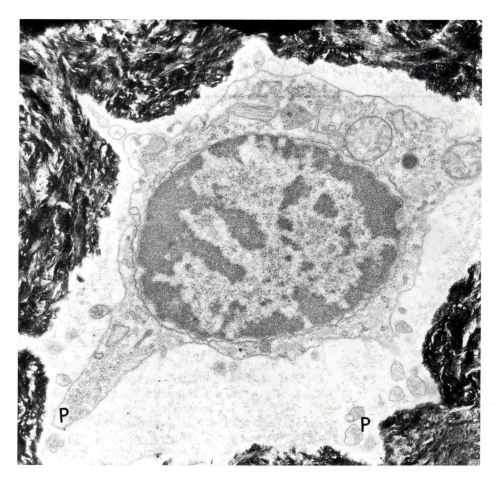

Figure 1-18. An osteocyte in its lacuna. This cell has a rather large nuclear-to-cytoplasmic ratio. The cytoplasm contains mitochondria, some rough-surfaced endoplasmic reticulum, and free RNA particles. Numerous cytoplasmic processes (P) leave the cell, cross the lacuna, and leave by way of canaliculi. (Original magnification × 16,200.) *(Reprinted, by permission, from Cooper et al.: 1966.)*

THE EXTRACELLULAR MATRICES

The matrix gives connective tissue its mechanical properties: tensile strength, stiffness, resiliency, and cohesiveness. Cells bind to the matrix and thereby to other cells; the matrix protects the cells and allows them to maintain the organization of complex tissues like growth plate and bone. Despite its formless or irregular appearance the matrix possesses a complex internal organization of macromolecules. This macromolecular framework holds fluid within the matrix yet allows diffusion of water, ions, and small molecules. Variation in the arrangement and amounts of the macromolecules and their relationship to the tissue fluid produce the profound differences in the different forms of skeletal connective tissue.

Composition

The matrix consists of tissue fluid, an organic molecular framework, and in bone, an inorganic matrix. The amount of tissue fluid differs in bone, tendon, and cartilage as shown in Figure 1–19. Hyaline cartilage has a relatively high water content, which contributes to its stiffness to compression, resiliency, and its ability to participate in joint lubrication. Dense fibrous tissues have less water, but their state of hydration still influences their mechan-

ical properties; bone has the least proportion of water. Since the matrices of connective tissues are not surrounded by membranes, the interaction of the water with the matrix molecules holds it within the matrix and controls its passage through the matrix.

Variations in the organic macromolecular framework give the connective tissues their special forms and properties. This framework consists of four classes of macromolecules: collagens, elastic fibers, proteoglycans, and structural glycoproteins. A high proteoglycan content (Fig. 1–19), the presence of type II collagen, a small protein called chondronectin, and possibly other molecules distinguish hyaline cartilage from the other tissues. Fibrocartilage and bone have similar organic matrices: high concentrations of type I collagen and small concentrations of proteoglycan. Connective tissue cells synthesize all four types of macromolecules from amino acids and carbohydrates. Variation in the amounts and arrangement of amino acids and carbohydrates creates the differences in these macromolecules.

The inorganic matrix found in bone and calcified cartilage consists of relatively insoluble calcium phosphate deposited in and around the collagen fibrils. In bone the inorganic matrix contributes the major share of the tissue (Fig. 1–19).

Procollagen

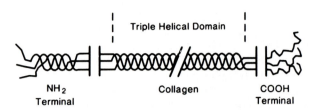

Figure 1–22. Diagrammatic representation of procollagen. At least two enzymes help convert procollagen to collagen: one enzyme to remove the NH₂-terminal peptide and the other to remove the COOH-terminal peptide.

They also have decreased levels of the enzymes necessary to convert procollagen to collagen. In animals with dermatosparaxis, minor trauma causes large sloughing wounds. Would infection and sepsis frequently cause death. These animals lack the enzyme necessary to cleave the terminal peptides from procollagen. Tropocollagen itself consists primarily of the triple helical region with 1000 amino acids per alpha chain. The rodlike form of the triple helix gives it great rigidity and strength (Fig. 1–22). The helical form places most of the peptide bonds within the helix, making them more resistant to attack by proteolytic enzymes. The nonhelical regions constitute only about 20 amino acids or 5 percent of the molecule, but they are the site of hydroxylysine cross-links that tend to stabilize the molecule. With time, cross-links form both within and between collagen molecules, strengthening and stabilizing the fibrils. The intramolecular cross-links derive from the lysine side chain. The extent of cross-linking varies with the function and age of the tissue. Stiffer tissues appear to be more highly cross-linked, whereas the more flexible tissues are less so. The importance of collagen cross-linking for matrix integrity is illustrated by the effects of β-aminoproprionitril, an agent that interferes with the cross-linking of collagen. Animals treated with this drug have extremely fragile connective tissue matrices, and develop skeletal deformities as well as dissecting aneurysms of the aorta.

Collagen is not a single type of molecule but rather a closely related family of molecules. At least ten distinct forms of collagen exist that differ in the amino acid composition of their alpha chains (Fig. 1–23) and thus must be coded for by different genes. The form and location of these collagens divides them into fibrillar interstitial collagens and nonfibrillar collagens. The nonfibrillar collagens may lie in close proximity to cells, may help form the external skeleton of the cell, and participate in the formation of the basement membranes. These collagens appear to form network or matlike structures rather than fibrils. Other nonfibrillar collagens may help organize and stabilize the extracellular matrix. Of the fibrillar collagens, type I is the most common and is found in skeletal connective tissues that resist tensile loads including tendon, ligament, joint capsule, and bone. Type II collagen has a higher hydroxylysine content, a higher degree of glycosylation, and smaller collagen fibrils. Type II is found in tissues with a high water and proteoglycan content that usually resist compressive loads; it forms the fibrillar matrix of hyaline cartilage and nucleus pulposus.

Elastic Fibers. Elastic fibers form the second fibrous component of the connective tissue extracellular matrix. Unlike collagen, they are not found in every tissue, but they can form a significant functional part of some tissue matrices such as elastic arteries, skin, and ligamentum flavum. Elastic fibers contribute relatively little to the macromolecular framework of skeletal connective tissue—less than 1 percent of the dry weight, with the exception of elastic cartilages and some ligaments like the nuchal ligament and ligamentum flavum (see Fig. 1–19). Elastic fibers in skeletal connective tissue tend to be cylindrical and lie parallel to the collagen fibrils (Fig. 1–24). They provide some tensile strength, though less than that of collagen. Their most distinctive property, unlike collagen or other mammalian proteins, is the ability to be deformed and then regain their original size and shape. Because of their relatively small amount, their contribution to most skeletal connective tissues remains uncertain.

Elastic fibers consist of two components: the protein elastin and a fibrillar glycoprotein. Elastin constitutes

Figure 1–23. A list of five collagen types divided into the interstitial fibrillar collagens and the pericellular basement membrane collagens. These collagens differ in amino acid composition, glycosylation, form, location, and function. Only five of the described collagens are shown.

COLLAGEN TYPES

INTERSTITIAL

Type	α Chains	Native Polymer	Distribution	Hydroxylysine Content Residues/1000	Carbohydrate Content % hydroxylysine glycosylated
I.	$[\alpha 1(I)]_2 \alpha 2$	Fibril	Skin. Tendon. Bone. Meniscus. Annulus	6 - 8	< 20
II.	$[\alpha 1(II)]_3$	Fibril	Hyaline Cartilage, Nucleus Pulposus. Vitreous Body	20 - 25	50
III.	$[\alpha 1(III)]_3$	Fibril	Skin. Blood Vessels. Granulation Tissue. Reticulin Fibers	6 - 8	15 - 20

PERICELLULAR & BASEMENT MEMBRANE

IV.	$[\alpha 1(IV)]_2$	Basement Lamina	Kidney Glomeruli. Lens Capsule	60 - 70	80
V.	$\alpha A(\alpha B)_2$ $(\alpha A)_3$ $(\alpha B)_3$	Unknown	Cell Surface. Pericellular Matrix	?	?

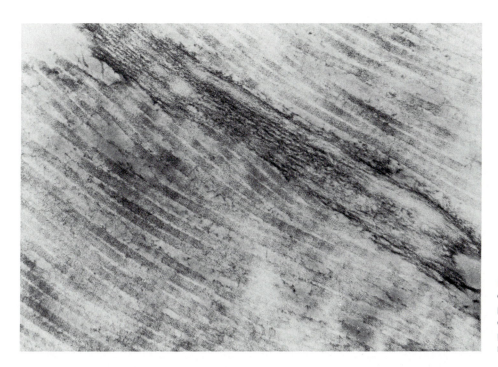

Figure 1-24. Electron micrograph of an immature elastic fiber lying parallel to collagen fibrils. The elastic fiber has fibrillar and amorphous components. (Original magnification × 16,000.)

more than 90 percent of the mature elastic fiber and has an amorphous appearance with electron microscopy. Microfibrils consist primarily of protein but do have some attached carbohydrates, although their exact structure remains unknown. Elastin has a unique composition. As in collagen, glycine contributes approximately one third of the amino acids, although not in a regular repeating sequence, and elastin is rich in proline. Unlike collagen, alanine forms a large part of the elastin molecules, and elastin has no hydroxylysine and little hydroxyproline. Two amino acids, desmosine and isodesmosine, synthe-

sized from four lysines, are found only in elastin and provide a distinctive marker.

The synthesis and formation of elastic fibers follows a complex sequence (Fig. 1–25). The cell synthesizes long chains of amino acids and forms them into an elastin precursor called tropoelastin. Tropoelastin contains no desmosine and less lysine than elastin. The cell secretes tropoelastin, and most of the elastin lysine residues condense to form cross-links creating the elastin macromolecule. Outside the cell elastin first appears among bundles of microfibrils. The amorphous component of the elastic

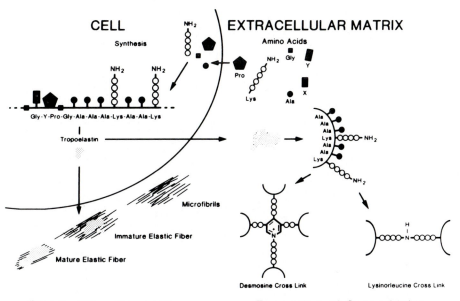

Elastic Fiber Formation   **Formation of Cross Links**

Figure 1-25. Diagrammatic representation of the synthesis of elastin and elastic fiber formation. The critical elastin cross-links form from lysine. Immature elastic fibers consist entirely of microfibrils. The amorphous elastin accumulates in the regions of these microfibrils, forming more and more of the fiber until the mature elastic fiber consists almost entirely of elastin.

fiber, elastin, increases until only remnants of the micro-fibrils can be seen. The microfibrils appear to be synthesized separately from elastin and are not an elastin precursor. Their function may be to help align the tropoelastin molecules precisely for cross-linking, thus serving as a scaffolding for the deposition and alignment of elastin.

Proteoglycans. Proteoglycans form the major macromolecule of the connective tissue ground substance. They form a significant portion of the hyaline cartilage matrix and make a much smaller contribution to bone and dense connective tissue (see Fig. 1–19). The composition and structure of cartilage proteoglycans have been well defined (Buckwalter and Rosenberg, 1982; Hascall and Hascall, 1981), but the less abundant bone and dense fibrous tissue proteoglycans have not been studied as extensively. Bone (Fisher et al., 1983) and dense fibrous tissue proteoglycans (Roughley et al., 1981) share their basic pattern with cartilage proteoglycans but have definite differences in size, form, and composition. Tissue-specific proteoglycans thus exist and may have different functions in different tissues. Unlike the fibrillar components of the connective tissue matrix, proteoglycans consist primarily of carbohydrate. In hyaline cartilage they contribute to the stiffness of the tissue to compression and to its resiliency. They also help maintain the hydration of the tissue and control the diffusion of ions and other molecules through the matrix. In the growth plate they may influence mineralization of the matrix.

Proteoglycans consist of about 95 percent polysaccharide and 5 percent protein. Unlike the formation of collagen from tropocollagen, proteoglycans are not assembled from identical subunits, rather their components vary in

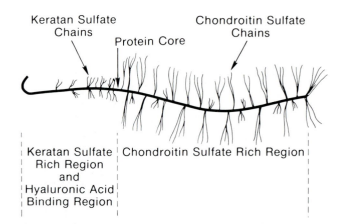

Figure 1–26. Diagrammatic representation of a cartilage proteoglycan subunit. Chondroitin sulfate and keratan sulfate chains are covalently bound to a protein core. The hyaluronic acid-binding region, the keratan sulfate-rich region, and the chondroitin sulfate-rich region form the three domains of the protein core. (*From Buckwalter JA: Articular cartilage. In: American Academy of Orthopaedic Surgeons: Instructional course lectures, Vol. XXXII, St. Louis, C. V. Mosby, 1983, with permission.*)

size and composition. They may be considered on two levels of organization: subunits, or monomers, and aggregates. The subunit is the basic unit of the cartilage proteoglycan; it cannot be reduced to smaller units without disruption of covalent bonds. It consists of a thin protein core with multiple covalently bound glycosaminoglycan chains (Fig. 1–26). The protein core and the glycosaminoglycan chains can be demonstrated by electron microscopy (Fig. 1–27). The protein core has three distinct

Figure 1–27. Electron micrograph showing the structure of a proteoglycan subunit in which the central filament represents the protein core and the projecting side arms consist primarily of chondroitin sulfate. (Original magnification × 60,000.) (*From Buckwalter JA: Articular cartilage. In: American Academy of Orthopaedic Surgeons: Instructional course lectures, Vol. XXXII, St. Louis, C. V. Mosby, 1983, with permission.*)

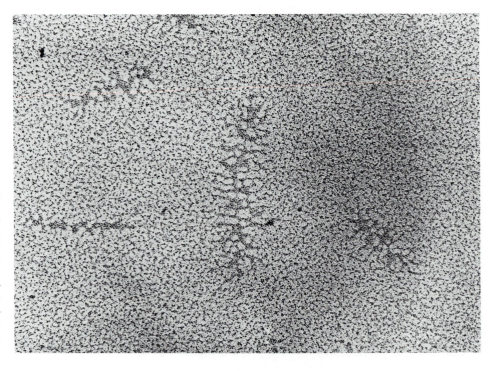

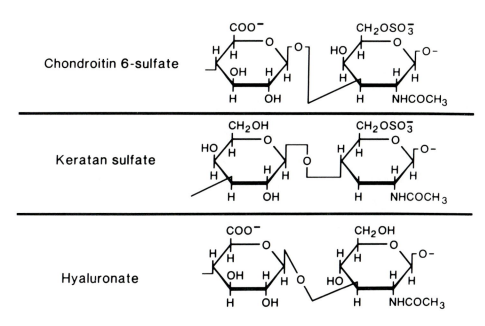

Figure 1-28. Diagrammatic representation of the structures of the glycosaminoglycans, chondroitin sulfate, keratan sulfate, and hyaluronate. Chondroitin sulfate has two negative changes per disaccharide, and others have one.

regions: a small globular hyaluronic acid–binding region, a keratan sulfate–rich region, and a chondroitin sulfate–rich region. The chondroitin sulfate–rich region of the protein core varies considerably in length and is believed to be responsible for most of the variability in proteoglycan composition and size. The glycosaminoglycans (chondroitin sulfate, keratan sulfate, and hyaluronic acid) consist of repeating disaccharide units of amino sugars (Fig. 1–28). Because the sugars contain carboxylate and sulfate groups, the molecules create long chains of negative charges. These negative charges tend to repel one another, thus holding the molecules extended in solution. This space-filling property allows them to occupy a volume of solution more than 50 times their dry weight. They also bind counterions and help retain water within the tissue. These properties may be important in providing articular cartilage with stiffness to compression, resiliency, and the abil-

ity to participate in joint lubrication. Loads applied to the tissue drive water from the domain of these proteoglycan molecules, forcing the negatively charged chains closer together, increasing their tendency to repel each other, and thus increasing the resistance to further compression (Fig. 1–29). Release of the pressure may allow the tissue fluid to return to the proteoglycan molecular domain and thus restore the tissue to its previous form.

Proteoglycan aggregates consist of long hyaluronic acid filaments associated with multiple subunits (Fig. 1–30). Electron microscopy shows their hyaluronate filaments and attached subunits (Fig. 1–31). Link proteins are small proteins of 40,000- to 50,000-molecular weight that spontaneously associate with both hyaluronic acid and proteoglycan subunits. The link proteins appear to stabilize the aggregates and may help direct their assembly. Aggregates form in the matrix and may have a role in

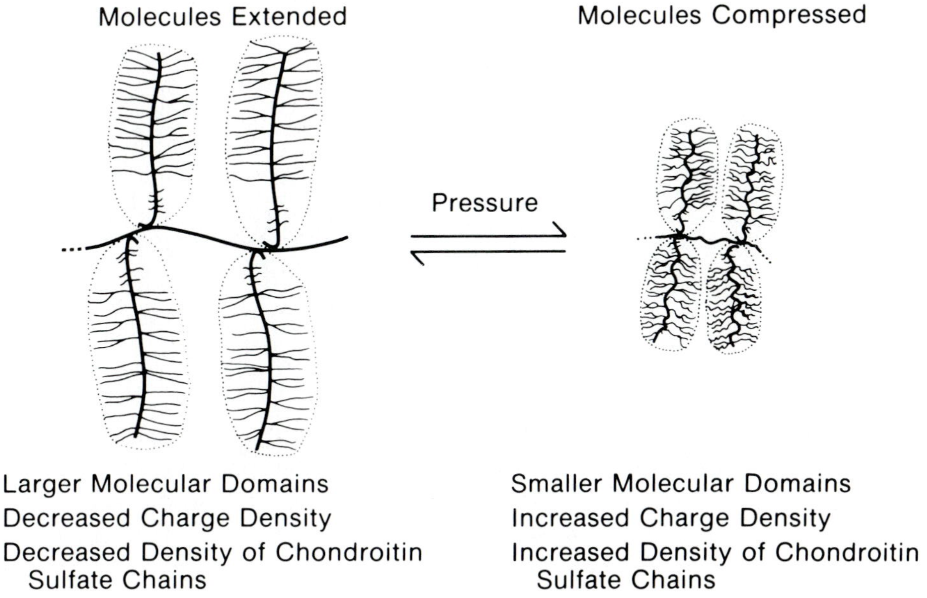

Molecules Extended   Molecules Compressed

Pressure

Larger Molecular Domains
Decreased Charge Density
Decreased Density of Chondroitin
    Sulfate Chains

Smaller Molecular Domains
Increased Charge Density
Increased Density of Chondroitin
    Sulfate Chains

Figure 1-29. Diagrammatic representation of the change in the proteoglycan domain in response to pressure. Loading drives the tissue fluid from the molecular domain and forces the negatively charged chondroitin sulfate chains together, thus increasing their resistance to further compression. *(From Buckwalter JA: The fine structure of human intervertebral disc. In: American Academy of Orthopaedic Surgeons Symposium on Idiopathic Low Back Pain. St. Louis, C. V. Mosby, 1982, with permission.)*

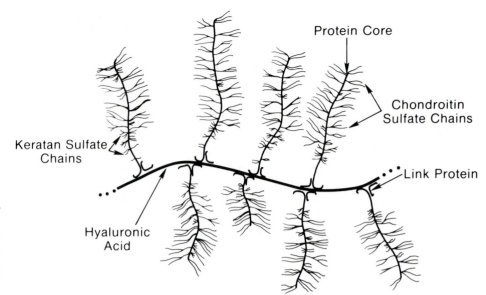

Protein Core

Chondroitin Sulfate Chains

Keratan Sulfate Chains

Link Protein

Hyaluronic Acid

Figure 1-30. Diagrammatic representation of proteoglycan aggregate structure. *(From Buckwalter JA: The fine structure of human intervertebral disc. In: American Academy of Orthopaedic Surgeons Symposium on Idiopathic Low Back Pain. St. Louis, C. V. Mosby, 1982, with permission.)*

immobilizing subunits within the matrix and directing their relationship with the other matrix macromolecules.

Noncollagenous Proteins and Glycoproteins. Glycoproteins and noncollagenous proteins contribute a unique group of molecules to the matrix macromolecular framework (Aplin and Hughes, 1982). They are perhaps the least well understood of the matrix macromolecules, and only recently have specific glycoproteins been isolated and characterized (Paulsson and Heinegård, 1984). They exist in the connective tissue extracellular matrix and in basement membranes associated with other macromolecules

and the surfaces of cells. Glycoproteins help organize, support, and connect the matrix macromolecules as well as attach the matrix macromolecules to cells. They thus stabilize the matrix, maintain the relationship of cells to the matrix, and may have other functions as well. All of them seem to have specific domains that bind other molecules or cells. Connective tissue cells synthesize the structural connective tissue glycoproteins and then secrete these molecules into the matrix where the glycoproteins form specific associations with the cell surface or the matrix macromolecules. Other glycoproteins exist in the serum, but these have distinct and separate functions. The struc-

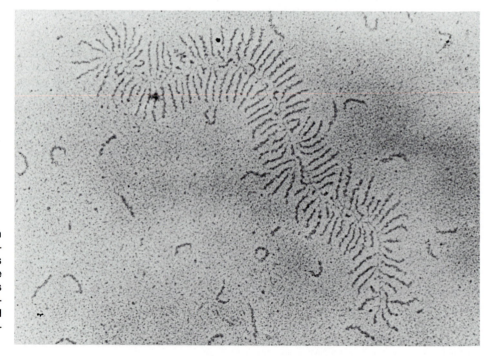

Figure 1-31. Electron micrograph showing a large proteoglycan aggregate. The central filament is hyaluronic acid; the side arms are proteoglycan monomers. In this preparation the chondroitin sulfate chains are collapsed around the protein core. (Original magnification × 28,000.)

	Associated Cells	Location	Binding	Molecular Weight
Fibronectin	Fibroblasts Endothelial cells Others	Extra cellular matrix Basement membranes	Cell Surface Collagen Fibrinogen Heparin Heparan Sulfate Hyaluronic Acid Actin DNA	420,000 to 500,000
Chondronectin	Chondrocytes	Cartilage matrix	Chondrocyte Surface Type II Collagen	180,000
Osteonectin		Bone Matrix	Collagen Hydroxyapatite	32,000
Laminin	Epithelial + Endothelial cells	Basement membranes	Type IV Collagen Cell Surface Heparin Heparan Sulfate	800,000

Figure 1-32. The characteristics of four skeletal connective tissue glycoproteins.

tural glycoproteins and other poorly characterized non-collagenous proteins form a variable amount of the matrix in different types of connective tissue (see Fig. 1–19).

In contrast to proteoglycans, glycoproteins consist primarily of protein. Recent work has identified at least five biochemically and functionally distinct connective tissue glycoproteins: link protein, fibronectin, chondronectin, osteonectin, and laminin; undoubtedly many more exist (Fig. 1–32). As discussed under proteoglycans, link protein stabilizes proteoglycan aggregates and may influence the assembly of aggregates (Buckwalter and Rosenberg, 1984). Fibronectin is widely distributed. It binds to cell surfaces, collagen, glycosaminoglycans, and fibrin. Frequently it forms a significant portion of the pericellular matrix. It appears to have several identifiable binding domains on its surface (Fig. 1–33). These distinct domains may allow it to participate in specific interaction with collagen and other matrix molecules. It can form fibrils in the matrix with or without collagen and is not limited to association with fibroblasts but rather is found with many different cell types. Fibronectin may also influence the cells. Under certain conditions fibronectin stimulates the transformation of chondrocytes into fibroblastlike cells (West et al., 1979). Chondronectin (Hewitt et al., 1982; Hewitt et al., 1983) found in the pericellular regions of cartilage binds specifically with chondrocytes, type II collagen, and cartilage proteoglycan. It associates with the cell surface rather than forming a significant matrix component and does not mediate fibroblast attachment. In contrast, fibronectin does not show a specificity for a collagen type, it does not mediate the attachment of chondrocytes to collagen, and it may form an important matrix component. Unlike fibronectin, chondronectin may help stabilize chondrocytes in their differentiated form. Osteonectin, a bone-specific glycoprotein, binds selectively to type I collagen and hydroxyapatite. This osteonectin collagen complex can nucleate mineral deposition from a metastable solution and may help initiate active mineralization in normal bone (Termine et al., 1981). Laminin along with type IV collagen and fibronectin forms part of the basement membranes. Adhesion of epithelial cells to basement membranes may be mediated by laminin. Although much remains to be learned about structural glycoproteins, it is clear that the interactions of cells, glycoproteins, and other matrix molecules are necessary for normal skeletal connective tissue structure and function.

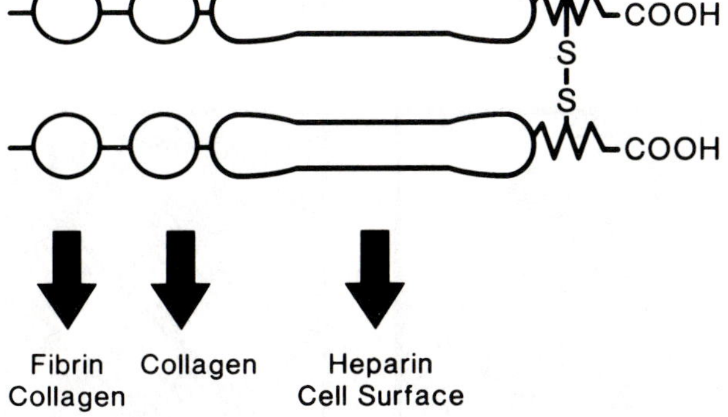

Synthesis and Assembly of Connective Tissue Macromolecules

The connective tissue macromolecules differ in composition, structure, distribution, and function. Nonetheless they share certain common features. The cells synthesize them from amino acids and sugars, and they follow essentially the same pathway through the cell from endoplasmic reticulum to Golgi membranes to secretion into the extracellular matrix (Fig. 1–34). A possible exception to this model is hyaluronate synthesis. Unlike collagens and proteoglycan monomers, hyaluronate may be synthe-

Figure 1-33. Diagrammatic representation of fibronectin showing its binding domains. The spherical and discoid regions are areas that bind specifically to certain molecules.

fields may change the cell membrane potential and cause ion fluxes, especially calcium and sodium, across the cell membrane. These ion fluxes may be responsible for the effects of electrical fields since blocking movement of the ions across the cell membrane eliminates the electrical effects (Rodan et al., 1978).

The connective tissue matrices make electromechanical transduction an important potential mechanism in the control of connective tissue function. These tissues do not actively propagate electrical signals like nerve and muscle. The matrix contains, however, a large volume of charged groups. Mechanical deformation of the matrix produces electrical potentials that may affect the cells like the externally applied electric fields. Electrical and mechanical influences may thus act through a common pathway: changing the cell membrane potential and altering ion fluxes across the membrane.

SUMMARY

The skeletal connective tissues assume three principal forms: bone; cartilage; and the dense fibrous tissue of tendon, ligament, and joint capsule. These tissues consist of cells and extracellular matrix. The cells originate from undifferentiated mesenchymal cells that assume highly differentiated forms and functions. They characteristically have relatively little direct cell-to-cell contact but an intimate and extensive contact with their extracellular matrix. These features distinguish them from epithelial cells. The matrix makes up the major volume of the skeletal connective tissues, and its composition and organization determine the function of the tissue. The matrix consists of tissue fluid, an organic macromolecular framework, and in bone, an inorganic matrix. The organic molecular matrix determines the properties of the tissue and consists of four classes of macromolecules: collagens, elastin, proteoglycans, and glycoproteins. Variation in the composition, organization, arrangement, and proportion of these macromolecules produces the differences in bone, cartilage, and dense fibrous tissue. Understanding of connective tissue cells and their matrices forms the foundation for study of the specific skeletal tissues and their properties as well as the processes of skeletal growth and development, degeneration, injury, and repair. Selective control of cell function has the potential to solve many of the most difficult musculoskeletal problems.

REFERENCES

Aplin JD, Hughes RC: Complex carbohydrates of the extracellular matrix structures, interactions and their biological roles. Biochim Biophys Acta 694:375, 1982.

Arcadi JA: Bull Hopkins Hosp 90:334, 1952.

Avery OT, MacLeod CM, McCarty M: Studies on the chemical nature of the substance inducing transformation of pneumococcal types. J Exp Med 79:137, 1944.

Belanger GF: Osteolysis: An outlook on its mechanism and causation in the parathyroid glands. In Galliard PJ, Talmage RV,

Budy AM (eds): The Parathyroid Glands. Chicago, University of Chicago, 1965, pp 137–143.

Brochet J, Mirsky AE: The Cell: Biochemistry, Physiology, Morphology. New York, Academic, 1959.

Buckwalter JA, Rosenberg LC: Electron microscopic studies of cartilage proteoglycans. J Biol Chem 257:9830, 1982.

Buckwalter JA, Rosenberg LC: The effect of link protein on proteoglycan aggregate structure. J Biol Chem 259:5361–5363, 1984.

Claude A, Porter KR, Fullam EF: A study of tissue culture cells by electron microscopy. J Exp Med 81:233, 1945.

Cooper R, Milgram JW, Robinson RA: Morphology of the osteon. J Bone Joint Surg 48-A (7):1239, 1966.

Danielli JF, Davson H: A contribution to the theory of permeability of thin films. J Cell Comp Physiol 5:495, 1935.

Deiss WP, Holmes LB, Johnston CC: Bone matrix biosynthesis in vitro. I. Labelling of hexosamine and collagen of normal bone. J Biol Chem 237:3555, 1962.

DeDuve C: Lysosomes, a new group of cytoplasmic particles. In Hayashi T (ed): Subcellular Particles. New York, Ronald, 1958, p. 128.

DeDuve C: The lysosome. Sci Am 208:64, 1963.

DeRobertis EDP, DeRobertis EMF: Cell Biology, 7th ed. Philadelphia, Saunders, 1980.

Dessau W, Von Der Mark H, Von Der Mark K, Fisher S: Changes in the patterns of collagens and fibronectin during limb-bud chondrogenesis. J Embryol Exp Morphol 57:51–60, 1980.

Dobele C: Antony Van Leeuwenhoek and His "Little Animals." New York, Dover, 1960.

Dudley HR, Spiro D: The fine structure of bone cells. J Biophys Biochem Cytol 11:627, 1961.

Fisher LW, Termine JD, Dejtes SW, et al: Proteoglycans of developing bone. J Biol Chem 288:6588–6594, 1983.

Folkman J, Moscona A: Role of cell shape in growth control. Nature 263:345–349, 1978.

Folkman J, Tucker RW: Cell configuration, substratum and growth control. In: Subtelny S, Wessells NK (eds): The Cell Surface: Mediator of Developmental Processes. New York, Academic, 1980, pp 259–275.

Fulmer HM: Enzymes in mineralized tissues. Clin Orthop 48:285, 1966.

Gillard GC, Reilly HC, Bell-Booth PG, Flint MH: The influence of mechanical forces on the glycosaminoglycan content of the rabbit flexor digitorum profundus tendon. Connect Tissue Res 7:37– 46, 1979.

Godman GC, Lane N: On the site of sulfation in the chondrocyte. J Cell Biol 21:353, 1964.

Golgi C: Sur la structure des cellules nerveuses des ganglions spinaux. Arch Ital Biol 30:278, 1898.

Grodzinsky AJ: Electromechanical and physicochemical properties of connective tissue. CRC Crit Rev Biomed Engineering 9:133–199, 1983.

Hancox NM, Boothroyd B: Motion picture and electron microscopic studies on the embryonic avian osteoclast. J Biophys Biochem Cytol 11:651, 1961.

Hascall VC, Hascall GK: Proteoglycans. In Hay ED (ed): Cell Biology of the Extracellular Matrix. New York, Plenum, 1981, pp 39–64.

Hay ED: Cell Biology of the Extracellular Matrix. New York, Plenum, 1981.

Hewitt AT, Varner HH, Silver MH, et al.: The isolation and partial characterization of chondronectin, an attachment factor for chondrocytes. J Biol Chem 257:2330–2334, 1982.

Hewitt AT, Varner HH, Silver MH, Martin GR: The role of chondronectin and cartilage proteoglycan in the attachment of chondrocytes to collagen. In: Limb Development and Regeneration. New York, Liss, 1983, pp 25–33.

Hooke R: Micrographia. R Soc London 1665.

Jacob F, Monod J: Genetic regulatory mechanisms in the synthesis of proteins. J Mol Biol 3:318, 1961.

Kornberg A: Active center of DNA polymerase. Science 163:1410, 1969.

Kosher RA, Church RL: Stimulation of in vitro somite chondrogenesis by procollagen and collagen. Nature 258:327–330, 1975.

Lehninger AL: How cells transform energy. Sci Am 205:62, 1961.

Lehninger AL: The mitochondrion: Molecular basis of structure and function. New York, Benjamin, 1964.

Lehninger AL: Biochemistry. New York, Worth, 1975.

Leung DYM, Glagov S, Matthews MB: A new in vitro system for studying cell response to mechanical stimulation. Exp Cell Res 109:285–298, 1977.

Mankin HJ: Orthopaedics in 2013: A prospection. J Bone Joint Surg 65A:1190–1194, 1983.

Martin JH, Matthews JL: Mitochondrial granules in chondrocytes, osteoblasts, and osteocytes. An ultrastructural and microincineration study. Clin Orthop 68:273, 1970.

Maurer PH, Hudack SS: Isolation of hyaluronic acid from callus tissue during early healing. Arch Biochem Biophys 38:49–53, 1952.

McKusick VA: Heritable Disorders of Connective Tissue (4th ed.). St. Louis, C.V. Mosby, 1972.

McLean FC, Urist MR: Bone. An introduction to the physiology of skeletal tissue. Chicago, University of Chicago, 1955.

Meselson M, Stahl FW: The replication of DNA in E. coli. Proc Natl Acad Sci USA 44:671, 1958.

Norton LA, Rodan GA, Bourrett LA: Epiphyseal cartilage cAMP changes produced by mechanical and electrical perturbations. Clin Orthop 124:59–68, 1977.

Nirenberg MW, Matthaei JH: The dependence of cell-free protein synthesis in E. coli upon naturally occurring or synthetic polyribonucleotides. Proc Natl Acad Sci USA 47:1588, 1961.

Nirenberg MW, Leder P: RNA codewords and protein synthesis. Science 145:1399, 1964.

Owen M: Cell population kinetics of an osteogenic tissue. J Cell Biol 19:19, 1963.

Owen M: Uptake of [³H]uridine into precursor pools and RNA in osteogenic cells. J Cell Sci 2:39, 1967.

Palade GE: A small particulate component of the cytoplasm. J Biophys Biochem Cytol 1:59, 1955.

Paulsson M, Heinegård D: Noncollagenous cartilage proteins. Coll Rel Res 4:219–229, 1984.

Poole AR, Pidoux I, Reiner A, Rosenberg L: An immunoelectron microscope study of the organization of proteoglycan monomer, link protein and collagen in the matrix of articular cartilage. J Cell Biol 93:921–937, 1982.

Reddi AH: Regulation of local differentiation of cartilage and bone by extracellular matrix: A cascade type mechanism. In: Limb Development and Regeneration. Part B. New York, Liss, 1983, pp 261–268.

Reid T, Flint MH: Change in glycosaminoglycan content of healing rabbit tendon. J Embryol Exp Morphol 31:489–495, 1974.

Revel JP, Hay ED: An autoradiographic and electron microscopic study of collagen synthesis in differentiating cartilage. Z Zellforsch 61:110, 1963.

Robertson JD: The ultrastructure of cell membranes and their derivatives. Biochem Soc Symp 16:1, 1959.

Robinson RA: Observations regarding compartments for tracer calcium in the body. In Frost H (ed): Bone Dynamics. Boston, Little, Brown, 1964, p 423.

Rodan GA, Bourrett LA, Norton LA: DNA synthesis in cartilage cells is stimulated by oscillating electrical fields. Science 199:690–692, 1978.

Roughley PJ, McNicol D, Buckwalter JA: The presence of a cartilage-like proteoglycan in adult human meniscus. Biochem J 197:77–83, 1981.

Siekevitz P: The organization of biologic membranes. N Engl J Med 283:1035, 1970.

Smith GN, Toole BP, Gross J: Hyaluronidase activity and glycosaminoglycan synthesis in the amputated newt limb. Dev Biol 42:221–232, 1975.

Termine JD, Kleinman HK, Whitson SW, et al.: Osteonectin: A bone specific protein linking mineral to collagen. Cell 26:99–150, 1981.

Toole BP: Glycosaminoglycans in morphogenesis. In Hay ED (ed): Cell Biology of the Extracellular Matrix. New York, Plenum, 1981, pp 259–294.

Toole BP, Gross J: The extracellular matrix of the regenerating newt limb: Synthesis and removal of hyaluronate prior to differentiation. Dev Biol 25:57–77, 1971.

Urist MR: Bone: Formation by autoinduction. Science 150:893, 1965.

Virchow R: Cellular Pathology. Churchill CF (trans). London 1859.

Watson JD, Crick FHC: Molecular structure of nucleic acids: A structure for deoxyribose nucleic acid. Nature 171:737, 1953.

Watson J, DeHass WG, Hauser SS: Effect of electric fields on growth rate of embryonic chick tibiae in vitro. Nature 254:331–332, 1975.

West CM, Lanza R, Rosenbloom J, et al.: Fibronectin alters the phenotypic properties of cultured chick embryo chondroblasts. Cell 17:491–501, 1979.

Woods JF, Nichols G: Collagenolytic activity in rat bone cells. Characteristics and intracellular location. J Cell Biol 26:747, 1965.

Young RW: Specialization of bone cells. In Frost H (ed): Bone Biodynamics. Boston, Little, Brown, 1964, p 117.

Zamecnik PC: Protein synthesis. Harvey Lect 54:256, 1960.

Chapter 2
Genetics

Stanley M. Elmore

The genes are becoming the focal point for our understanding of what disease is and how it works.

    —Z. Harsanyi and R. Hutton, *Genetic Prophecy: Beyond the Double Helix*

The generation of new knowledge of genetics since the discovery of the internal structure of DNA by Crick and Watson in 1952 has created a revolution in the biologic sciences. The ability now to isolate single genes and manipulate recombinant DNA has created a new science of genetic engineering that has practical as well as commercial value. It has created heretofore unimagined dilemmas in philosophy, religion, politics as well as science. Genetic material from two different species can now be recoupled so as to create new DNA that can be directed to either serve mankind or lead to its destruction. The ethical debates continue but genetic technology marches onward.

    DNA can be enzymatically cut, spliced, and repaired so as to deliberately manufacture desirable proteins that have clinical value. Human genetic material selected as a blueprint is inserted into the DNA of fast-growing yeast or bacteria, causing them to produce quantities of human growth hormone, interferon, insulin, antihemophiliac factor, serum albumin, streptokinase, and endorphins for commercial sale. Using viruses, the same gene-splicing techniques can be made to produce vaccines against some types of herpes and hepatitis.

    The field of sociobiology, exploring many of the common threads that make us human, is applying the science of genetics to their discipline. Some recent theories are indeed provocative in declaring that much human behavior is shaped by genes as well as culture. The notion that genes construct a brain organized in such a way as to process certain kinds of information in certain ways is a premise that is supported by the following observations. Anthropologic studies show that smiles and expressions of grief and joy have the same meaning in every society. Also our visual apparatus and brain are genetically programmed to see 440 nm of wavelength light; therefore, the human species perceives color universally as discrete colors of red, green, yellow, and blue. All other shades are products of particular cultural bias. Other social traits that seem to have universality are phobias to dangerous natural phenomenon, avoidance of incest, and a propensity to instruct children.

    Animal studies have shown that brains may be receptive to learning some specific social behaviors at very specific times under rigid environmental conditions. When that "window of learning" is closed, that specific information cannot be learned later. This is a slightly higher level of brain activity than instinct, which is fundamental to animal behavior and is widely accepted as being preordained by genetic makeup. Individual species do react to their environment in predictable and uniform ways; yet there are numerous instances that reveal that lower animals and insects are capable of controlled environmentally influenced learning that can be later transferred within the species to influence behavior in less predictable activity. Somewhere in the genes of animals is the instinct to learn, but the content and storage of learning is rigidly controlled by the genetically organized brain.

Neural pathways that control some of this learning behavior are now being revealed and are bringing together the sciences of neurobiology, genetics, sociobiology, and anthropology.

HISTORY

Before 1900, classical science thought of heredity as a blending process, a mixing of traits of parents yielding an offspring who was something in between the two, possessing no firm qualities of either parent. In 1866 Mendel reported his discovery of the principle of genetics using the garden pea but received no recognition of it from contemporary scientists. His work was essentially rediscovered in 1900 when the universal nature of this type of inheritance was recognized, and it became the foundation of modern genetics.

Mendel's most significant contribution was the recognition of the particulate nature of inheritance and the ultimate pairing of these particles into individual sets. Using the garden pea, he crossed pure lines differing in seven clearly identifiable characteristics and followed these traits through two generations. He found that original traits reappeared in unaltered form in the second generation, disproving the possibility of blending. He explained his results in terms of units that individually carried a specific trait or characteristic. These units are now called genes. He recognized that these units were paired in the individual plant and that they separated into single units in the pollen and were reunited or paired again in different combinations, independent of other genes, at the time of fertilization to form a new individual.

He also formulated the concept of one unit being dominant or recessive to the other member of the pair, e.g., when tall plants and short plants were crossfertilized, the first generation were all tall plants, proving dominance of the tall gene over the short gene. However, self-pollination of this second generation of tall plants produced approximately one fourth short plants, which confirmed the unitary nature of genetic transmission from generation to generation as well as confirming the mathematic probability of paired (tall and short, heterozygous) dissimilar units recombining to produce a short individual in 25 percent of the offspring.

The universal nature of this Mendelian type of inheritance was finally recognized in 1900, and its application to medical genetics was made complete in 1902 by Garrod, who reported alkaptonuria (a recessive trait) as the

first example of Mendelian inheritance in man and recognized the significance of parental consanguinity in the same case. He later described all of the clinical and genetic features of three other recessive diseases—cystinuria, pentosuria, and albinism.

Archibald Garrod, professor of medicine at Oxford, in the first decade of this century was the first to develop ideas of the chemical individuality of diseases and deduced that genes controlled products of metabolism by directing the synthesis of the protein (enzyme) that controls it. He anticipated the discovery of enzymes in 1923 and even the individual characteristic responses to drugs, now a special field of interest known as pharmacogenetics. He coined the term "inborn errors of metabolism" and regarded "freaks of metabolism" as analogous to congenital malformation. He pioneered the concept of one gene, one enzyme as causes of hereditary disorders and suggested the molecular rather than cellular basis of human heterogeneity and evolution. He was the first to say, "There are special proteins for every species, and indeed for every individual in a species" (Childs, 1970). He recognized that "the chromosome germinal cells are the starting points of mutations great and small" (Childs, 1970). In 1929 he said, "Each one of us differs from his fellows, not only in bodily structure and the proteins which enter into his composition, but apart from or rather in consequence of such individualities, men differ in mental outlook, character and ability" (Childs, 1970). Remarkably Garrod's solid clinical works as well as his prophetic concepts were largely ignored until the beginning of the modern biologic revolution in 1950. In 1927 Muller discovered the mutagenic effects of x-radiation on cellular material. In 1941 Beadle and Tatum, using irradiated (mutated) bread mold in a series of intricate experiments, concluded that one important gene function was to control the structure of enzyme protein. In 1944 Avery and McCarty showed that specific heritable genetic traits could be transferred from one strain of bacteria to another and revealed the material responsible for this to be deoxyribonucleic acid. The biochemical nature of gene action was then established.

Avery's work influenced Chargaff to use paper chromatography to search for chemical differences among nucleic acids. In 1950 he discovered that DNA could be structured with an almost infinite number of nucleotide sequences while noting that the proportion of adenine to thymine and guanine to cytosine were always approximately equal in the DNA of bacteria, yeast, domestic animals, and human beings. These findings later proved to be the key to solving the three-dimensional structure of DNA.

NUCLEIC ACIDS

The well-known double helical structure of chromosomal DNA was worked out by Watson and Crick in 1953. They deduced an inward arrangement of the base pairs of guanine and cytosine and adenine and thymine attached to a double spine of deoxyribose and phosphate that would explain the transfer of genetic information through a process of meiosis and mitosis with a low probability of error (Fig. 2–1). They showed how all the important properties of genes could be explained by the physical structure of the DNA molecule. The theory also gave a clear understanding of how mutation may occur through pairing error or base-pair substitution.

The order of base pairs contained in the DNA molecule has a specific genetic effect in that it determines which enzyme or protein is produced by the cell; it also determines the genetic specificity transmitted from generation to generation. This order (genetic code) seems to be a triplicate, or three-letter, code of any combination of base pairs. In this system adenine (A) associates only with thymine (T) and guanine (G) only with cytosine (C). With this triplicate any combination of these pairs may carry the genetic message. Thus, a paired sequence such as A-T, A-T, G-C presumes the complementary linear sequence in the daughter strand of DNA after mitosis or meiosis

yielding A, A, G and T, T, C components, which will replicate into the same original sequence. Each of 20 different amino acids is known to be specified by one or more particular sequences of these bases in the DNA molecule. This, of course, is the universal essence of heredity, the ability to reproduce its own molecular structure (Fig. 2–2).

Jacob and Monod in 1961 were the first to show that DNA does not produce protein synthesis directly. They suggested that protein synthesis begins with the transcription of the sequence of base pairs of DNA onto ribonucleic acid (RNA), or messenger RNA (mRNA). RNA replicated in the same manner as DNA, except wherever adenine occurred in the DNA molecule, uracil substituted for thymine in the RNA molecule. The coded message of the DNA was thus transcribed into the RNA by a coded sequence of base pairs (Fig. 2–3).

More recent research has revealed some significant and startling changes in the mechanics of genetic information transfer within the cell nucleus. New evidence indicates that the gene is "no longer a single, stable unit"

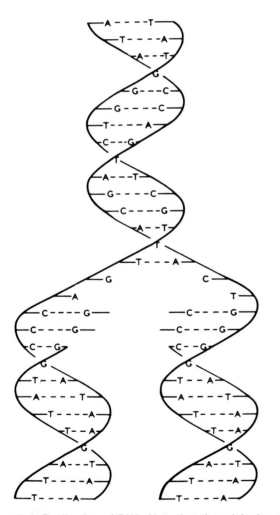

Figure 2-1. Replication of DNA. Note that the original molecule (top) unwinds and the halves separate. As the double-stranded parent unwinds, the separated strands serve as templates for the alignment of nucleotides (A–T and C–G), which combine to form new strands complementary to the new molecule. *(From Sutton, 1975, with permission.)*

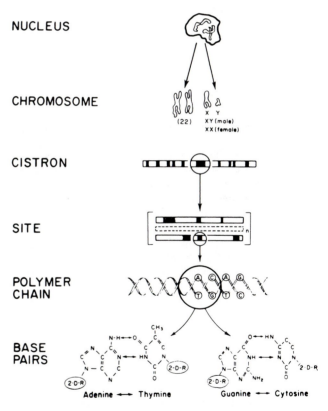

Figure 2-2. Diagrammatic representation of the various configurations of the "genetic material." All cells contain 22 pairs of autosomal chromosomes and 1 pair of sex chromosomes. The XX form represents the normal female, whereas the XY form represents the normal male. A number of different segments exist in each chromosome; within each segment there are progressively smaller units called loci and sites. Each of these is mutable. The smallest mutable unit is composed of a single base (purine–pyrimidine) pair. *(From Milch and McKusick, 1964, with permission.)*

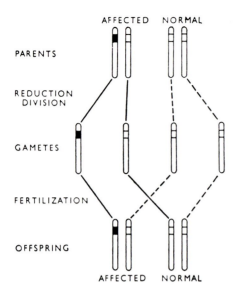

Figure 2-5. Chromosome diagram showing the transmission of the genes in the mating to a normal of a person heterozygous for a dominant trait. *(From Roberts, 1973, with permission.)*

laxity. The sex chromosome abnormalities of Turner's (XO) and Klinefelter's (XXY) syndromes are occasionally seen by an orthopaedist because of the musculoskeletal abnormalities associated with them.

Chromosome abnormalities of clinical significance occur 3 to 5 times in 1000 births. The incidence is nine to ten times as great in the conceptus, but most of these are eliminated as spontaneous abortions. In general, chromosomal disorders produce structural changes in multiple-organ systems and frequently result in individuals who are

stillborn or who die in the first year of life. These disorders are classified as genetic because they result from a deficiency or a change in the DNA content of chromosomes, but they do not follow the normal genetic mechanisms of inheritance. In fact, most instances of chromosomal aberration occur sporadically. Down's syndrome is perhaps the most predictable, occurring with greater frequency in older mothers or younger translocation carriers. More is known about the sex chromosomes than any of the 22 pairs of autosomes because they can be more easily identified and paired in a karyotype. Two kinds of sex chromosomes can now be identified—X chromatin and Y chromatin.

A high proportion of female nuclei contain a sex chromatin body, known as the Barr body, on the inner surface of the nuclear membrane (usually a buccal smear). Only cells with more than one X chromosome (Lyon principle) will have a Barr body, which represents the inactivated X chromosome (Fig. 2–10). The F body represents the Y chromosome in a nucleus and is visualized by a fluorescent staining technique. The number of F bodies in a nucleus represents the number of Y chromosomes in a cell, whereas there will always be one less Barr body than the total number of X chromosomes in a cell.

In 1961 Lyon hypothesized that in females, at a very early stage of embryonic development, one of the two normal X chromosomes becomes functionally inactive in all somatic cells and is visualized as the Barr body. The inactivation of one of two X chromosomes in any given cell at this stage of zygotic differentiation is a random process and independent of events in other cells. Once inactivated that particular X chromosome remains inactive during subsequent development. This leads to the interesting conclusion that most if not all females are genetic mosaics and helps explain many of the phenotypic variations in sex-linked diseases. The male, having only one X chro-

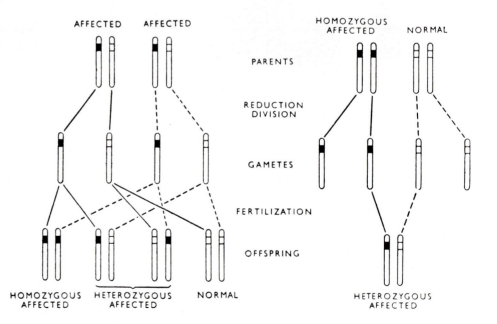

Figure 2-6. A. Chromosome diagram showing the transmission of the genes in the mating of two persons heterozygous for a dominant trait. **B.** Chromosome diagram showing the transmission of the genes in the mating to a normal of a person homozygous for a dominant trait. *(From Roberts, 1973, with permission.)*

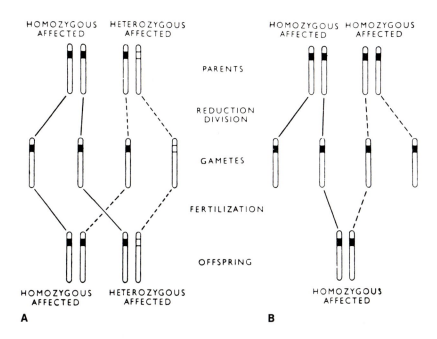

Figure 2-7. **A.** Chromosome diagram showing the transmission of the genes in the mating of two persons respectively homozygous and heterozygous for a dominant trait. **B.** Chromosome diagram showing the transmission of the genes in the mating of two persons homozygous for a dominant trait. *(From Roberts, 1973, with permission.)*

mosome, always received from the mother, and one Y chromosome, received from the father, will manifest all the genetic traits received on the X chromosome because there is no comparable genetic locus on the Y chromosome to form an allele. This condition is termed hemizygous. Hence, one can understand why there is no male-to-male transmission of sex-linked disease. Likewise, the genetic mosaicism of the female allows us to understand the subclinical condition of some females who carry X-

linked diseases such as vitamin D–resistant rickets, hemophilia, and muscular dystrophy. Male offspring of such maternal mosaics will receive a full dose of the abnormal gene and will be phenotypically abnormal, whereas the female mosaics may range from being phenotypically normal to having a mild to moderate form of the disease. Careful muscle testing and enzymatic studies may be necessary to detect female carriers of a disease such as muscular dystrophy.

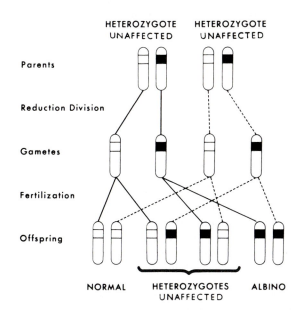

Figure 2-8. Chromosome diagram showing the transmission of the genes in the mating of two persons heterozygous for a recessive trait; the mating from which the great majority of affected persons are born. *(From Roberts, 1973, with permission.)*

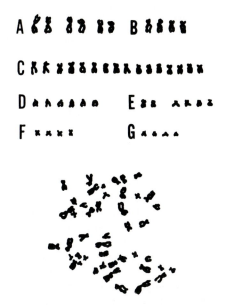

Figure 2-9. The normal karyotype of a 35-year-old woman with Maffucci's syndrome. Forty of fifty cells counted had a normal modal number of 46. Nine karyotypes were made and showed no chromosomal abnormality. *(From Elmore and Cantrell, 1966, with permission.)*

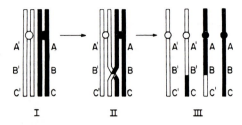

Figure 2-13. Diagrammatic illustration of crossing over: (I) synapsis or pairing of replicated homologous chromosomes to form tetrad; (II) exchange of chromosome regions bearing *C* gene between two chromotids; (III) chromosomes that will be carried by the four resulting gametes. Two of the four chromosomes carry rearranged genes. *(From Nance et al., 1965, with permission.)*

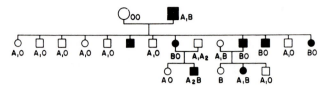

Figure 2-14. Pedigree illustrating dominant inheritance of the nail-patella syndrome and close linkage of the gene determining this disorder to the ABO blood group locus. In this family, the nail-patella gene is carried on the same chromosome as the B blood group gene. All males (■) and females (●) who inherited the blood group gene also inherited the nail-patella syndrome. The nail-patella gene is not associated with any particular ABO gene, and in other families it may be linked to the A gene, the O gene, or the AB genes. *(From Nance et al., 1965, with permission.)*

dividuals will manifest only one or two of these traits and may show a wide variety of bone fragility. This phenomenon is called pleiotropy and implies that one gene produces several effects.

It is also recognized that several genes, presumably at different loci, can produce similar effects. The three common types of muscular dystrophy (Duchenne's, sex-linked recessive; limb-girdle, autosomal recessive; and facioscapulohumeral, autosomal dominant) are all genetically determined muscular dystrophies caused by different genes producing a similar muscular effect. This is an example of genetic heterogeneity. The recent discovery of introns and exons and the split-gene theory previously described may better explain this phenomenon, but application to these diseases awaits confirmation by further research.

It is interesting to consider the time of action of genes. Obviously all of an individual's genes are present from the time of fertilization, but they may not become operative until later in life. In fact, the presence of some genes cannot be detected until adulthood, e.g., limb-girdle muscular dystrophy, which does not appear before puberty, or Huntington's chorea, which rarely appears before 30 years of age. Conversely, some genes undoubtedly are operative only during embryogenesis and cease to function for the remainder of a person's life. The controller genes are not well understood, especially the mechanisms of turning them off and on; this is the subject of much current research.

If genes are located on different chromosomes, they sort and recombine independently, but if genes are located close together on the same chromosome, they often travel together during the first stage of meiosis and are said to be linked. Linked genes are an exception to Mendel's law of independent assortment. The ABO blood group and the nail-patella syndrome genes are two well-studied linked autosomal genes (Fig. 2–14). Linked genes have been a valuable tool in mapping the true loci of genes on chromosomes. So far about 1700 human genes have been mapped.

This information has proved useful in isolating specific genes with restriction enzymes. The gene once isolated can then be decoded by cutting the strands of DNA into ever shorter segments and reading the sequence of nucleotides. The genetic codes of some defective genes can now be worked out in this way. A method of detecting the presence of sickle cell anemia from cells taken at amniocentesis and treating it with restriction enzymes allows detection of the disease before birth. The ultimate hope in using these methods is to be able to detect abnormal genes early in life and eventually substitute a corrected or normal gene. Hence gene mapping is a valuable step in breaking the genetic code and is fundamental to the principles of genetic engineering now and for the future.

Mutation

Genes that change their characteristics, giving rise to new genes, are called mutations. Fortunately mutations are relatively rare events because most are considered harmful. Nevertheless, they provide the basis of evolution in which natural selection acts to favor certain characteristics. On a molecular level, this is the basis for the theory of survival of the fittest. Mutations in germ cells are transmitted to the next generation; they can be induced by a variety of environmental hazards. The best known mutagens include ionizing radiation and certain chemicals. Mutations of somatic cells have no effect on future generations but may have significance to the individual who carries them. The mutation of somatic cells has been implicated as one possible mechanism to explain the cause of cancer.

Mutations occurring in the germ cells of previously normal parents give rise to genetically affected offspring. Diseases such as neurofibromatosis (autosomal dominant), osteogenesis imperfecta (autosomal dominant), and achondroplasia (autosomal dominant) are three common genetic diseases that result from higher-than-average mutation rates in parental germ plasm.

INHERITANCE PATTERNS

Single-Gene Disorders

There are more than 2300 phenotypically recognizable genetic disorders. Many of these diseases follow the classical pattern of inheritance established by Mendel. Most diseases are either autosomal dominant or recessive in their inheritance pattern. Only a few diseases are associated with the unique properties of X chromosome inheritance. It is perhaps best to recognize that discovery of most genetic diseases begins with a single individual usually called a propositus, or proband. Investigation of a proband's family tree or pedigree will usually confirm the suspicion of genetic disease in the proband by finding similar traits in his kindred. The pattern of inheritance across generations will usually be a strong clue as to the type of genetic disease being studied. For example, Figure 2–15 shows the presence of an identifiable phenotype in at least three consecutive generations, typical of the dominant gene. Figure 2–16 is typical of a recessive gene because of a lack of continuity between generations, indicating the likelihood of heterozygous parents forming a homozygous offspring.

Each of the four basic types of inheritance patterns has its own unique characteristics, which can be used to help identify the pattern present for any given disorder (Table 2–1). These include the following:

1. Autosomal dominant inheritance
   a. Every affected person will have at least one affected parent (except when there is mutation of parental germ plasma).
   b. Affected persons mating to normal persons will have approximately 50 percent affected children (a 50-50 chance with each pregnancy) (see Fig. 2–5).
   c. If both parents are heterozygous for the same gene, 75 percent of the offspring will be affected (see Fig. 2–6).
   d. Sexes will be equally affected.
   e. Normal children of affected parents will have normal children.
   f. The trait will be directly transmitted through three or more generations in the absence of consanguinity (see Fig. 2–15).
   g. In general, dominant traits tend to cause structural deformities with less functional loss than recessive traits.
2. Autosomal recessive inheritance
   a. Affected persons usually have normal parents who are heterozygous for a single mutant gene. Two abnormal genes, one from each parent, must combine to produce an abnormal offspring (see Fig. 2–8).
   b. Twenty-five percent of the offspring of heterozygous parents will be affected.
   c. Sexes are equally affected.
   d. The rate of consanguinity is high.
   e. Fifty percent of the offspring of heterozygous parents will be heterozygous carriers of the gene but will not be affected (see Fig. 2–8).
   f. Pedigree studies indicate a horizontal form of inheritance with only siblings being affected (see Fig. 2–16).
   g. In general, the defects constitute a more severe threat to normal life and function than those caused by dominant genes. The effects tend to result from a single-enzyme deficiency.
3. Sex-linked dominant inheritance (Fig. 2–17)
   a. There is no male-to-male transmission; there is only one known abnormal gene passed from father to son, namely, hairy ears. Fathers transmit only to daughters.
   b. There will be more affected females than males in pedigree studies.
   c. Affected females who are homozygous will transmit to all their children.
   d. Affected females who are heterozygous will transmit to 50 percent of their children.
4. Sex-linked recessive inheritance (Fig. 2–18)
   a. There will be a predominance of affected males in pedigree studies.
   b. There is no male-to-male transmission.
   c. Traits are passed from affected fathers to all daughters who will transmit it to half their sons.
   d. Female carriers may be phenotypically normal.

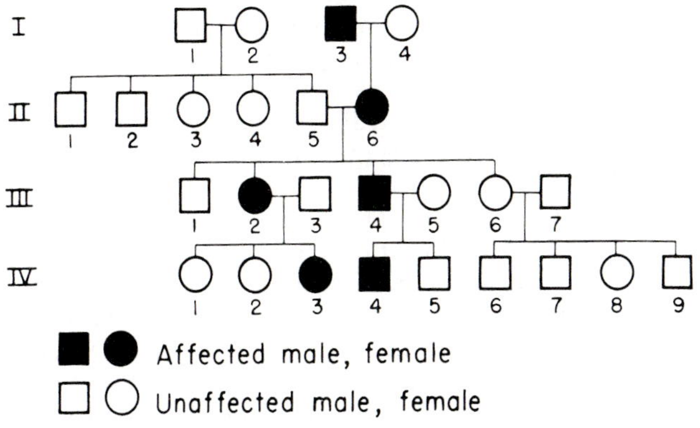

Figure 2-15. Idealized pedigree pattern of a rare autosomal dominant condition. *(From Milch and McKusick, 1964, with permission.)*

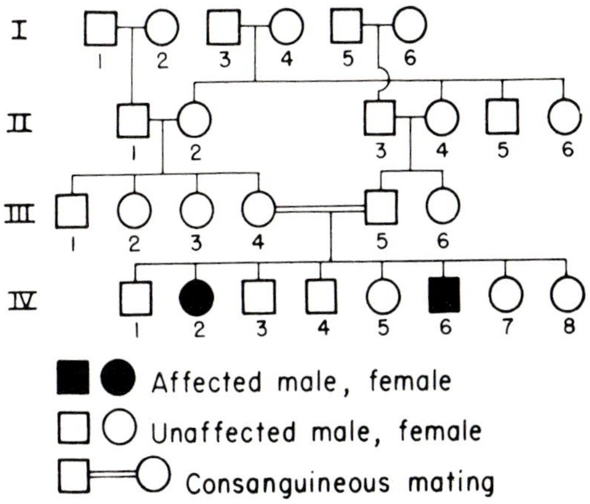

Figure 2-16. Idealized pedigree pattern of a rare autosomal recessive condition. Note that the parents of the affected individuals are first cousins. *(From Milch and McKusick, 1964, with permission.)*

Multifactorial Inheritance

Congenital malformations occur in 2 or 3 percent of all live births. They probably represent the largest category of disease caused by a combination of environmental in-

TABLE 2–3. PROPORTION OF FIRST-, SECOND-, AND THIRD-DEGREE RELATIVES AFFECTED WITH SOME COMMON MALFORMATIONS—RELATIVE TO THE INCIDENCE IN THE GENERAL POPULATION

	Congenital Dislocation of Hip		Talipes Equinovarus	Anencephalus and Spina Bifida
	All Patients	Female Relatives of Female Patients		
Population incidence (approximate)	0.001	0.0018	0.001	0.005
Monozygotic twins	×500	×300	325	—
First-degree relatives	×40	×35	20	8
Second-degree relatives	×4	×3	5	—
Third-degree relatives	×$1\frac{1}{2}$	×2	2	2

(From Carter, 1965, with permission.)

dentical twins. Pedigree studies indicate a higher incidence of acetabular dysplasia in near relatives and 40 to 50 times the normal incidence of congenital dislocation of the hip in siblings. These data support a genetic basis for congenital dislocated hip; yet there is good evidence for environmental influence. This evidence includes the fact that 50 percent of children affected with congenital dislocation of the hip are firstborn and 16 percent are breech births. In addition, the ratio of congenital dislocation of the hip in winter compared to summer is 1.6:1. Cultures that swaddle their infants with the hips in extension such as Laplanders or the American Navajo show an increased incidence of congenital dislocation of the hip compared with Eskimos who carry their infants with the hips in abduction and flexion.

Clubfoot. Clubfeet occur in association with a variety of other congenital malformations such as spina bifida, cerebral palsy, arthrogryposis, and congenital dislocation of the hip, but there are types of clubfeet that occur independently of other diseases. One form is talipes equinovarus, with an incidence of 1 per 1000 births and a male-to-female ratio of 2:1. Identical twin concordance is 35 percent, whereas nonidentical twin concordance is only 3 percent. In parents of affected children, the incidence of clubfoot is 10 times that of the general population, and in siblings it is 20 times. The incidence is, however, only slightly greater in second- and third-degree relatives than in the normal population, suggesting a polygenic type of inheritance influenced by environmental factors (Table 2–3).

Idiopathic Scoliosis. Adolescent idiopathic scoliosis remains the predominant form of spinal curvature in North America that concerns orthopaedic surgeons. The many population studies on the epidemiology and incidence of idiopathic scoliosis vary as to evaluation and examination techniques, which yields a wide discrepancy in incidence rates. The best of these studies shows a general population incidence of 1.8 to 4.5 percent of adolescent idiopathic scoliosis in the general population. Unfortunately, scoliosis in children is commonly associated with many other congenital, acquired, and genetic diseases. Diseases such as cerebral palsy, poliomyelitis, neurofibromatosis, mus-

cular dystrophy, and vertebral anomalies must first be ruled out.

All studies show a predominate female incidence of adolescent idiopathic scoliosis, especially for curves of 20 degrees or more. The sex ratio has been variously reported to be 5.4:1 to 7:1, female to male. Lower sex ratios of 1.2:1.0, female to male, occur if any curve at all is recorded, but few of these lesser curves progress or require treatment. Some studies have shown that 20 percent of females with curves of 20 degrees or more did not progress and 3 to 20 percent showed spontaneous improvement. On the other hand, larger curves seem to progress with the degree of curvature. Maternal age over 30 is associated with a slightly higher incidence of adolescent scoliosis in females. This information clearly indicates environmental influence, yet the evidence for genetic factors is more compelling.

Pedigree studies of index cases all show a greater-than-normal incidence of idiopathic scoliosis in first-, second-, and third-degree relatives. One study of 320 index cases revealed that one third of family members had curves greater than 10 degrees, and the defect was traced through four generations in some. In another study of 413 index cases, the incidence of scoliosis in first-, second-, and third-degree relatives was 6.6, 1.6, and 1.0 percent respectively. If both parents of index patients are normal, the risk to a subsequent brother is 2 percent and to a sister 7 percent; however, if only one parent has idiopathic scoliosis, the risk to a subsequent brother is 7 percent and to the sister 42 percent! Clearly a genetic disposition exists in such pedigrees.

Cumulative twin studies are limited by a small number of cases but do show a 73 percent incidence of scoliosis in monozygotic compared with 50 percent incidence in dizygotic twins.

This information is suggestive of an autosomal dominant mode of inheritance with incomplete penetrance and variable expressivity. Some studies have suggested an X-linked dominant form with incomplete penetrance, but other studies have been able to identify a father-to-son inheritance, that, although rare, rules out an exclusive X-linkage mode of inheritance. More recent studies have shown a significant association of idiopathic scoliosis with asymmetries in the vestibular apparatus and abnormal electroencephalograms (EEGs), which points toward a polygenic and multifactorial inheritance pattern. The current data on idiopathic scoliosis indicate that it does not result from a single genetic abnormality, but it tends to be transmitted like an autosomal dominant gene with variable expressivity and incomplete penetrance with multifactorial qualities.

Some biochemical studies have suggested that abnormal protein metabolism such as increased excretion of certain amino acids and hydroxyproline is associated with idiopathic scoliosis. Some have theorized that abnormal collagen cross-linkage and increased collagen type 1 content explain the loss of structural integrity of the spine, but most of this speculation is based on tissue taken from scoliosis already established or in progress and does not yet give any real support to a single-gene cause for idiopathic scoliosis.

Cancer. The cause of cancer remains a mystery, yet more of the mechanisms and sequences that produce a cancer are now revealed with the discovery of oncogenes in 1981. Specific genes identified as oncogenes are present in all of our normal body cells all our lives. These are identified with specific forms of cancer including breast, lung, bladder, and bowel. Oncogenes usually remain harmless and may have served a useful function earlier in life, especially at times of normally rapid growth as in embryonic development and the growth spurts of childhood. A carcinogen or external agent such as a chemical, radiation, or a virus may cause chromosomes to break and rearrange themselves so that an oncogene moves to a more active region of another chromosome. Here it begins an accelerated production of abnormal DNA that may be the genesis of a cancer. Chromosomal breaks have long been regular features of cancer cells. It is now recognized that normal human chromosomes have several fragile sites, identified with regularity, that are susceptible to breaks and translocation. The physical rearrangement of the oncogenes on different chromosomes is the key to understanding cancer in this decade.

Each oncogene is now recognized as bracketed by a sequence of DNA on each side that travels with the oncogenes and seems to act as a regulator or control for the oncogene in its new location. This particular DNA is known as a long term repeat (LTR). The oncogene, once stimulated, seems to have the ability to speed up a normal cellular function without any ability to stop the process once begun. The discovery of oncogenes now gives a certain unity to the theory of cancer pathogenesis and may allow a concentrated effort toward more effective cancer treatment. It is the single most important breakthrough in cancer research to date.

Sporadic Cases
The appearance of offspring with genetic disease in the previously unaffected family can be very disconcerting to the parents and kindred who take pride in their family trees. Assuming no extramarital or consanguineous mating, sporadic cases can be understood to have occurred for any one of the following reasons: it may arise from the combination of recessive homozygous genes in both parents or from a mutation of parental germ plasm. If males are affected, it may indicate a sex-linked recessive disease with a maternal carrier state, or it may be the result of a dominant gene that was nonpenetrant in the parent. Finally, a phenocopy must be considered as a possible mimic of an abnormal genotype.

GENETIC COUNSELING

Genetic counseling falls beyond the purview of the orthopaedic surgeon. Although orthopaedic surgeons should have more than a casual acquaintance with the genetic aspects and recurrent risks of the common musculoskeletal disorders, they cannot be expected to act as the final authority for families and individuals afflicted by heritable disorders. A medical geneticist or a genetic clinic should be used to answer questions concerning why a disorder occurred, what the chances are that a disorder will recur, or whether a child is likely to transmit the disorder to his or her children.

The advent of amniocentesis offers some hope of detecting diseases such as neural tube defects, sickle cell anemia, and hemophilia in the fetus but raises harsh ethical, legal, and political dilemmas as well.

Some generalizations are helpful in considering genetic risk. Chromosomal abnormalities occur at a rate of 5600 per million live births or 0.5 percent. Three percent of live births will show a major congenital abnormality of multifactorial origin. Every individual alive probably carries five to seven recessive genes in their genotype. When the family history is negative for heritable disorders, there is a one percent risk that any pregnancy will produce an affected child.

SELECTED REFERENCES

Books
Akeson WH, Bornstein P, Glimcher MJ: AAOS Symposium on Heritable Disorders of Connective Tissue. St. Louis, C.V. Mosby, 1982.
Bailey JA: Disproportionate Short Stature. Philadelphia, Saunders, 1972.
Goodman RM, Gorlin RJ: The Face of Genetic Disorders. St. Louis, C.V. Mosby, 1970.
Harris H: The Principles of Human Biochemical Genetics, 2nd ed. New York, Elsevier Science, 1975.
Harsanyi Z, Hutton R: Genetic Prophecy: Beyond the Double Helix. New York, Rawson Wade, 1981.
Lumsden CJ, Wilson EO: Genes, Mind and Culture: The Coevolutionary Process. Cambridge, Mass, Harvard University, 1981.
McKusick VA: Human Genetics. Englewood Cliffs, NJ, Prentice-Hall, 1964.
McKusick VA: Heritable Disorders of Connective Tissue, 4th ed. St. Louis, C.V. Mosby, 1972.
McKusick VA: Mendelian Inheritance in Man; Catalogues of Phenotypes, 1st–6th eds. Baltimore, Johns Hopkins University, 1982.

McKusick VA, Clairborne R (eds): Medical Genetics. New York, H P, 1973.

Roberts JAF: An Introduction to Medical Genetics, 6th ed. London, Oxford University, 1973.

Smith DW: Recognizable Patterns of Human Malformation: Genetic, Embryologic and Clinical Aspects. Philadelphia, Saunders, 1970.

Stern C: Principles of Human Genetics, 3rd ed. San Francisco, Freeman, 1973.

Sutton EH: An Introduction to Human Genetics, 2nd ed. New York, Holt, Rinehart & Winston, 1975.

Thompson JS, Thompson MW: Genetics in Medicine, 2nd ed. Philadelphia, Saunders, 1973.

Wynne-Davies R: Heritable Disorders in Orthopaedic Practice, London, Blackwell, 1973.

Wynne-Davies R, Fairbank TJ: Fairbank's Atlas of General Affections of the Skeleton, 2nd ed. Edinburgh, London, and New York, Churchill Livingstone, 1976.

General References

Bishop MJ: Oncogenes. Sci Am March, 1982.

Carter CO: The inheritance of common congenital malformations. Prog Med Genet 4:59, 1965.

Chedd G: Genetic Gibberish in the Code of Life. Science 2:50, 1981.

Childs B: Sir Archibald Garrod's conception of chemical individuality: A modern appreciation. N Engl J Med 282:71, 1970.

Current concepts in genetics. N Engl J Med 294:17, 381, 480, 706, 823, 883, 1976.

Duthie RB, Townes PL: The genetics of orthopaedic conditions. J Bone Joint Surg 49B:229, 1967.

Elmore SM, Cantrell WC: Maffucci's syndrome. J Bone Joint Surg 48A:1607, 1966.

Fialkow PJ: The origin and development of human tumors studied with cell markers. N Engl J Med 291:26, 1974.

James JIP: The etiology of scoliosis. J Bone Joint Surg. 52B:410, 1970.

James JIP, Wynne-Davies R: Genetic factors in orthopaedics. In Apley AG (ed): Recent Advances in Orthopaedics. Baltimore, Williams & Wilkins, 1969, p 1.

Jones HW. (ed): Symposium of congenital defects. Am J Obstet Gynecol 90:7, 1964.

Menkes JH: Prospects for biochemical treatment of genetic disorders. South Med J 64 (Suppl 1):96 1971.

Milch RA, McKusick VA: Genetics of congenital deformity. Clin Orthop 33:3, 1964.

Nance WE, Elmore SM, Hillman JW: Genetics and orthopaedics. J Bone Joint Surg 46A:1260, 1965.

Riseborough ES, Wynne-Davies R: A genetic survey of scoliosis in Boston, Massachusetts. J Bone Joint Surg 55A:974, 1973.

Rogala ES, Drummond DS, Gunn J: Scoliosis: Incidence and natural history. J Bone Joint Surg 60A:173, 1978.

Saldanha PH: Frequency of congenital malformation in mixed populations of southern Brazil. In: Congenital Malformations, 2nd International Conference. New York, International Medical Congress, 1964.

Stelling FH: General affections of the skeletal system. Pediatr Clin North Am 14:359, 1967.

Wynne-Davies R: The genetics of some common congenital malformations. In Emery A (ed): Modern Trends in Human Genetics. New York, Appleton-Century-Crofts, 1972, p 316.

Yunis JJ: The chromosomal basis of human neoplasia. Science 221:227, 1983.

Chapter 3

Prenatal Development and Growth of the Musculoskeletal System

John A. Ogden and Dennis P. Grogan

The overall development and growth of the vertebrate musculoskeletal system are divided arbitrarily into prenatal (embryonic and fetal) and postnatal segments, with most basic or applied research being directed toward the prenatal phase since this period obviously contains the most striking changes. It must be appreciated, however, that significant changes beyond progressive growth and enlargement continue throughout the postnatal maturation of the musculoskeletal system. The period of time until skeletal maturity is reached may range from a few weeks in small mammals (mouse, rat) to several years (primates, man). Accordingly, postnatal changes may develop rapidly or may extend over a lengthy period. This time factor obviously affects the consequences of both congen-

ital deformities as well as acquired ones (i.e., injuries resulting from trauma or infection, metabolic or hematologic disorders).

This chapter will introduce basic concepts of chondro-osseous development and the specific aspects of *prenatal* development and growth. The subsequent chapter will deal with *postnatal* development and growth through the attainment of skeletal maturity.

Chondro-osseous development refers to the complete structural and functional maturation of the component tissues of the musculoskeletal system as well as those elements of the nervous system integral to this maturation process. The chief characteristic of development is cumulative, progressive change, with each component act and subsequent result losing significance unless viewed against what has proceeded, what follows, and what occurs concomitantly and integrally in related systems. Most micromorphologic and macromorphologic changes achieved during any given time sequence, especially in the early phases of prenatal development, are in anticipation of later functions or are a response to functional demands (e.g., biochemically or biomechanically oriented modeling and remodeling of trabecular and cortical bone). Developmental changes contrast sharply with recurrent, nonprogressive physiologic changes concerned with maintenance of the skeletal components, changes that characterize the constant remodeling of the mature skeleton throughout adult years, and the pathologic remodeling associated with arthritic changes.

Development proceeds concomitantly with growth, which can be defined as an increase in the mass of previously differentiated cellular, tissue, and organ components over a period of time. This can be accomplished by several means: (1) differentiation or modulation of connective tissue cells into a skeletogenic mode (the pleuripotential mesenchymal cell); (2) mitotic increase of already differentiated cartilaginous and osseous component cells; (3) increased intracellular synthesis of structural proteins; (4) increased intracellular water uptake, with accompanying shifts of water content between the intracellular and extracellular spaces; and (5) elaboration of increasing amounts of extracellular substances and water. The last method of growth is particularly characteristic of the skeletal system in which large amounts of extracellular matrix materials and hydration must be formed and accumulated in both the cartilaginous (chondroid) and osseous (osteoid) phases.

Based upon external and internal morphologic criteria, Streeter et al., (1951) divided the human embryonic period into 23 stages, each of which was termed a horizon (Table 3–1). These horizons described development relative to the embryonic period, which, in the human, comprises approximately the first 8 weeks of development. At

TABLE 3-2. AGE-LENGTH RELATIONSHIPS IN FETAL STAGE

Age of Embryo (Lunar Months)	Crown-Rump Length (mm)
3	56
4	112
5	160
6	203
7	242
8	277
9	313
10	350

the end of this time period, virtually all the major differentiation processes affecting the forming skeleton are completed. The remainder of gestation, the fetal period, is primarily characterized by growth of the differentiated chondro-osseous, neural, and muscular components and is defined by crown-rump length, with the accepted length of the full-term fetus being 360 to 370 mm (Table 3–2) (Scammon and Calkins, 1929).

Congenital defects may result from aberrations in either the developmental stage, the growth stage, or both. For example, hemimelia may result from a primary failure to form the fibrous or cartilaginous anlage (developmental error), a primary failure to chronologically synthesize appropriate quantities of those collagen or glycosaminoglycan (mucopolysaccharide) moieties that will allow further cellular changes (growth error), or the subsequent growth failure, resulting from abnormal biochemical syntheses, after a normal or relatively normal primary differentiation (e.g., a skeletal dysplasia in which the basic components are all present, but one or more time-dependent or biochemically dependent phases of progressive chondro-osseous maturation are adversely affected). Once a developmental error has been introduced into the sequential developmental pattern of the skeleton, numerous associated abnormalities may ensue because of these interrelated patterns of development of each of the skeletal components. Musculoskeletal defects having origin in the embryonic phase have a greater likelihood of associated multisystem abnormalities, and those occurring in the fetal period tend to be more localized abnormalities.

HISTORY

The concept that a cartilaginous skeleton preceded the osseous skeleton was commonly accepted in anatomic writings by the fifteenth and sixteenth centuries, but actual scientific observations concerning bone growth did not become significant until the early eighteenth century. Although Nesbitt (1736) postulated that some bones formed without cartilaginous antecedents, Haller (1763) substantiated the cartilaginous primordium concept. Bell (1823) argued that the osseous skeleton was separate in origin from the cartilaginous primordium and that the latter

TABLE 3-1. AGE AND LENGTH OF STAGE 12 TO 23 EMBRYOS (HUMAN)

Stage (Horizon)	Age (Postovulatory Days)	Usual Length (mm)
12	26	3–5
13	28	4–6
14	32	5–7
15	33	7–9
16	37	8–11
17	41	11–14
18	44	12–17
19	48	16–19
20	50	18–23
21	52	22–24
22	54	23–28
23	56	27–31

Modified from Gardner, 1970, with permission.

served as the replaceable scaffolding for the former. J. Muller and Sharpey (1836) histologically corroborated these concepts. A more detailed description of the provisional nature of cartilage and its gradual but total replacement by bone was advanced by H. Muller (1858). Loven (1863) first described the primary bone collar surrounding the cartilaginous precursor, and Ranvier (1875) described the adjacent perichondrial ring and its relationship to the growth plate. Fell (1925) detailed the development of zones within the cartilaginous primordia.

Concepts of bone growth and structural development paralleled the aforementioned studies. Hales (1729) described differential bone growth at each end in his treatise, "Vegetable Staticks," citing an experiment in which he introduced marker lines in a chick and observed the lines were the same distance apart in the grown chicken. Duhamel (1739) made use of intermittent madder feedings to show the periosteum was osteogenic. Not until 1770, however, did Hunter, using similar madder-feeding techniques, evolve the concept of metaphyseal bone remodeling; he showed that new bone was added at both metaphyseal ends and under the diaphyseal periosteum and that bone was absorbed around the outer metaphysis and inner diaphysis. Berard (1835) and Humphrey (1861) showed unequal longitudinal growth contributions from each end.

Van Leeuwenhoek (1674) first described blood vessels in bones, and Clopton Havers (1691) published his observations on vascularity of bone, especially in the marrow. Volkmann (1863) described additional vessels within the cortical bone. As will be discussed later, much of the subsequent detailed work on bone vascularity has been conducted by Trueta, Rhinelander, and Brookes.

Delpech first introduced the concept of biologic plasticity of cartilage, but this was not fully explored and substantiated until the works of Heuter and Volkmann in the 1860s. The microscopic response of bone to stress was presented by Wolff (1870). D'Arcy Wentworth Thompson in the early part of this century extensively studied comparative morphologic properties in relation to mechanical and species-specific factors and extensively used Cartesian transformations to show how the morphology of an individual bone could vary significantly from species to species by selective growth rate alterations in limited areas.

The introduction of improved microscopic techniques led to descriptions of bone formation by a specific cell, the osteoblast (Goodsir, 1845; Virchow, 1860; Gegenbaur, 1864). Kölliker (1873) described cellular events in bone remodeling, especially the presence of multinucleated giant cells that he termed osteoclasts. Ranvier, and later Lacroix, added considerably to the understanding of the histology of bone growth, especially in the epiphyseal and physeal regions.

Bernays (1878) published one of the earliest sequential studies of the prenatal development of the human skeleton, concentrating on the progressive changes in the knee. Rambaud and Renault (1864) published a detailed atlas of the developing skeleton. Hammar (1892) and Lubosch (1910) presented more detailed studies concerning the histology of joint development. More recently, Gardner, Gray, and O'Rahilly have vastly extended knowledge of prenatal skeleton development.

GENERALIZED PRENATAL DEVELOPMENT

Embryonic development proceeds through a series of replacement events wherein one molecular type or cell state is replaced by the next more complex state. Such replacement does not occur instantaneously nor does it necessarily involve a completely different moiety. The molecules or cells taking part in these replacement events are both similar and yet distinctly different. These different types are called isoforms. The most obvious cellular isoform is the replacement of a chondrocyte by an osteoblast. Both cell types synthesize and elaborate an extracellular matrix providing variably rigid structural support during embryonic and fetal growth. These isoforms arise during discrete developmental stages in which molecular and cellular demands are changing or are a result of genetic programming (Caplan et al., 1984).

All bones begin as mesenchymal condensations during the early embryonic period (Gardner, 1970). These mesenchymal cells are derived from the primary germ layers, usually under the mechanical or chemotactic influence of another tissue structure such as the notochord, neural tube, or apical ectodermal ridge. Some of these cellular condensations subsequently become fibrocellular and directly ossify to form the membranous bones of the cranial and facial skeleton and the clavicle. Most of the axial and appendicular skeleton components, however, are derived from the transformation of the mesenchymal model into a cartilaginous model and subsequently into an ossified structure by two discrete processes: (1) the formation of a primary osseous collar around the cartilage and subsequent vascular invasion to form the primary ossification center, which enlarges to become the diaphysis and metaphysis; and (2) a subsequent vascular-mediated ossification within the epiphyseal cartilage to form the secondary ossification center. This latter process of secondary ossification is almost always a postnatal phenomenon in the human (the distal femoral ossification center is the usual exception, its presence being indicative of a full-term pregnancy).

Selected areas of cartilage, termed growth plates or physes and capable of rapid growth, develop between the primary ossification center and epiphysis (Siegling, 1941; Sissons, 1971). This gradual replacement of the preexistent cartilage model by osseous tissue is termed endochondral ossification. These two types of bone formation, membranous and endochondral, refer only to the primary pattern of development. Subsequent growth after this initial differentiation may involve selected and juxtaposed areas of both patterns. Endochondrally derived bones have membranous ossification with appositional growth from the periosteum. Similarly, membranous bones may undergo subsequent growth by a modified endochondral process (e.g., clavicle). The basic concept of these two developmental and growth patterns will be discussed in the ensuing sections and will be elaborated upon in those sections specifically concerned with axial and appendicular skeletal formation.

Bones and joints are relatively self-differentiating structures once beyond the initial anlage establishment phase (Murray and Huxley, 1925). This certainly does not mean that they are independent from external influence or environment, but rather that the attainment of the initial form (anlage), which is often very similar in contour to the final, mature shape, is a result of factors intrinsic to the developing cell mass. This capacity exists through the primary mesenchymal stage, after which stabilization factors render the ensuing cartilaginous or osseous stages much more dependent upon joint movements and pressures from adjacent, growing, and increasingly functional parts. Such regions become even more mechanically dependent during the postnatal phase as the child begins ambulation and progressively increased physical activity.

Skeletogenesis poses two basic questions: (1) how does the development of a bone commence?, and (2) what determines where a particular bone will develop?

The first sign that skeletogenesis is imminent is condensation of mesodermal or ectomesenchymal cells to form the anlage (primordium) of the bone. The position of the condensation within the embryo defines the subsequent position and spatial relationships of the bone at the end of skeletal maturation. The shape of the condensation defines only the subsequent basic shape of the bone. Adverse surrounding tissue forces or forces external to the embryo–fetus can significantly alter the basic and developing shape of any of these biologically plastic skeletal precursors (Noback, 1944). The condensing mesodermal or ectomesenchymal cells either arise locally in the position that the bone will eventually occupy (as in the formation of the vertebra, limbs, or certain skull bones), or they migrate from elsewhere in the embryo to the site wherein skeletogenesis occurs (as in migration of mesodermal cells to form the mandible or the migration of ectomesenchymal cells from the neural crest to form parts of the skull). The specific factors responsible for the various cellular condensations are largely unknown, although cell adhesion and chemical interaction must play a role.

The position of the condensed mesoderm or ectomesenchyme as well as the shape, size, and rate of growth of the cellular condensations (fields) are all determined by interaction with adjacent ectoderm (the epithelial-mesenchymal interactions) (Ede, 1971). These interactions may involve bidirectional interchange between a stationary layer of ectoderm and adjacent mesoderm, as in the formation of the amniote limb, or they may involve establishment of an association between mobile (migrating) mesoderm and ectoderm (as in tooth formation). Other mesodermal cells adjacent to the specialized ectodermal fields, but outside the specific reacting mesodermal condensation, have the capacity to form skeletogenic tissue, but only the tissues subsequently arising within the mesodermal condensation do form skeletal tissues. To illustrate such a concept, during the formation of the cartilaginous primordia of the long bones of the embryonic chick, any mesodermal cell in the limb bud is intrinsically

capable of producing either cartilage or muscle up to stage 24 (approximately 4½ days of incubation). After this stage, however, only the cells within the central condensed mesoderm form cartilage, and these are the cells most closely associated with the specialized apical ectodermal ridge. Thus, up until certain stages any mesenchymal cell is potentially capable of producing more than one skeletal tissue, and during early development local environmental factors (especially inductive epitheliomesenchymal interactions) stabilize the genome of cells in specific fields for skeletogenesis and thereby influence what type of skeletal tissue will eventually form (Haines, 1969, 1975; Lacroix, 1951; Lucas and Schoch, 1980; Madderson, 1975; Rang, 1969; Ricqlès, 1968, 1969, 1972; Romer, 1942, 1963, 1972; Schaffer, 1961; Thompson, 1942).

Hall suggests that the combination of inductive influences from both notochord and central nervous system direct mesoderm to endochondrally ossify, whereas induction only from neural tissue directs the cells to membranous ossification (Bradamante and Hall, 1980; Hall, 1970, 1971; Mereel, 1967). Certainly somatic mesoderm destined to form the axial skeleton (vertebra) requires the combined influence of the developing spinal cord and the notochord before commencing chondrogenesis.

The second question concerns what determines the size and shape of the skeleton. Once chondro-osseous cellular differentiation commences, a three-dimensional structure develops. At first the cells within the condensing mesoderm are randomly arranged. As the cells elaborate extracellular matrix and differentiate further, however, they align themselves to the longitudinal axis of the condensation and thus initiate pattern and direction to the growth and shape of the anlage. From this point in the development of the skeletal anlage, factors other than the genome of the tissue become influential (i.e., genetic factors are superseded by epigenetic factors).

The attainment of the fundamental form (the basic three-dimensional morphology) of any chondro-osseous anlage is initially independent of any functional demands and thus under strong genetic control (Alexander, 1975; Bardeen, 1905; Bock and Von Wahlert, 1965). For example, if the mesodermal anlage of a bone (or even after chondrogenesis or early osteogenesis) is grafted onto the chorioallantoic membrane or transplanted subcutaneously, intramuscularly, or intracranially, the fundamental three-dimensional configuration develops. This is the expression of inherent rates of cell division, hypertrophy, and extracellular matrix elaboration.

Once the fundamental form develops, modification of features such as ridges for muscular attachments, tuberosities, etc., become increasingly contingent upon functional demand and thus can be structurally modified by the environment (the epigenetic factors) (Mereel, 1967). The minor morphologic changes thus determine the final, rather than fundamental, form of the bone. The continued application of mechanical factors is necessary to maintain that form.

The evolutionary consequences of such concepts concerning bones would be that a change in the morphogenetic processes responsible for the basic three-dimensional morphology of the skeleton would require considerable integrated alteration in the genome and, therefore, would be a relatively slow phylogenetic process. In contrast, changes in the minor elements could occur quite rapidly as ontogenetic modifications within the phases of prenatal and postnatal skeletal maturation of the individual.

Integrated genomic alteration obviously occurs in the human in the multitude of skeletal dysplasias that affect the fundamental form and specific segments of the various endochondral and membranous formative processes. Such fundamentally deformed bone is much more susceptible to epigenetic mechanical deformation. For example, the bone in achondroplasia is fundamentally short, whereas the development of coxa vara and genu varum are epigenetic phenomena. Both the fundamental expression of the specific genetic alteration and the epigenetic biologic response have considerable variation among affected individuals.

Skeletal development thus can be divided into two major stages—the morphogenetic phase and the cytodifferentiation phase. The morphogenetic phase is characterized by cellular movements and cellular interactions that determine the eventual location and shape of each skeletal component, whereas the cytodifferentiation phase is concerned with the establishment of the multiple cellular components and modulation of pleuripotential cells. In chondro-osseous tissues this phase is further featured by the elaboration of and changes in the extracellular matrix, which is composed principally of water, hyaluronic acid, chondroitin sulfate–protein complexes, and collagen. Essential to mesenchyme-cartilage-bone modulations are two important changes on the molecular level—the appearance of the enzyme hyaluronidase and the quantitative increase in chondroitin sulfate. Quantitatively there appears to be an inverse relationship between hyaluronic acid and chondroitin sulfate in the prenatal extracellular matrix. The earliest phases of the morphogenetic (mesenchymal) stage are characterized by hyaluronic acid production, but as cellular differentiation continues, chondroitin sulfate becomes the primary intercellular molecule of the cartilaginous stage, and hyaluronic acid is removed by increased hyaluronidase production. Hyaluronic acid appears necessary for cellular aggregation and may be essential to the accumulation of a sufficient number of precartilage cells to precipitate the transition from the morphogenetic phase to the cytodifferentiation phase (Milaire, 1962, 1963; Pritchard, 1952; Toole, 1974).

The effects of hyaluronic acid can be antagonized by some growth-promoting hormones, especially thyroxine, but the effects at this early stage of development are poorly understood (Canalis, 1983; Chalmers, 1965; Cruess, 1985; Daimon, 1973; Medoff, 1967; Trueta, 1968). As will be discussed, quantitative deficiencies of specific chemical moieties may prolong cellular transition and lead to skeletal reduction deformities.

The collagen molecular types appear to go through a similar spatial and temporal transition. The characteristic collagen molecule of adult bone has two α-1(I) and one α-2 units and is designated type I. In contrast, the collagen molecule of hyaline cartilage has three α-1(II) chains and is designated type II. Furthermore, the α-1 chains of both types of collagen appear to have slightly different amino acid sequences (therefore, the designations α-1[I] and α-1[II]). Additionally, there are translational changes that can occur in the molecules through the mechanisms of cross-linkage and subtle chemical differences in the extent of the hydroxylation of proline and lysine and the glycosylation of hydroxylysine. Collagen of the precartilage (mesodermal) stage appears similar to adult bone, namely type I. But when cartilage differentiates, type II appears but is restricted to the central core, whereas the outer regions (i.e., the presumptive periosteum and bone collar) still contain the type I collagen molecule. Type I collagen is certainly the main constituent of endochondral osteoid. More recently a specific type of collagen (type III) has been demonstrated in the lacunae of the hypertrophic zone of the physis. Von der Mark and Von der Mark (1977) divide the zones of the physis as follows: type II in the uncalcified and calcified cartilage, type III in the hypertrophic zone where it is being replaced by the invading perivascular tissue, and type I in the osteoid of the primary spongiosa.

Schmid and Linsenmayer (1983) have recently described a short-chain collagen (SC or type X) specifically synthesized by the physeal hypertrophic cells. This molecule, on the basis of immunofluorescent studies, is not found in any other zones of the physis. Thus, within a single-cell type (i.e., a chondrocyte), it appears there are subpopulations of cells with qualitative and quantitative biologic and biochemical differences. Such differences may be important conceptually when one considers potential changes in homogeneous cell populations produced by such diverse stimuli as tissue interactions, cell-matrix interactions, and response to injury.

Thus, there exists a timing element, the onset of a specific cartilage collagen in the anlage, and a spatial element, the separation of different collagen types within the mesenchyme that will eventually become cartilage, bone, fibrous tissue, and muscle. A similar differentiation of collagen components also appears during later stages of development. The collagen of osteoid tissue appears to have a higher degree of hydroxylation of lysine than the collagen in mature (lamellar) bone matrix. It is important to realize that each of these changes in collagen types parallels changes in structure and function.

The rationale for the appearance and turnover of the three (or more) genetically distinct types of collagen during bone development is not clear, nor has a knowledge of these structural molecular differences led to a conclusive explanation of functional differences of the collagen types. However, increasing interest in the differing types and distribution of collagen has led to the demarcation of various subtypes of osteogenesis imperfecta.

The third extracellular molecular component is chondroitin sulfate (types A and B), which complexes with various proteins to form glycosaminoglycans (previously referred to as mucopolysaccharides). These various glycosaminoglycan moieties interact with collagen. This interaction seems important to morphogenesis and to the

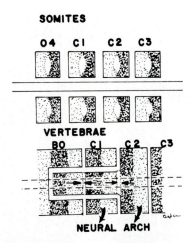

Figure 3-14. Schematic formation of upper cervical spine from the fourth occipital to third cervical somites. The odontoid process (dens) is derived from portions of the O4, C1, and C2 somites, whereas the ring of the C1 vertebra is derived from the C1 and C2 somites. A part of the C1 somite forms the basiocciput with O4.

play an integral role in the structural formation of the basicranium. Cellular components from the fourth occipital somite fuse with some of the cellular material of the first cervical somite to form, in lower vertebrates, the proatlas. In humans, this same somite fusion contributes to the ligaments extending from the skull to the odontoid process (dens) and also contributes to the cranial end of the odontoid process (the portion that eventually will ossify to become the os terminale).

The major cell mass composing the odontoid process (dens) is derived from the first and second cervical somites. This same C1-C2 somite amalgamation contributes to the formation of the anterior arch (centrum) of C1 and some of the supporting ligaments connecting C1 to the odontoid process. In rat embryos, the odontoid still has a centrally located notochordal remnant, which corroborates the centrum origin of the odontoid. In mouse embryos, a cartilage bridge may form between the anterior arch of C1 and the odontoid process, but usually disappears before birth. In one particular mouse genetic strain termed "undulated" (Un/Un), this bridge persists and may even ossify, leading to C1-C2 fusion.

The centrum of C2 is derived from portions of the second and third cervical somites. The aforementioned developmental processes explain the origin of the C1 nerve root between the skull and the C1 vertebra.

Completion of the sclerocoele might be the cause of congenital pseudarthrosis between C2 and the odontoid process. Failure of the C1 centrum to separate into anterior arch and odontoid in association with complete sclerocoele formation in the second cervical somite might be the cause of absence or hypoplasia of the odontoid process, especially in patients with skeletal dysplasia. Trauma, however, may be a more likely factor in the causation of the os odontoideum in otherwise normal children.

Notochord. The notochord becomes totally encased by the migrating mesenchymal cells of the paired sclerotomes as they coalesce in the midline (Williams, 1908). As the vertebral column continues to differentiate, the enclosed notochord gradually regresses, although embryonic cells may transiently persist within the vertebral body as the mucoid streak (Fig. 3–15). However, between the vertebral bodies, the notochordal cells undergo mucoid change to form the gelatinous nucleus pulposus. Cells from the sclerocoele region form the perichordal ring, thus bridging the space between the resegmented somites. Eventually this perichordal tissue becomes the annulus fibrosus. In the adult, remnants (cell rests) of the notochord may persist in either the basisphenoid region or the coccygeal region where they subsequently may form a chordoma with the characteristic mucoid-containing physaliphorous cells.

Neural Arch Formation. A second mass of cells of sclerotomal origin migrates dorsally, juxtaposed to the neural tube, to form the neural (vertebral) arch (Fig. 3–16). The majority of precursor cells appear to originate in the caudal half of each sclerotome. Sclerotomic resegmentation of the posterior arches comparable to the anterior process of the vertebral centra formation does not occur to any significant degree. Further, the neural arch does not begin formation until after the anterior somite–centrum resegmentation process is almost completed. The neural arches alternate with the spinal ganglia and thus are situated intersegmentally with respect to the myotomes such that each neural arch is connected to two successive myotomal segments. Experimental evidence suggests that the dorsal root ganglia precede the neural arches in developmental sequence and probably play a role in inducing neural arch development. For example, in the salamander embryo, somite transplantation to increase the number of somites unilaterally leads first to the formation of extra dorsal root ganglia, although not necessarily equal to the number of transplanted somites. An induced neural arch then appears between successive ganglia. Some vertebral anomalies may therefore be due to primary neurologic defects that induce maldevelopment of the associated vertebral centrum, neural arch, or both.

Neural Arch Defects. Midline defects of the axial skeleton are relatively common. Research on various genetic defects supports an early onset of these abnormalities in the primitive streak, notochord, somite formation, or resegmentation phases rather than in the subsequent chondrification or ossification stages. Simple osseous defects in which the paired ossification centers of the neural arch fail to fuse posteriorly are quite common (especially involving the L5 and S1 vertebra), with some studies giving an incidence of as much as 20 percent in the general population (Fig. 3–17). This condition, spina bifida occulta, is rarely accompanied by significant primary neurologic defects. Larger areas of spina bifida occulta may involve the sacrum, culminating in failure to form the spinous process(es), and can predispose the individual to the congenital

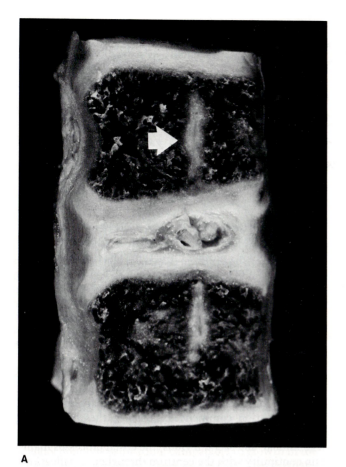

A

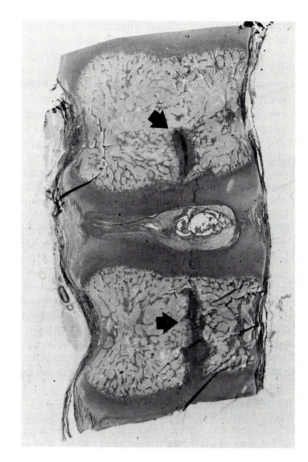

B

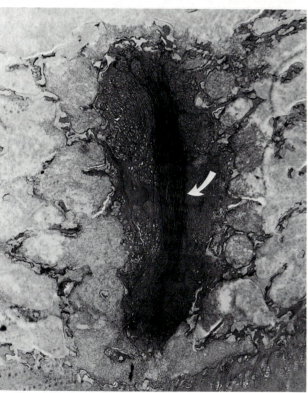

C

Figure 3-15. Sagittal section **(A)** and histologic section **(B)** of thoracic vertebrae from a human infant (approximately one year of age) showing retention of notochord tissue (arrows). **C.** Higher-power view of notochord remnant showing fibrocellular core (arrow) surrounded by irregular cartilaginous clones.

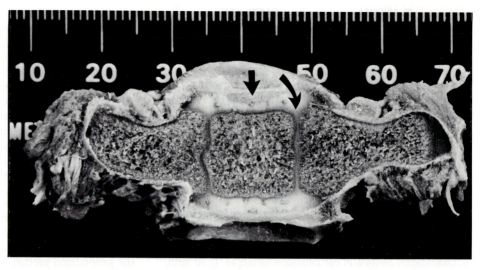

A

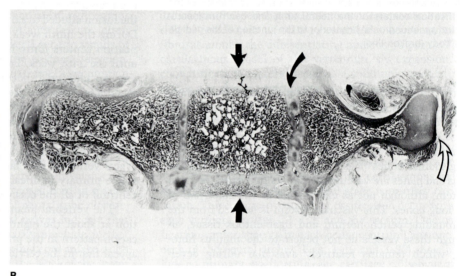

Figure 3-20. Morphologic **(A)** and histologic **(B)** appearance of end plate formation in a lumbar vertebra from a neonatal seal. Note the neurocentral synchondroses (curved solid arrows) separating the posterior and centrum ossification centers. Secondary ossification centers are present inferiorly and superiorly (straight solid arrows). The transverse processes have a cartilaginous epiphysis (open arrow).

B

first unite (postnatally) with the ossification center in the centrum in the upper lumbar region and progress both craniad and caudad.

The patterns of formation of the primary ossification centers in the centra and neural arches vary significantly. The cartilaginous centra exhibit early development of a cartilage canal (vascular) system and begin endochondral ossification analogous to the development of a secondary (epiphyseal) ossification center of a long bone. Because of this particular pattern, there can be no periosteum until the ossification center expands to the peripheral margins of the centrum. The centra are surrounded only by perichondrium during the fetal period and early infancy (Figs. 3–19 and 3–20). In contrast, the neural arches develop a primary bone collar, periosteum, and primary ossification center in a manner analogous to primary ossification center formation in tubular (longitudinal) bones.

Fusion between the primary ossification centers of the anterior centrum and posterior arches occurs anterior to the anatomic pedicle at the site of the original neurocentral synchrondrosis (Fig. 3–23). This rarely occurs before birth. Accordingly, these regions are very evident in a radiograph of the neonatal spine and must not be interpreted as either congenital deformity or trauma.

There is no pattern of ossification center development in the lumbar neural arches to suggest that the pars articularis defect in spondylolisthesis or spondylolysis is the congenital result of a failure of fusion of the posterior primary ossification centers. The normal site of ossific fusion of the centrum with the neural arches is well anterior to the pathologic defect, *within* the vertebral body. Accordingly, the pars defect must be an acquired, undoubtedly traumatically incurred failure within the primary ossification center of the neural arch (Ogden, 1982).

Development of the Ribs and Sternum
The ribs develop from costal processes derived from the caudal portion of the sclerotome forming the neural arch.

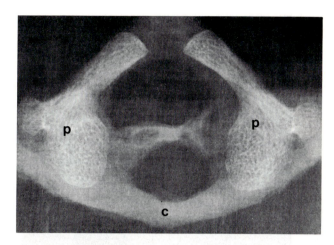

Figure 3-21. Neonatal view of C-1 (roentgenograph). Note the paired posterior element (P) ossification, which extends anterior to the facet joints. The centrum (C) has not commenced primary ossification.

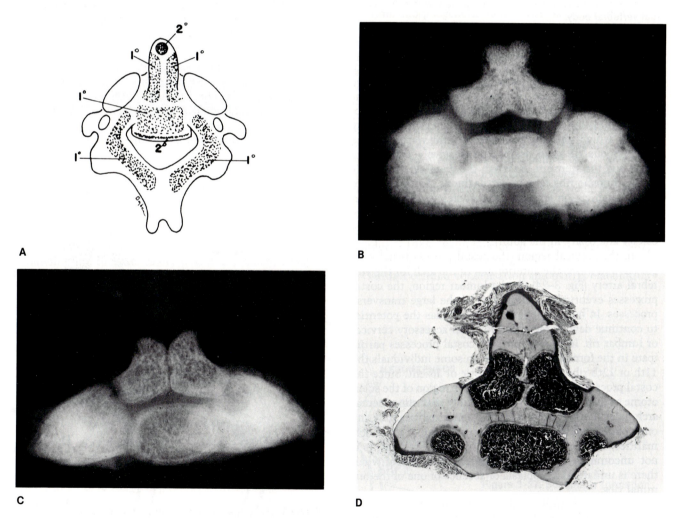

Figure 3-22. A. Primary (first degree) and secondary (second degree) ossification centers of the second cervical vertebra. Note the bilateral centers in the odontoid. **B.** Roentgenograph of fused odontoid centers at term. **C.** Roentgenograph of bifid odontoid ossification centers at full term. **D.** Histologic section of bifid centers.

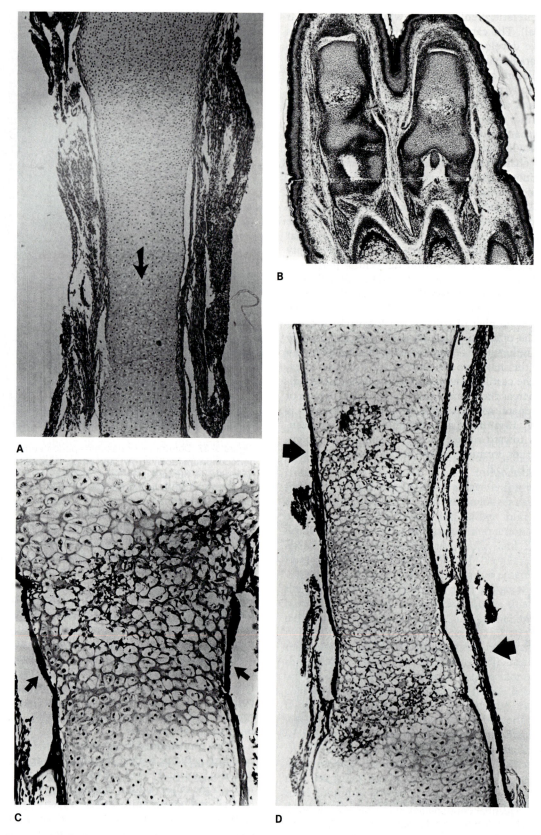

Figure 3-38. A. Early cartilaginous anlage of the femur. This cell population is relatively homogeneous, although some cell hypertrophy and lacuna formation is evident (arrow). **B.** Further central hypertrophy in the phalanges. Note the absence of a bone collar. **C.** Formation of bone collar (arrows) around the hypertrophic cells. **D.** Specimen showing bipartite hypertrophic regions (arrows).

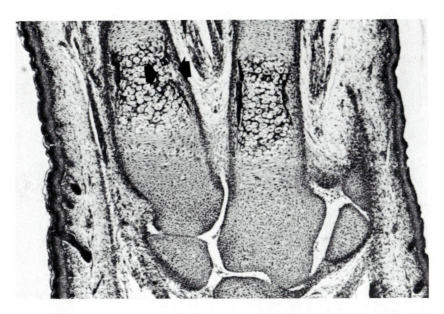

Figure 3–39. Developing metacarpals showing the primary bone collar around the central zone of hypertrophied chondrocytes and an area of vasoformative irruption (arrow). (×20)

(Burkus and Ogden, 1982). This vessel, which becomes the nutrient artery, enters the anlage at right angles to the longitudinal axis and maintains this orientation during most of prenatal development. The primary ossification center contains osteoblastic and angioblastic tissue and does not exhibit any hematopoietic function (this occurs later, after extensive remodeling of the diaphysis).

The onset of primary ossification occurs in all the major long bones toward the end of the second gestational month (Gardner, 1970; O'Rahilly and Gardner, 1972). The humerus is usually the first to ossify (horizons 21–22), followed by the radius (horizons 21–23). The femur, tibia, and ulna all ossify at approximately the same time (horizons 22–23), whereas the fibula is usually the last to ossify (horizon 23).

Once the initial ossification center has formed and the nutrient artery is established, further ossification progresses rapidly toward each end as the variably developed cartilage of the phase 1 to 4 zones begins more rapid maturation to phase 5 (hypertrophic, calcified) cartilage. This sequential replacement of cartilage by bone is endochondral ossification. The bone first formed is a loose trabecular network that fuses with the multilayered periosteal shell (Fig. 3–41). This initial ossification process extends at relatively equal rates toward each end of the bone, with new cartilage formation also occurring at approximately the same rate for each end. Postnatally, however, there often is a significant difference in the rates of growth for each epiphysis and physis within a given bone (Haines, 1974; Ogden et al., 1975; Ogden and Southwick, 1976).

As the primary ossification process approaches each end, the cartilage compacts and begins to more closely resemble the definitive growth plate. This usually occurs by the end of the third or early in the fourth gestational month. As the primary ossification center progresses toward the cartilaginous ends, the primary periosteal col-

lar also extends toward these regions, but always slightly ahead of the endochrondral ossification center. Once the physis is established (usually after 70 to 80 percent of the cartilage has been replaced by primary ossification), the periosteal ring stops further extension toward the epiphysis and remains level with the zone of hypertrophic cartilage (with which it continues growth in an integrated fashion), although it may extend further as osteoid tissue to reach the germinal zone (Fig. 3–42). The association of periosteal ring, peripheral physis, and fibrovascular tissue is referred to as the zone of Ranvier, which is an important area of diametric expansion (to be discussed in detail in the next chapter concerning postnatal development). The

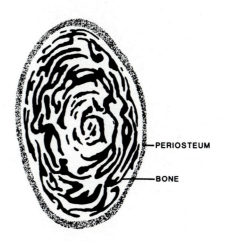

Figure 3–40. Schematic of multilayered bone collar derived primarily from periosteal membranous bone formation. Note the similarity to ring formation in trees. This bone will be modified extensively during the postnatal period by ostean formation (Haversian bone).

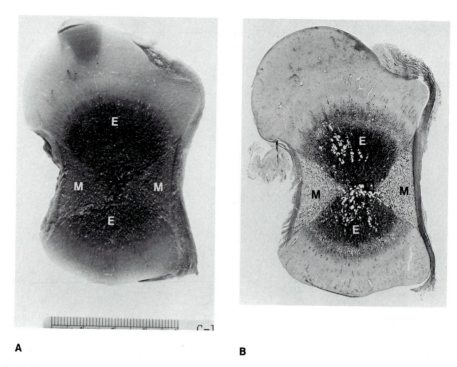

Figure 3–41. Morphologic **(A)** and histologic **(B)** sections of humerus from a fetal humpback whale showing juxtaposition (fusion) of two bone types. E, endochondral; M, membranous (periosteal).

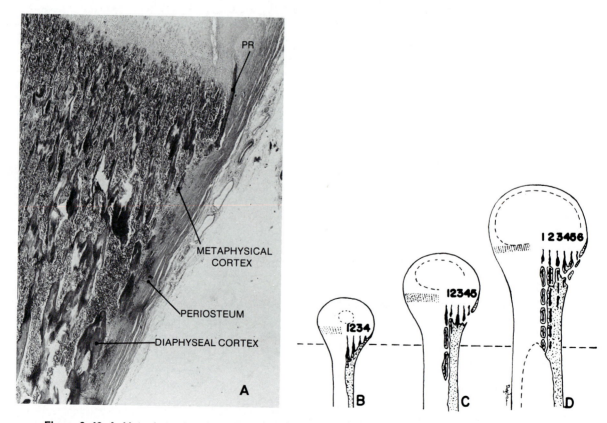

Figure 3–42. A. Metaphyseal cortex in a 2-month-old female (postnatal) showing the periosteal ring (PR) and the porous metaphyseal cortex. (×7.50) **B, C, D.** Schematic of remodeling, longitudinal, and diametric growth.

periosteal ring does not always extend to the zone of hypertrophy, especially in the smaller bones (metacarpals), and may not completely surround the physis in every bone (Burkus and Ogden, 1984; Pratt, 1959).

Active remodeling occurs in two areas of the metaphysis—central and peripheral. Bone is removed from the peripheral cortical surface, and new bone is added to the endosteal surface (Fig. 3–42). The endosteal bone will become contiguous with the diaphyseal cortical bone. Bone modeling and remodeling is so active that the metaphyseal cortex is relatively porous. This porous bone is easily penetrated by an osteomyelitic abscess originating in the metaphysis, allowing it to reach the subperiosteal space (or joint, if this region happens to be intraarticular as in the proximal femur). The central part of the metaphysis may remodel by a process that causes bone to "flow" centripetally and toward the diaphysis. Although controversial, such flow may play a role in metaphyseal narrowing (Johnson, 1966).

While remodeling is occurring in the metaphysis, the diaphysis is steadily increasing in diameter by appositional (membranous) bone deposition and endosteal remodeling. The endosteal surface is the site of both new bone formation and osteoclastic osteolysis, with replacement of primary spongiosa by secondary spongiosa. Remodeling varies from bone to bone, even within a bone, and is intimately related to vascular changes (Albu et al., 1973). If it fails to occur properly, the bone ends may become more flared. This can be seen in several bone dysplasias such as osteopetrosis, Gaucher's disease, and Englemann's disease.

By birth, the long bones consist primarily of trabeculae that are oriented longitudinally and cylindrically, with secondary trabeculae intermittently spanning the intervening spaces. These trabeculae contain coarse-fibered or woven bone. There is only a small marrow cavity; however, near term, lamellar (i.e., compact or osteonal) bone develops, although extensive formation of this fine-fibered type is principally a postnatal phenomenon (and will be discussed in the next chapter). Cortical thickness and trabecular orientation within this new, lamellar bone will form in accord with intraosseous stress patterns. This is known as Wolff's law. Basically this law states that bone formation will increase in areas of compression and decrease in areas of tension. The trabeculae will similarly orient along major stress lines and will form secondary trabeculae that act as struts or tie beams (Chamay and Tschantz, 1972; Enlow, 1968; Ogden, 1982, 1984).

Limb Deformation. The pathomechanics of limb deformities are not as well understood as those of the axial skeleton, but as in the axial skeleton, it appears that most transverse and intercalary reduction and duplication deformities occur very early in development (Amprino, 1965; Frantz and O'Rahilly, 1961; Grüneberg, 1963; Jaffe, 1972; Mitolo, 1973; Ogden, 1976, 1979, 1982; Ogden et al., 1976; Ogden et al., 1978; Ogden et al., 1976; O'Rahilly, 1951; Scott et al., 1980; Swinyard, 1969; Warkany, 1971). Further, it seems likely that most deformities are mesodermal defects. Primary ectodermal defects appear to be rare. When supposed ectodermal (apical ectodermal ridge [AER]) defects have been detected, they appear to be a consequence of related mesodermal defects; either the lateral-plate mesoderm fails to induce differentiation of the AER, or once the ectoderm is formed, the mesoderm fails to produce those maintenance factors that allow continued differentiation.

The only proven primary AER defect is the wingless mutant in chickens. The ectoderm is defective and fails to form an AER in response to the lateral-plate mesoderm; thus, the limb bud cannot differentiate further. However, if normal ectoderm (from an unaffected embryo) is transplanted over the mesoderm, the limb bud does have the intrinsic capacity to differentiate normally.

A pathomechanism that appears particularly characteristic of limb abnormalities is cellular competition. When the available mesenchymal material within the distally differentiating limb bud is quantitatively reduced, the skeletal components compete to recruit cells such that a large, vigorously growing section may recruit blastemal cells normally intended for another region, which is rendered "weak" by genetic or teratogenic action. The continuity of the early blastemal cells allows this competition to occur. If recruitment is extensive, the weaker area will be progressively reduced in size and may even fall below a threshold cell population sufficient to allow subsequent differentiation and independent development. This cellularly weaker region may fuse with adjacent elements, may become hypoplastic or fibrotic, or may transfer the remaining blastemal cells distally where the excess blastemal material is quantitatively sufficient to develop into extra digits, even though not quantitatively sufficient to form the original skeletal element (e.g., the frequent association of tibial hemimelia with polydactyly).

Scott et al., (1980) suggested that a delay in the onset of physiologic necrosis in the AER led to the subsequent induction of preaxial polydactyly. In the absence of cell death and release of inhibiting substances, the AER continues to function and influence further digital development (polydactyly or polyphalangia).

Mesodermal defects have been studied in many animals. As in the human, manifestation of each specific defect varies considerably, and different genes appear responsible for similar skeletal deformities. Maldevelopment of the tibia is an excellent example. This defect is infrequent in humans, but when present, it is highly variable (Fig. 3–43). The deformity may also occur in chickens and is relatively common in mice. The genes for each of these variants in mice, although expressing grossly similar tibial defects, appear to be carried on more than one chromosome.

Deformities in mice generally show reduction of more distal elements, with preservation of more proximal regions if any portion remains. In contrast, reduction deformities in chickens (especially those involving the radius) tend to affect the proximal region and leave the distal end intact. In humans, the former appears to be the most common pattern, although infrequently there may be absence of a proximal segment of a bone. In animals, postaxial hemimelia (i.e., involvement of ulna and

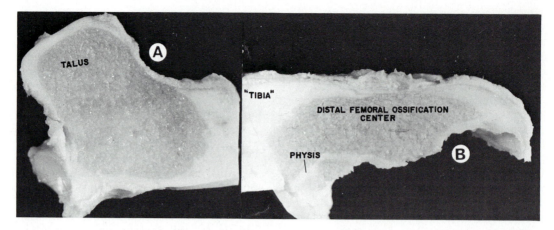

Figure 3-43. Reconstructed specimen from a 6-year-old girl with absent tibia. There was no knee or ankle joint, and a large, poorly differentiated piece of cartilage included both distal femoral and talar ossification centers.

fibula) is much less common than preaxial hemimelia, whereas in humans, preaxial (radial) hemimelia is most common in the upper extremity, and postaxial (fibular) hemimelia is more common in the lower extremity.

Although most abnormalities affect the early mesoderm, it is possible to alter differentiation at subsequent stages. In the brachypod mouse (bp^H), the femur and tibia are normal, but the fibula is small and remains cartilaginous throughout fetal development, not showing initial signs of primary ossification until 2 weeks after birth. Interestingly, the morphologic defect appears due to a quantitative chemical deficit. The aforementioned phase formation in the cartilaginous model is related to secretion of a hyaline organic matrix, the two major components of which are type II collagen and the acid glycosaminoglycans (chondroitin sulfates A and C). Collagen appears to act as the stabilizing factor within the chondrogenic matrix, and critical quantitative levels of synthesis and accumulation of collagen appear necessary for the effective transition of osseous tissue. Further, the relative levels of collagen to chondroitin sulfate also influence whether a tissue will have a chondrogenic or os-

teogenic expression. In the bp^H mouse fibula, the collagen molecule is normal, but the rates of both synthesis and degradation are abnormal, whereas the rate of synthesis of chondroitin sulfate is normal, but the total amount and rate of degradation are abnormal. This combination leads to the formation of cartilaginous tissue that lacks phase formation at the time sequence appropriate for ossification. However, the quantitative thresholds are finally attained postnatally, and primary ossification then commences. Nonetheless, the absence of a normal-sized, mechanically efficient fibula has a detrimental effect on subsequent postaxial development. This similar phenomenon of postnatal formation of a primary ossification center in a previously radiologically absent bone can be encountered in reduction deformities in man (Fig. 3-44).

Postaxial deformities, although infrequent in laboratory animals, can be induced by chemical compounds (Ogden et al., 1978; Ogden et al., 1976). The administration of acetazolamide to pregnant rats during the 10th to 12th days of gestation causes variably severe ulnar deficiencies (Fig. 3-45). Interestingly, although the drug is a potent carbonic anhydrase inhibitor and theoretically should be ter-

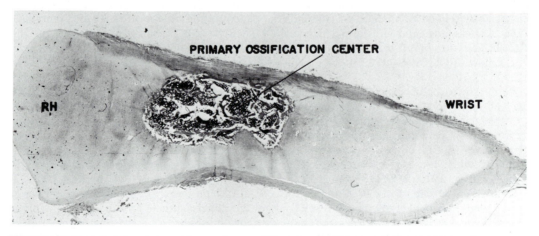

Figure 3-44. Absent radius removed from a 4-year-old boy. A rudimentary radial head (RH) has formed. The ossification center is eccentric. The cartilage has no canalicular (vascular) system. (×2.50)

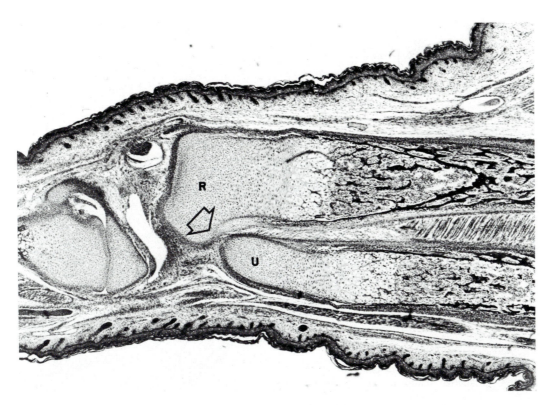

Figure 3–45. Hypoplastic ulna (U) from a newborn rat from a mother treated with acetazolamide during pregnancy. The distal end of the ulna is deformed and incompletely separated (arrow) from the radius (R). (×17)

atogenic through this chemical mechanism, there is no histochemical evidence of carbonic anhydrase activity at the susceptible embryonic stage (this may reflect an inability to detect it in the quantity present).

Development of Joints

As previously discussed, the blastemal appendicular skeleton initially forms as a continuous structure, with no gaps separating the differentiating major anlagen from each other. But as the mesenchymal model begins chondrification, concomitant changes occur in the region of the presumptive joint to create the interzone. This structure has three layers—two parallel chondrogenic layers and an intermediate, less dense layer (Figs. 3–46 and 3–47). The primitive joint capsule differentiates at the same time. It is derived from that interface of intermediate and deep mesoderm that gave rise to perichondrium and periosteum, thus establishing continuity of the joint capsule with the soft tissues of the adjacent bones (Gray and Gardner, 1950; Gray et al., 1957; Ogden, 1974).

The more peripheral regions of the interzone intermediate layer form synovial tissue. Blood vessels penetrate the evolving joint capsule to reach the blastemal synovium, but they do not usually penetrate the central joint regions. The intra-articular structures (e.g., menisci and cruciate ligaments) appear as further cellular condensations in the intermediate mesenchyme (Clark and Ogden, 1983). The remaining undifferentiated cells of the intermediate layer become associated with the two chondrogenic layers. Once the basic articular contours and

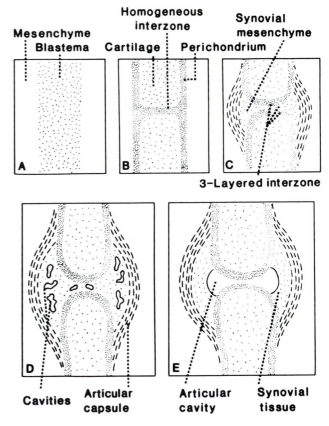

Figure 3–46. Schematic depiction of progressive stages of interzone formation leading to a synovial joint.

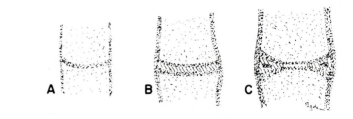

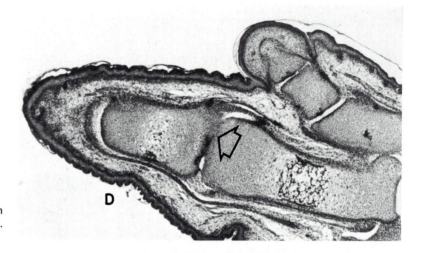

Figure 3-47. Partial formation of a joint between the phalanx and the metacarpal (open arrow). Thumb joint formation is already complete.

intra-articular structures are established, minute spaces appear in the intermediate zone. These spaces coalesce to form the joint cavity. Cavitation is probably an enzymatic process that appears initially independent from joint motion. The chondrogenic layers establish the contours of the opposing joint surfaces, taking along cells of the intermediate layer that will form synovium in the recesses. Cavitation quickly expands to firmly establish most joints spaces by ten weeks of gestation.

Joints are relatively self-differentiating structures that attain their basic form through factors presumably intrinsic to the interzone cells and possibly some inductive influence from juxtaposed skeletal blastema (Haines, 1947). If a joint primordium is removed from the differentiating limb bud and grown in culture, it has only a limited capacity for self-differentiation (Hall, 1972), that is, a joint-like structure will form, but will be morphologically limited in its overall developmental potential. If a small amount of adjacent skeletal blastema is included in the explant, however, more complete differentiation occurs. When a presumptive joint region is excised from the mesenchymal skeleton, the remaining tissue can redistribute and reform the interzone to create a normal joint. However, resection of the interzone after chondrification has commenced results in fusion of the juxtaposed anlagen and a complete lack of a joint (chondrification is equated with stabilization of independent self-differentiating capacity).

Some diarthrodial (synovial) joints differ in the basic developmental patterns. Small joints in the hands and feet may show considerable delay between interzone formation and cavitation, with the contiguous skeletal elements sometimes proceeding to the ossification stage before a definitive joint is established. The distal interphalangeal

joint and some carpal and tarsal joints may not go through the homogenous three-layer zone; instead, they form a joint directly from the layer of dense cartilage between the developing bones. Synchondroses form in a fashion similar to that of diarthrodial joints, except that no intermediate zone develops (in the ribs) or the interzone becomes fibrocartilage (symphysis pubis).

Because of concomitant development of innervated muscle, some motion can begin early. This enhances joint

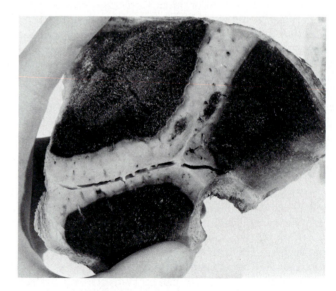

Figure 3-48. Elbow joint from a pygmy sperm whale (*Kogia breviceps*) showing the limited joint space with multiple transarticular blood vessels.

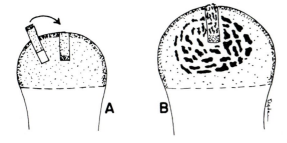

Figure 3-49. Schematic of hyaline–articular cartilage reversal experiment. See text for details.

modeling in utero (Drachman and Sokoloff, 1966; Meikle, 1975; Murray and Drachman, 1969). Postnatally, joint motion and joint reaction forces become more consequential to the final joint contours attained by skeletal maturity.

Fusion between small joint surfaces (e.g., carpal or tarsal coalitions) probably occurs because of segmentation failure during the cavitation stage, but it seems more likely that major joint fusions occur at an earlier stage, probably resulting from defective lateral-plate differentiation of the initial mesenchymal anlage cells.

Failure to form joints occurs in many congenital deformities. In Apert's syndrome, although there may be radiographic separation between the phalanges, a true joint often fails to form. Other joints such as the sacroiliac have virtually no motion (syndesmosis). Certain animals offer interesting analogues to both these abnormal and normal situations. Cetaceans have minimal to nonexistent motion in joints distal to the shoulder. The elbow joint in the pygmy sperm whale (*Kogia breviceps*) has articular surfaces, but has vessels crossing it (Fig. 3–48). In the interphalangeal joints of the pilot whale (*Globicephala macrorhynchus*) vessels also cross the presumptive joint, which has fibrous tissue connecting the adjacent epi-

physes. Variations of joint formation such as these offer interesting areas for morphologic research into skeletal development.

When the hyaline cartilage of the chondroepiphysis first forms, there is no significant histochemical or histologic difference between the cells of the joint surface (derived from the chondrogenic layer of the interzone) and the remainder of the hyaline cartilage. At some point, however, the articular cartilage stabilizes and differentiates from the rest of the epiphyseal cartilage. Although techniques are not yet available to detect any significant early biochemical differences, an interesting experiment has firmly established that these two cartilage types are different functionally (and, by implication, biochemically). If a core of articular and underlying epiphyseal cartilage is removed, turned 180 degrees, and reinserted, the transposed epiphyseal cartilage will form bone at the joint surface, but the articular cells will remain cartilaginous and will be completely surrounded by the enlarging secondary ossification center (Fig. 3–49) (McKibbin and Holdsworth, 1967). Articular cartilage does not appear capable of significant ossification. As skeletal maturity is reached, a tide mark develops near the articular cartilage; this appears to be a boundary between these two cartilaginous cell regions.

The articular cartilage, like physeal cartilage, must be able to respond to joint reaction forces, both physiologic and pathologic. Pathologic increases in compression forces retard physeal growth. The reaction in articular cartilage differs. The compressed cells undergo histochemical modulation (probably by altered prostaglandin and cathepsin release) that dissolves the intercellular matrix and allows migration of cells away from the abnormal pressures where they reform lacunae and matrix. Migration of large numbers of cells, however, yields lacunae containing multiple cells (Fig. 3–50). The subchondral bone adjacent to these

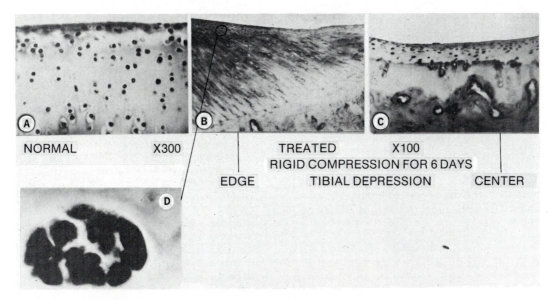

Figure 3-50. Effect of prolonged compression and immobilization on articular cartilage from a rat knee joint. Note the cartilage narrows centrally, whereas peripherally, lacunae become filled with migrating chondrocytes **(D)**.

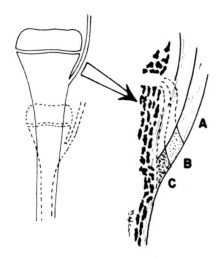

Figure 3–51. Schematic of growth region of a tendon or ligament inserting into the metaphysis or diaphysis. **A.** Germinal and resting cells. **B.** Metabolically active cells. **C.** Cellular region blending with periosteum and capable of migration integrated with metaphyseal and diaphyseal growth.

multicellular regions appears to increase, leading to osteophyte formation. As described for physiologic epiphyseodesis, it also appears that articular cartilage, after skeletal maturation, may become capable of some degree of calcification and ossification.

Development of Ligaments and Tendons

Some ligaments and tendons attach to the diaphysis or metaphysis. These structures must have a means to accommodate to overall bone growth. As one elongates, the site of insertion of the tendon or ligament must be progressively displaced away from the central reference point (nutrient artery foramen). Major tendons (such as the iliopsoas) appear to adapt by retaining part of the original physis (in the fetal stage the lesser trochanter is a part of the large proximal femoral epiphysis; in postnatal life it becomes a separate structure). This allows longitudinal displacement of the tendinous iliopsoas as new bone is formed and older bone is remodeled.

Recent experimental data have shown that ligaments and tendons without associated, localized physes also possess a similar, albeit histologically different, growth mechanism (Videman, 1970). The distal tendon or ligament has three major regions—a zone of cellular proliferation, a zone of maturing cells synthesizing intercellular matrix, and a zone of bone formation. The growth of each of these areas seems fully integrated with the associated physis. The new bone that is formed is replaced by the normal process of remodeling (Fig. 3–51).

SUMMARY

The prenatal development of the appendicular and axial skeleton and the related neurologic and musculotendinous components is an extremely complex, diffusely integrated process. Whenever developmental abnormalities

occur, the final result will always be manifest in the osseous skeleton, even though the defect may have commenced in one of the antecedent, nonosseous phases. The possibility also must be considered that a gene may actively disturb cellular processes common to successive phases of development, affecting both blastemal and cartilaginous phases, thus compounding the defects. This is not the same as the formation of a mesenchymal defect that is perpetuated in abnormally shaped cartilage (the cartilage is normal, but the structural framework is not).

Developmental abnormalities, whether genetically, biochemically, or virally induced, must potentially affect a phase of skeletal development, but need not necessarily do so in the entire embryo to the same extent or at the same time. Some cells or groups of cells may be more sensitive than others, whereas some cells may be susceptible only during a certain phase of their life cycle; this sensitive phase may not occur in all of them simultaneously. Therefore, although many conditions are potentially systemic, the distribution of affected cells may be relatively localized. In contrast, if the defect does not manifest itself until the final stage of a cell type (i.e., chondroblast or osteoblast), an abnormality not obvious at birth may increase in severity with subsequent postnatal chondro-osseous maturation. This type of defect appears dependent upon threshold levels of abnormal cell products to begin manifestation of the disorder (e.g., mucopolysaccharide disorders, Gaucher's disease). Finally, the sensitive phase may be transient, leading to a steady state that may eventually allow progression from one cellular type to another, but in a severely retarded time sequence that also affects the ability to form normal structures.

REFERENCES

The available literature concerning normal and abnormal limb development is voluminous, and a complete listing is certainly beyond the intent of this book. Instead, references have been chosen because of historical perspective, extensive literature reviews, excellent summaries of the title-described topics, and comprehensive subject treatment. It is recommended that the interested reader consult these for additional references on specific items.

Albu I, Georgia R, Stoica E, et al.: Le système des canaux de la couche compacte diaphysaire des os longs chez l'homme. Acta Anat 84:43, 1973.

Alexander R McN: Evolution of integrated design. Am Zool 15:419, 1975.

Amprino R: Aspects of Limb Morphogenesis in the Avian Embryo. In Dehaan C, Ursprung W (eds): Organogenesis. New York, Winston, 1965.

Bale PM: A congenital intraspinal gastroenterogenous cyst in diastematomyelia. J Neurol Neurosurg Psychiatry 36:1011, 1973.

Bardeen C: Studies of the development of the human skeleton. Am J Anat 4:265, 1905.

Bateman N: Bone Growth: A study of the grey-lethal and microphthalmic mutants in the mouse. J Anat 88:212, 1954.

Bell E, Kaighn L, Fessenden L: The role of the mesodermal and ectodermal components in the development of the chick limb. Dev Biol 1:101, 1959.

Berrill N: Morphogenetic fields, their growth and development. Dev Biol 7:342, 1963.

Bock W: Kinetics of the avian skull. J Morphol 114:1, 1964.

Bock W, von Wahlert G: Adaptation and the form-function complex. Evolution 19:269, 1965.

Bowen V, Cassidy JD: Macroscopic and microscopic anatomy of the sacroiliac joint from embryonic life until the eighth decade. Spine 6:620, 1981.

Bradamante Z, Hall BK: The role of epithelial collagen and proteoglycan in the initiation of osteogenesis by avian neural crest cells. Anat Rec 197:305, 1980.

Bremer JL: Dorsal intestinal fistula; accessory neurenteric canal; diastematomyelia. Arch Pathol 54:132, 1952.

Burkus J, Ogden J: Bipartite primary ossification in the embryonic human femur. J Pediatr Orthop 2:63, 1982.

Burkus J, Ogden J: Development of the distal femoral epiphysis: A microscopic morphological investigation of the zone of Ranvier. J Pediatr Orthop 4:661, 1984.

Canalis E: Effect of hormones and growth factors on alkaline phosphatase activity and collagen synthesis in cultured rat calvariae. Metabolism 32:14, 1983.

Caplan AI, Fiszman MY, Eppenberger HM: Molecular and cell isoforms during development. Science 221:921, 1983.

Chalmers J: A study of some of the factors controlling growth of transplanted skeletal tissue. In Richelle LJ and Dallemagne MJ (eds): Proc 2nd Eur Symp Calcified Tissues. Coll des Colloq de l'Univ de Liege, 1965, p 177.

Chamay A, Tschantz P: Mechanical influences in bone remodeling. Experimental research on Wolff's law. J Biomech 5:173, 1972.

Chen J: Studies on the morphogenesis of the mouse sternum. J Anat 86:387, 1952.

Clark C, Ogden J: Development of human knee joint menisci: Relationship to childhood meniscal injury. J Bone Joint Surg 65A:538, 1983.

Cohen J, Sledge CB: Diastematomyelia. An embryological interpretation with report of a case. Am J Dis Child 100:257, 1960.

Crelin E, Koch W: An autoradiographic study of chondrocyte transformation into chondroclasts and osteocytes during bone formation in vitro. Anat Rec 158:473, 1967.

Crock HV: The Blood Supply and the Lower Limb Bones in Man. London, Livingstone, 1967.

Cruess, RL: Binding sites in fetal and growth plate cartilage. J Orthop Res 3:109, 1985.

Daimon T: Effects of large dose of insulin on the chondrogenesis of the tibiotarsus in developing chick embryos. 1. A light microscopic study. Acta Histochem Cytochem 6:280, 1973.

Dodds G: Row formation and other types of arrangements of cartilage cells in endochondral ossification. Anat Rec 46:385, 1930.

Dodds G: Osteoclasts and cartilage removal in endochondral ossification of certain mammals. Am J Anat 50:97, 1932.

Dommisse GF: The Arteries and Veins of the Human Spinal Cord from Birth. New York, Churchill Livingstone, 1975.

Drachman D, Sokoloff L: The role of movement in embryonic joint development. Dev Biol 4:401, 1966.

Ede D: Control of form and pattern in the vertebrate limb. Symp Soc Exp Biol 25:235, 1971.

Elliot GB, Tredwell SJ, Elliot KA: The notochord as an abnormal organizer in production of congenital intestinal defect. AJR 110:628, 1970.

Enlow D: Wolff's law and the factor of architectonic circumstance. Am J Orthod 54:803, 1968.

Fell H: The osteogenic capacity in vitro of periosteum and endosteum isolated from limb skeleton of fowl embryos and young chicks. J Anat 66:157, 1932.

Fell H: Skeletal development in tissue culture. In Bourne G (ed): The Biochemistry and Physiology of Bone. New York, Academic, 1956.

Felts W: The prenatal development of the human femur. Am J Anat 94:1, 1954.

Felts W: Transplantation studies of factors in skeletal organogenesis. I. The subcutaneously implanted immature long-bone of the rat and mouse. Am J Phys Anthropol 17:201, 1959.

Felts W: In vivo implantation as a technique in skeletal biology. Int Rev Cytol 12:243, 1961.

Frantz C, O'Rahilly R: Congenital skeletal limb deficiencies. J Bone Joint Surg 43A:1202, 1961.

Frost HM: A chondral modeling theory. Calcif Tissue Int 28:181, 1979.

Gardner E: The embryology of the clavicle. Clin Orthop 58:9, 1968.

Gardner E: Osteogenesis in the human embryo and fetus. In Bourne G (ed): The Biochemistry and Physiology of Bone. New York, Academic, 1970.

Gardner E, Gray D: The prenatal development of the human femur. Am J Anat 129:121, 1970.

Gray D, Gardner E: Prenatal development in the human knee and superior tibiofibular joints. Am J Anat 86:235, 1950.

Gray D, Gardner E, O'Rahilly R: The prenatal development of the skeleton and joints of the human hand. Am J Anat 101:169, 1957.

Grüneberg H: The Pathology of Development: A Study of Inherited Skeletal Disorders in Animals. New York, Wiley, 1963.

Haines R: Cartilage canals. J Anat 68:45, 1933.

Haines R: The development of joints. J Anat 81:33, 1947.

Haines R: Epiphyses and sesamoids. In Gans C (ed): Biology of the Reptilia. New York, Academic, 1969, p 81.

Haines R: The pseudoepiphysis of the first metacarpal in man. J Anat 117:145, 1974.

Haines R: The histology of epiphyseal union in mammals. J Anat 120:1, 1975.

Hall, B: Cellular differentiation in skeletal tissue. Biol Rev 45:455, 1970.

Hall B: Histogenesis and morphogenesis of bone. Clin Orthop 74:249, 1971.

Hall B: Immobilization and cartilage transformation into bone in the embryonic chick. Anat Rec 174:391, 1972.

Hall B, Jacobson H: The repair of fractured membrane bones in the newly hatched chick. Anat Rec 181:55, 1975.

Hall BK: Viability and proliferation of epithelia and the initiation of osteogenesis within mandibular ectomesenchyme in the embryonic chick. J Embryol Exp Morphol 56:71, 1980.

Harris H: The vascular supply of bone, with special reference to the epiphyseal cartilage. J Anat 64:3, 1929.

Holtrop M: The origin of bone cells in endochondral ossification. In Third European Symposium on Calcified Tissue. New York, Springer-Verlag, 1966, p 32.

Horstadius S: The Neural Crest. London, Oxford, 1950.

Irving M: The blood supply of growth cartilage. J Anat 98:631, 1964.

Jaffe H: Metabolic, Degenerative and Inflammatory Diseases of Bones and Joints. Philadelphia, Lea & Febiger, 1972.

Johnson L: The Kinetics of Skeletal Remodeling. In Structural organization of the Skeleton. Birth Defects, Vol. 2, No. 1. National Foundation March of Dimes, 1966.

Johnson M: A radioautographic study of the migration and fate of cranial neural crest cells in the chick embryo. Anat Rec 156:143, 1966.

Kember N: Patterns of cell division in the growth plates of the rat pelvis. J Anat 116:445, 1973.

Lacroix P: The Organization of Bones. Philadelphia, Blakiston, 1951.

Lash J: Chondrogenesis: Genotypic and phenotypic expression. J Cell Physiol 72 (Suppl 1):35, 1968.

Lucas SG, Schoch RM: Cope, marsh and the type specimen of *Lystrosaurus "frontosus,"* a mammal-like reptile from the Triassic of South Africa. Discovery 15:29, 1980.

McKibbin B, Holdsworth F: The dual nature of epiphyseal cartilage. J Bone Joint Surg 49B:351, 1967.

MacConaill M: Calcospheritic calcification of cartilage. J Anat 115:23, 1973.

MacEwen GD, Winter RB, Hardy JH: Evaluation of kidney anomalies in congenital scoliosis. J Bone Joint Surg 54A:1451, 1972.

Maderson P: Embryonic tissue interactions as the basis for morphological change in evolution. Am Zool 15:315, 1975.

Mathews M: Comparative biochemistry of chondroitin sulphate–proteins of cartilage and notochord. Biochem J 125:37, 1971.

Medoff J: Enzymatic events during cartilage differentiation in the chick embryonic limb bud. Dev Biol 16:118, 1967.

Mereel M: Recherches sur la relation inductrice entre chondrocytes et périoste dans le tibia embryonnaire du poulet. Arch Biol 78:145, 1967.

Meikle M: The influence of function on chondrogenesis at the epiphyseal cartilage of a growing long bone. Anat Rec 182:387, 1975.

Milaire J: Histochemical aspects of limb morphogenesis in vertebrates. Adv Morphogen 2:183, 1962.

Milaire J: Étude morphologique et cytochemique du développement des membres chez la souris et chez le taupe. Arch Biol (Liege) 74:129, 1963.

Mitolo V: A model approach to some problems of limb morphogenesis. Acta Embryol Morphol Exp 3:323, 1973.

Moore W: Muscular function and skull growth in the laboratory rat (*Rattus norvegicus*). J Zool (London) 152:287, 1967.

Murray P: The fusion of parallel long bones and the formation of secondary cartilage. Aust J Zool 2:364, 1954.

Murray P, Drachman D: The role of movement in the development of joints and related structures: The head and neck in the chick embryo. J Embryol Exp Morphol 22:349, 1969.

Murray P, Huxley J: Self-differentiation in the grafted limb-bud of the chick. J Anat 59:379, 1925.

Noback C: The developmental anatomy of the human osseous skeleton during the embryonic, fetal and circumnatal periods. Anat Rec 88:91, 1944.

Ogden J: The anatomy and function of the proximal tibiofibular joint. Clin Orthop 101:186, 1974.

Ogden J: Development of the epiphysis. In Ferguson AB Jr (ed): Orthopaedic Surgery in Infancy and Childhood, 5th ed. Baltimore, Williams & Wilkins, 1982.

Ogden J: Ipsilateral femoral bifurcation and tibial hemimelia. J Bone Joint Surg 58A:712, 1976.

Ogden J: Proximal fibular growth deformities. Skeletal Radiol 3:223, 1979.

Ogden J: Chondro-osseous development and growth. In Urist M (ed): Fundamental and Clinical Bone Physiology. Philadelphia, Lippincott, 1981.

Ogden J: Anomalous multifocal ossification of the os calcis. Clin Orthop 162:112, 1982.

Ogden J: Skeletal Injury in the Child. Philadelphia, Lea & Febiger, 1982.

Ogden J: Dynamic pathobiology of congenital hip dysplasia. In Tachdjian MO (ed): Congenital Hip Disease. New York, Churchill Livingstone, 1982.

Ogden J: The uniqueness of growing bones. In Rockwood CA, Wilkins KE, King RE (eds): Fractures, Vol 3, Children. Philadelphia, Lippincott, 1984.

Ogden J, Conlogue G, Bronson M, Jensen P: Radiology of postnatal skeletal development. II. The manubrium and sternum. Skeletal Radiol 4:189, 1979.

Ogden J, Conlogue G, Phillips S, Bronson M: Sprengel's deformity. Radiology of the pathological deformation. Skeletal Radiol 4:204, 1979.

Ogden J, Hempton R, Southwick W: Development of the tibial tuberosity. Anat Rec 182:431, 1975.

Ogden J, Hempton R, Weil U: Developmental humerus varus. Clin Orthop 116:158, 1976.

Ogden J, Pais M, Murphy M, Bronson M: Ectopic bone secondary to avulsion of periosteum. Skeletal Radiol 4:124, 1979.

Ogden J, Southwick W: Contraposed curve patterns in monozygotic twins. Clin Orthop 116:35, 1976.

Ogden J, Southwick W: Osgood-Schlatter's disease and development of the tibial tuberosity. Clin Orthop 116:180, 1976.

Ogden J, Southwick W: Congenital and infantile scoliosis in triplets. Clin Orthop 136:159, 1978.

Ogden J, Vickers T, Tauber J, Light T: A model for ulnar dysmelia. Yale J Biol Med 51:193, 1978.

Ogden J, Watson H, Bohne W: Ulnar dysmelia. J Bone Joint Surg 58A:467, 1976.

O'Rahilly R: Morphological patterns in limb deficiencies and duplications. Am J Anat 89:135, 1951.

O'Rahilly R, Gardner E: The initial appearance of ossification in staged human embryos. Am J Anat 134:291, 1972.

O'Rahilly R, Gardner E, Gray D: The ectodermal thickening and ridge in the limbs of staged human embryos. J Embryol Exp Morphol 4:254, 1956.

O'Rahilly R, Meyer DB: The timing and sequence of events in the development of the human vertebral column during the embryonic period proper. Anat Embryol 157:167, 1979.

O'Rahilly R, Muller F, Meyer DB: The human vertebral column at the end of the embryonic period proper. 1. The column as a whole. J Anat 131:565, 1980.

Owen R, Goodfellow J, Bullough P: Scientific Foundations of Orthopaedics and Traumatology. Philadelphia, Saunders, 1980.

Pratt C: The significance of the "perichondral zone" in a developing long bone of the rat. J Anat 93:110, 1959.

Pritchard J: A cytological and histochemical study of bone and cartilage formation in the rat. J Anat 86:259, 1952.

Pritchard J, Ruzicka A: Comparison of fracture repair in the frog, lizard and rat. J Anat 84:236, 1950.

Rang M: The Growth Plate and Its Disorders. Baltimore, Williams & Wilkins, 1969.

Ricqlès A de: Recherches paléohistologiques sur les os longs des tétrapodes. I. Origine du tissu osseux plexiforme des dinosauriens sauropodes. Ann Paléontol 54:133, 1968.

Ricqlès A de: Recherches paléohistologiques sur les os longs des tétrapodes. II. Quelques observations sur la structure des os longs des teriodontes. Ann Paléontol 55:3, 1969.

Ricqlès A de: Recherches paléohistologiques sur les os longs des tétrapodes. III. Titanosuchiens, dinocéphales et dicynodontes. Ann Paléontol 58:17, 1972.

Rivard CH, Narbaitz R, Uhthoff HK: Congenital vertebral malformations: Time of induction in human and mouse embryo. Orthop Rev 8:135, 1979.

Romer A: Cartilage an embryonic adaptation. Am Nature 76:394, 1942.

Romer A: The ancient history of bone. Ann NY Acad Sci 109:168, 1963.

Romer A: The vertebrate as a dual animal—somatic and visceral. Evol Biol 6:121, 1972.

Saunders J: The proximo-distal sequence of origin of the parts of chick wing and the role of the ectoderm. J Exp Zool 108:363, 1948.

Saunders J, Cairns J, Gasseling M: The role of the apical ridge of ectoderm in the differentiation of the morphological structure and inductive specificity of limb parts in the chick. J Morphol 101:57, 1957.

Saunders J, Gasseling M, Saunders L: Cellular death in morphogenesis of the avian wing. Dev Biol 5:147, 1962.

Scammon R, Calkins L: The Development and Growth of the External Dimensions of the Human Body in the Fetal Period. Minneapolis, University of Minnesota, 1929.

Schaffer B: Differential ossification in the fishes. Trans NY Acad Sci 23:501, 1961.

Schmid TM, Linsenmayer TF: A short chain (pro) collagen from aged endochondral chondrocytes. J Biol Chem 258:9504, 1983.

Schowing J: Influence inductrice de l'encéphale embryonnaire sur le développement du crâne chez le poulet. I. Influence de l'excision des territoires nerveux antérieurs sur le développement crânien. J Embryol Exp Morphol 19:9, 1968.

Schowing J: Influence inductrice de l'encéphale embryonnaire sur le développement du crâne chez le poulet. II. Influence de l'excision de la chorde et des territoires encéphaliques moyen et postérieur sur le développement crânien. J Embryol Exp Morphol 19:23, 1968.

Schowing J: Influence inductrice de l'encéphale embryonnaire sur le développement du crâne chez le poulet. III. Mise en evidence du róle inducteur de l'encéphale dans l'ostéogenèse du crâne embryonnaire du poulet. J Embryol Exp Morphol 19:83, 1968.

Scott WJ, Ritter EJ, Wilson JG: Ectodermal and mesodermal cell death patterns in 6-mercaptopurine riboside–induced digital deformities. Teratology 21:271, 1980.

Searls R: The role of cell migration in the development of the embryonic chick limb bud. J Exp Zool 166:39, 1967.

Searls R, Janners M: The stabilization of cartilage properties in the cartilage forming mesenchyme of the embryonic chick limb. J Exp Zool 170:365, 1969.

Sensenig E: The early development of the human vertebral column. Contrib Embryol 33:21, 1949.

Siegling J: Growth of the epiphyses. J Bone Joint Surg 23:23, 1941.

Sissons H: The growth of bone. In Bourne G (ed): The Biochemistry and Physiology of Bone. New York, Academic, 1971.

Smith RG, Appel SH: Extracts of skeletal muscle increase neurite outgrowth and cholinergic activity of fetal rat spinal motor neurons. Science 219:1079, 1983.

Streeter G, Henser C, Corner G: Development horizons in human embryos. Contrib Embryol 2:166, 1951.

Swinyard C: Limb Development and Deformity: Problems of Evaluation and Rehabilitation. Springfield, Ill, Thomas, 1969.

Tanaka T, Uhthoff HK: Significance of resegmentation in the pathogenesis of vertebral body malformation. Acta Orthop Scand 52:331, 1981.

Tanaka T, Uhthoff HK: The pathogenesis of congenital vertebral malformations. A study based on observations made in 11 human embryos and fetuses. Acta Orthop Scand 52:413, 1981.

Thompson DW: On Growth and Form. Cambridge, Mass, Cambridge, 1942.

Toole B: Extracellular events in limb development. In Skeletal Dysplasias. New York, Symposia Specialists, 1974.

Trueta J: Studies of the Development and Decay of the Human Frame. Philadelphia, Saunders, 1968.

Tschumi P: The growth of the hind limb bud of *Xenopus laevis* and its dependence upon the epidermis. J Anat 91:149, 1957.

Videman T: An experimental study of the effects of growth on the relationship of tendons and ligaments to bone at the site of diaphyseal insertion. Doctoral dissertation, University of Helsinki, 1970.

Von der Mark K, Von der Mark H: The role of three genetically distinct collagen types in endochondral ossification and calcification of cartilage. J Bone Joint Surg 59B:458, 1977.

Wake D, Lawson R: Developmental and adult morphology of the vertebral column in the Plethodontid salamander *Eurycea bislineata*, with comments on vertebral evolution in the amphibia. J Morphol 139:251, 1973.

Warkany J: Congenital Malformations. Chicago, Year Book Med. Pub., 1971.

Watson AG: The phylogeny and development of the occipito–atlas-axis complex in the dog. Doctoral dissertation, Cornell University, 1981.

Williams L: The later development of the notochord in mammals. Am J Anat 8:251, 1908.

Wolpert L: Positional information and the spatial pattern of cellular differentiation. J Theor Biol 25:1, 1969.

Wyburn G: Observations on the development of the human vertebral column. J Anat 78:94, 1944.

Yasuda Y: Differentiation of human limb buds in vitro. Anat Rec 175:561, 1973.

Zwilling E: Limb morphogenesis. Adv Morphol 1:301, 1961.

Zwilling E: Morphogenetic phases in development. Dev Biol 2 (Suppl):184, 1968.

As discussed in the preceding chapter, the basic musculoskeletal and neural elements all are morphologically and histologically defined prenatally. The postnatal stage primarily consists of progressive chondro-osseous maturation and growth at the cellular level and is especially concerned with (1) the continued replacement of expanding epiphyseal cartilage by bone and (2) the biomechanically directed maturation of woven (laminar) bone to the constantly remodeling osteon (lamellar) bone that characterizes most of the cortical bone of the mature skeleton. Although significant morphologic changes are unusual in the postnatal period, the joint contours are modified, physeal contours progressively respond to changing biomechanics, becoming undulated rather than transversely planar, and certain areas such as the proximal femur develop final adult shapes moderately different from the morphology present at birth.

TYPES OF GROWTH MECHANISMS

The physis, which is the essential mechanism for endochondral ossification, is the major mechanism for enlargement of all components of the axial and appendicular skeleton. As initially described in the preceding chapter, the physis assumes characteristic cytoarchitectural arrangements by the fourth prenatal month, at which time the ossification center has expanded to occupy approximately 60 to 70 percent of the anlage length and compacted the differentiating physeal cells between metaphysis and epiphysis (Fig. 4–1). The basic cellular zones of each physis are thus well defined at birth.

Morphologically there are two basic types of growth plates—planar and spherical. Primary growth plates arising as a consequence of the formation of the primary ossification center of a long bone are planar (Fig. 4–2). They are characterized initially by a relatively flat (discoid) area of rapidly differentiating and maturing cartilage that grades imperceptibly into the remainder of the hyaline cartilage of the chondroepiphysis. The primary function of the planar physis is longitudinal growth, but it also contributes significantly to circumferential expansion of the bone through the zone of Ranvier. All planar physes change from flat to variably undulated structures as the bone elongates (Ogden, 1982b; Speer and Pitt, 1982).

The spherical physis, in contrast, does not contribute to longitudinal growth; instead, it is a constantly enlarging region at the interface of the undifferentiated epiphyseal cartilage and the secondary ossification center and may be properly termed a secondary growth plate. The spherical growth plate and ossification center also are found in the bones of the carpus and tarsus (Fig. 4–3). In such bones the endochondral ossification process is analogous to ossification within the epiphysis; however, it is difficult to term such ossification either primary or secondary because some of these small bones regularly develop another ossification center (e.g., calcaneus), whereas others do so less regularly (e.g., os trigonum of the talus and accessory navicular of the tarsal navicula). In other species such as

the cetaceans primary and secondary ossification is common in multiple carpal bones.

By progressive centrifugal expansion the spherical physis gradually assumes the contours of the epiphysis, carpal bone, or tarsal bone, although it does not reach the peripheral margins until late in skeletal maturation; therefore, an enveloping perichondrium, rather than periosteum, is present on the nonarticular surfaces. Thus, the initially spherical nature of these physes progressively changes to shapes mandated by the morphology of the epiphysis within which they are contained. The joint surface contours, the undulations of the primary growth plate, and the intervening epiphyseal contours all gradually delimit the shape of the secondary physis.

Histomorphology of the Growth Plate

The physis has a characteristic and virtually unchanging cytoarchitectural structure from early fetal life until the growth slowdown phase immediately preceding skeletal maturation (Dodds, 1930; Rang, 1969). The major differences among the various growth plates can be found in the relative amounts of cells in each zone, the overall heights of the physis (these two factors being reflections of growth rates), and cellular modifications such as replacement of the zone of hypertrophy with a zone of fibrocartilage (i.e., an area classically described as an apophysis). These basic patterns can be characterized on the basis of either histologic or functional (physiologic) criteria (Fig. 4–4).

Conceptualization of the anatomic regions of the physis is rendered by a terminology that implies discrete structural and functional zones when, in reality, there is a gradual transition of cellular components, extracellular components such as the continuous interspersed collagenous framework, and functional morphogenetic roles.

The zone of growth is concerned with both longitudinal and diametric expansion of the bone. It is the area where cellular addition and mitosis occur. The resting cells are intimately associated with the blood vessels that supply this region (the epiphyseal vessels). These small arterioles and capillaries also may be instrumental in providing undifferentiated cells from the perivascular regions that are subsequently added to the pool of resting chondrocytes. Additional cells also are elaborated peripherally through a specialized area of the perichondrium, the zone of Ranvier.

The next stage in the zone of growth is active cell division, which occurs principally in a longitudinal direction and leads to cell column formation. In an active growth plate, the cell columns may comprise half the overall height of the physis. The randomly dispersed collagen of the resting and dividing regions becomes more longitudinally oriented between the cell columns, which may be referred to as clones.

The next functional area is the zone of cartilage formation. In this zone, increased extracellular matrix is formed and undergoes the several significant biochemical changes necessary for eventual ossification. The matrix becomes histologically metachromatic and calcifies, and the chondrocytes become hypertrophic, a reflection of their increased metabolic activity. The eventual fate of

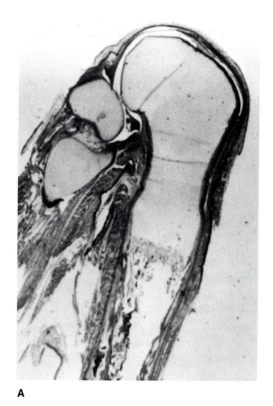

A

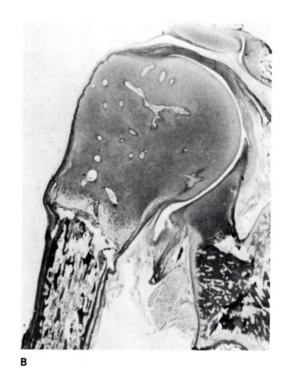

B

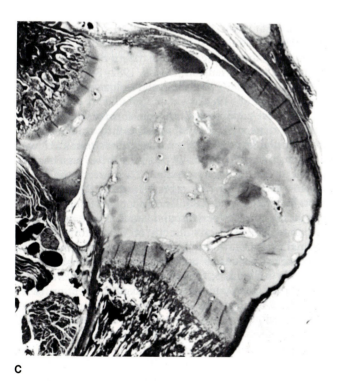

C

Figure 4-1. Prenatal development of the proximal humerus showing the gradual replacement of the cartilaginous anlage to define the epiphysis and physis. **A.** Four months. **B.** Six months. **C.** Full term.

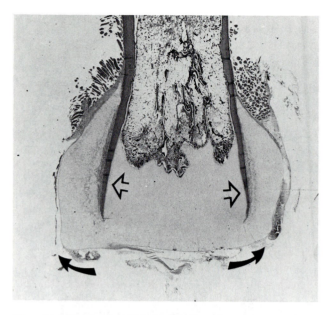

Figure 4-5. Frog's distal femur demonstrating the accentuated osseous ring of Lacroix (open arrows) and overlapping of the epiphysis and zone of Ranvier peripheral to the osseous ring (solid arrows).

primarily above the region of densely packed cells, do not contribute to formation of the osseous ring, but their exact role is unknown. Various histochemical and radioactive labeling experiments suggest that these cells may be cartilaginous precursors whose main function is appositional enlargement of the growth plate periphery.

The mechanism of growth in this area has only been partially defined and certainly requires further experimental analysis. Both appositional and interstitial growth occurs throughout a developing long bone in the earliest stages. Once central endochondral ossification begins (9 weeks), then chondrogenic interstitial and appositional growth becomes regionally restricted to the epiphyses. After 14 weeks of gestation, chondrogenic activity continues within the perichondrium, largely restricted to the area of loosely packed cells in the groove of Ranvier. The multipotential mesenchymal elements differentiate into chondrocytes that may be incorporated into the adjacent germinal region of the growth plate and thus provide increased latitudinal growth by apposition. With further differential growth, the area of loosely packed cells is no longer in direct apposition to the germinal region of the growth plate after birth. This area continues to decrease in size postnatally and by 2 years has completely disappeared as a distinct cytologic structure within the perichondrium. The size and activity of this area also has been correlated with the overall growth rates of the developing long bone. The early accelerated growth rate is associated with a large area of loosely packed cells, suggesting a significant appositional component of physeal growth. The decelerating fetal growth rates after 5 months' gestation were associated with a decrease in the size of this cellular area, suggesting a decreased appositional component to growth.

Collagen Patterns

The collagenous framework of a developing bone is produced by fibroblasts, chondroblasts, and osteoblasts to form an integrated architectural system of cells and collagen fibers that traverse or define the limits of the histologic zones classically defined by bright-field microscopy. These multiple collagen fiber systems, which contain diverse collagen types, groupings, and cross-linkage patterns (some of which may show subtle variations in different species), form an interdigitating fabric or microskeleton with significant tensile vector responsiveness.

Speer (1982) identified five major orientation patterns of collagen fibers: transphyseal (longitudinal), perichondrial-periosteal (longitudinal), epiphyseal (radial), perichondrial ring (circumferential), and metaphyseal bone (circumferential).

Transphyseal collagen fibers extend from the longitudinally oriented calcified cartilage in the metaphysis (primary spongiosa) completely across the physis and into the epiphyseal cartilage or secondary ossification, contingent upon the degree of maturation of the latter. These transphyseal fibers interdigitate with the radially oriented epiphyseal fibers located between the germinal and resting physeal zones and the developing secondary ossification center. This radial collagen fiber orientation is associated with a similar radial or spokelike orientation of the epiphyseal and physeal cells when viewed in the transverse plane. The longitudinal fiber orientation in the periosteum extends in a similar pattern toward the histologically similar periochondrium and also curves into the zone of Ranvier.

Many of the biomechanical properties and morphogenetic constraints of the physis are contingent upon the content, tensile strength, and organization of these various collagen fibers. The spatial orientation (architecture) of collagen fiber groups is a critical determinant of their biomechanical competence.

The perichondrial groove, of which the perichondrial osseous ring of Lacroix is an integral component, is a triangular cellular area encircling the physis and is bounded by the perichondrial-periosteal collagen fibers, by the peripheral extension of the radial epiphyseal collagen fibers, and by the most peripheral transphyseal collagen fibers.

The perichondrial ring comprises circumferential collagen fibers that morphologically create a cylindric collar surrounding the physis and adjacent metaphysis. Even in different bones of the same species, this ring may be either fibrous or osseous and may vary considerably in longitudinal extent. There is also a preponderance of circumferential collagen fibers in the periosteum and endochondral bone of the metaphysis.

Lappet Formation

The peripheral zone of Ranvier is the first region to change the planar or transverse morphology of the physis (Fig. 4–6). Usually within the first year in most physes this region progressively turns toward the metaphysis to create a circumferential overlapping of the entire zone. This introduces an initial intrinsic stability into the physeal-metaphyseal interface. With further growth such lappet formation becomes a dominant feature, although with variation from epiphysis to epiphysis. In certain regions such as the proximal femur the overlap may vary considerably, and the absence anteriorly in some patients may represent a mechanical predisposition to slipped capital femoral epiphysis (Ogden, 1981c). In other areas lappet formation is necessary for the formation of a joint extension (e.g., distal tibiofibular or distal radioulnar articulations) (Ogden, 1982b, 1983; Ogden et al., 1981).

DEVELOPMENT OF THE AXIAL SKELETON

The postnatal development of the axial skeleton comprises the development of the characteristic curves, growth of the vertebral body, the development of the ring apophysis, and changes in the longitudinal relationships between the vertebrae and the spinal cord, especially in the lumbar region (Schultz et al., 1984; Verbout, 1985; Watson and Lowery, 1954).

Curve Patterns

The spinal column of the neonate is extremely flexible, without any of the characteristic fixed curves eventually attained by skeletal maturation. The relatively stable curvatures typical of the older child and adult gradually become apparent and well established during late infancy and early childhood. Initially these curves can be straightened easily, but they progressively become permanent (i.e., structural) because of differential bone growth of the vertebral bodies, particularly in the lumbar region.

The neonatal spine normally is flexed (anteriorly concave) throughout its entire course, a reflection of intrauterine position; however, by the third postnatal month when the infant raises his or her head, the posteriorly con-

cave curvature of the cervical spine develops. At about 1 year of age a similar posteriorly concave curve develops in the lumbosacral spine, principally because of the increased assumption of an upright posture. These two primary curve introductions are associated with the concomitant development of a thoracic dorsal flexure and a forward tilting of the pelvis.

Because of congenital spinal differentiation errors or postnatal growth discrepancies (such as tumor or infection), accentuated anterior (kyphosis) or lateral angulation (scoliosis) may be superimposed upon these developing basic curve patterns. Other acquired conditions such as spondylolysis or spondylolisthesis may cause progressive loss of the normal lumbar lordosis or contribute to the development of scoliosis.

When there have been segmentation failures such as hemivertebrae or unilateral unsegmented bars, the consequent abnormal curve development becomes contingent upon where specific growth plates develop (Nasca et al., 1975; Taylor, 1983; Winter et al., 1968; Winter et al., 1973). Radiologically similar-appearing deformities may behave very differently because of the presence or absence of areas capable of longitudinal growth. A hemivertebra may be fused to the adjacent vertebra and thereby have a growth plate only on one surface. In such a situation the angular deformity present at birth may not increase rapidly; however, if the hemivertebra is independent and has a growth plate superiorly and inferiorly, a more rapid progression of the deformity is likely. Similarly, a progressive deformity is more likely if the hemivertebrae involve the centrum. If only the posterior element is involved, rapid progression is less likely because of the minimal contribution of the posterior elements to longitudinal growth. Progression is also more likely if the deformity is unbalanced. There may be a thoracic hemivertebra on the left side and a lumbar hemivertebra on the right side, with the two regions de-

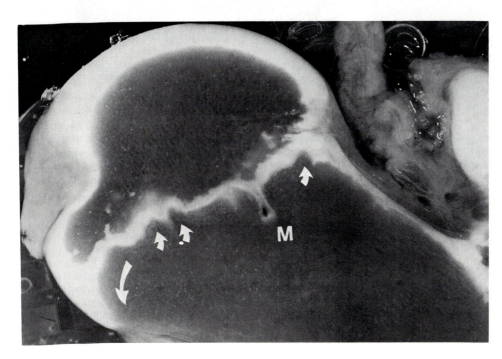

Figure 4-6. Proximal femur from an 11-year-old human showing undulations (small arrows), a mammillary process (M), and lappet formation medially (large arrow).

112

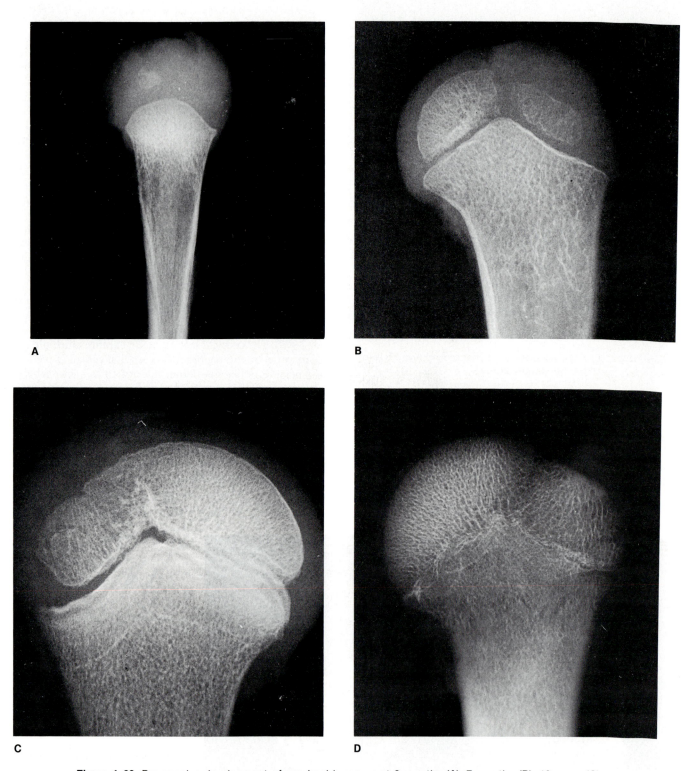

Figure 4-23. Progressive development of proximal humerus at 2 months **(A)**, 7 months **(B)**, 10 years **(C)**, and 16 years **(D)**.

Basic Patterns of Postnatal Growth

To demonstrate the various aspects of postnatal development and growth in the human, representative epiphyseal-physeal-metaphyseal units from the upper and lower limbs will be discussed. The proximal humerus, which contributes significantly to the length of the upper limb, demonstrates major contour changes in the physis and also develops multifocal secondary ossification in the chondroepiphysis. The distal tibia and fibula demonstrate less dramatic physeal contour changes while illustrating the necessity of integrated growth in paired epiphyses and physes. Detailed studies of the morphologic development of other regions may be consulted (Birch et al., 1984; Greulich and Pyle, 1959; McCarthy and Ogden, 1982a, 1982b; Ogden, 1983, 1984c; Ogden et al., 1978).

Proximal Humerus

The epiphyseal ossification center is not usually present at birth except in its early formative stage (i.e., cartilaginous hypertrophy within the preossification center). The secondary ossification center of the humeral head appears within the first 6 months, although 20 percent of neonates may have the center present (Ogden et al., 1978).

By 2 to 3 months the ossification center of the capital humerus is radiographically evident (Fig. 4–23). Interestingly, the contour of the physis at this stage resembles the proximal femur, with prominence of the medial portion. The metaphyseal cortex is thin and is composed of trabecular rather than osteon bone.

An additional secondary ossification center for the greater tuberosity is present by 1 year in the female and 2 years in the male, with fusion of the two secondary centers by the 6th year. The physis and metaphysis progressively form the characteristic conical or pyramidal contour. The trabecular pattern in the humeral head reflects the compression and tension regions of the capital humerus and tuberosity. The lateral metaphyseal cortex is thicker and extends almost to the physis as dense cortical (osteon) bone, whereas the medial cortex is still trabecular.

By 10 years, the dense metaphyseal cortex matures and extends toward the physis. This extension is more evident laterally than medially, which may be a factor in the tendency to have a large medial fragment in the type 2 growth mechanism injury known as the Thurstan and Holland sign (Ogden, 1981a, 1982b, 1982e).

As skeletal maturation approaches, the cartilaginous component of the humeral head (along the articular surface) thins, and ossification in the tuberosity replaces the remaining cartilage. Commensurate with cessation of growth, the physis thins and disappears. This process begins centrally.

The articular surface covers both the capital humeral portion of the epiphysis as well as part of the medial metaphysis; however, the physeal contour turns distally in the most medial portion (lappet formation) such that an epiphyseal cartilage or secondary ossification center is always present beneath the articular cartilage, separating it from the metaphysis. At no time during the developmental sequence is the articular cartilage ever directly apposed to metaphyseal bone.

Distal Tibia and Fibula

At birth the distal tibial physis is transverse. As the physis matures, undulations develop, and lappet formation occurs peripherally (Fig. 4–24). Although the initial distal tibial physeal contour in the infant is transverse, an anteromedial undulation develops within the first 18 to 24 months. This structural change effectively divides the distal tibial epiphysis into lateral and medial areas and may have an effect upon fracture patterns (Ogden, 1983).

Lappet formation occurs circumferentially around the physeal periphery. It is quite prominent at the medial malleolus, as well as laterally, where the epiphysis and articular cartilage curve proximally to form the distal tibiofibular articulation.

Secondary ossification in the distal tibia begins centrally and expands to fill the area over the tibial plafond. Laterally the tibial ossification center may be wedge shaped. If the child walks with a calcaneovalgus posture, this triangular contour may be maintained for several years and should not be misconstrued as abnormal or impaired development; however, myelomeningocele or cerebral palsy patients may have retarded lateral development through chronic valgus ankle posturing such that the wedge shape remains through skeletal maturation. The margin adjacent to the medial malleolus often is irregular and may show peripheral foci of ossification. By 7 to 8 years, the secondary center extends into the medial malleolus and usually is complete by 10 to 11 years. The malleolar tip may exhibit accessory ossification.

Within the secondary ossification center the trabecular bone progressively thickens and orients in characteristic patterns. Curvilinear trabecular orientation is evident along the periphery of the medial malleolus. Transverse orientation characterizes areas, primarily laterally, over the articular surface and adjacent to the physis.

Occasionally the medial malleolus develops a separate (accessory) distal center of ossification. Such accessory ossification may be referred to as the os subtibiale or talus accessorius and fuses to the main distal tibial ossification center during adolescence. From the few specimens available for histologic examination there is complete continuity of the surrounding cartilage, even though there is radiographically apparent discontinuity of bone.

By 14 to 15 years, the entire distal tibial epiphysis including the malleolus has ossified. Physiologic epiphysiodesis to the metaphysis occurs from 12 to 14 years in girls and from 15 to 18 years in boys. Closure of the distal tibial physis has a fairly characteristic pattern. Epiphysiodesis initially involves the medial portion, including the aforementioned anteromedial undulation. Closure then proceeds along the posterior margin. The anterolateral portion is the last to undergo fusion. This medial-to-lateral pattern may occur over a 1½-year period. This pattern of closure predisposes to fracture of the lateral portion of the

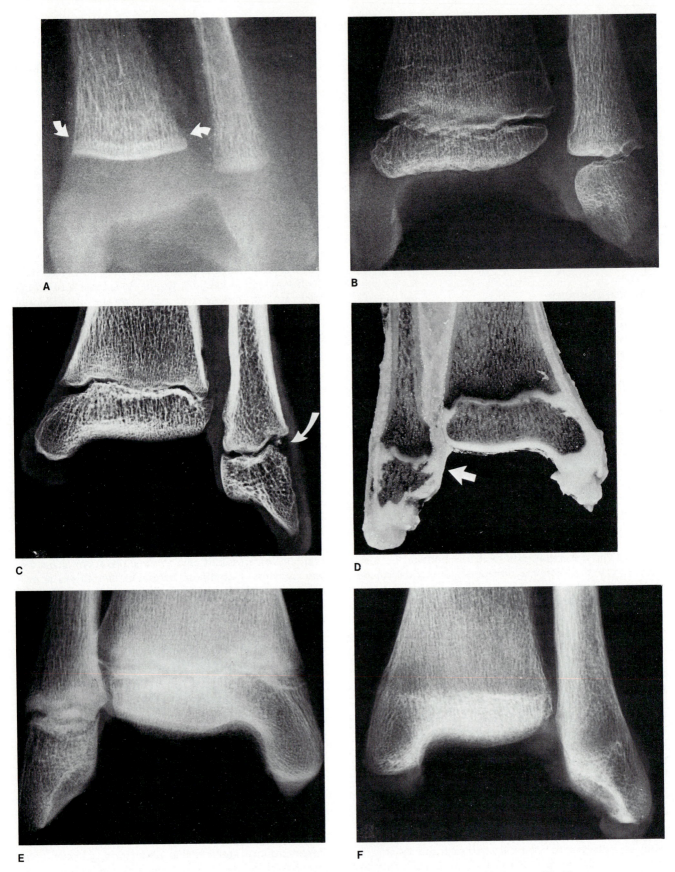

Figure 4-24. Progressive development of the distal tibia and fibula at 2 months **(A)**, 7 years **(B)**, 10 years **(C,D)**, 14 years **(E)**, and 16 years **(F)**. In **A** the arrows indicate a growth slowdown line. In **C** and **D** the arrows indicate irregular margins of the ossification centers.

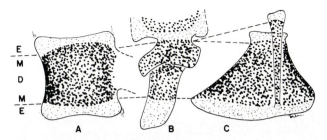

Figure 4-25. Schematic similarity of nontubular bones to the basic endochondral ossification pattern (E, epiphysis; M, metaphysis; D, diaphysis). **A.** Vertebral body (midsagittal section). **B.** Neural arch (vertebral body at top). **C.** scapula.

distal tibial epiphysis (fracture of Tillaux) as well as to triplane fractures.

The distal fibula usually develops an ossification center during the second to third years (6 months to 3 years). The distal fibular epiphysis also may exhibit irregular ossification at the tip, referred to as the os subfibulare.

Extensive undulation and lappet formation in the distal fibula is a biologic response to the shear stresses as well as the variable rotation the fibula undergoes to accommodate the different anterior and posterior widths that the talus presents to the ankle joint during dorsiflexion and plantar flexion. Within these regions of physeal overlap there may be small areas of accessory ossification (both medially and laterally).

The articular surface curves onto the lateral side of the distal tibia to form an articulation with the lateral malleolus (distal tibiofibular joint and syndesmosis). A similar articular surface extension occurs along the medial side of the fibula. These surfaces extend proximally to form a recess extending to the level of the distal tibial physis. This minimally mobile joint, which allows external rotation of the fibula as the ankle is dorsiflexed, is the syndesmosis.

The distal tibiofibular relationships are such that the distal fibular physis is most often level with either the tibial articular surface or the subarticular limits of the tibial ossification center (i.e., the subchondral plate). The distal fibular physis usually closes commensurate with the lateral side of the distal tibia.

Nontubular Bones

On superficial examination, nontubular bones seemingly differ from the characteristic pattern of endochondral ossification in the longitudinal bones, but when they are schematically analyzed, it is evident that each bone is still undergoing the basic endochondral growth process, albeit reorganized to conform to the specific contours of the bone.

Ossification of the vertebral centrum closely resembles a tubular bone, and the neural arch grows principally by periosteal appositional growth in the postnatal period; however, early growth of the neural arches is analogous to longitudinal bone growth, with the two neurocentral and

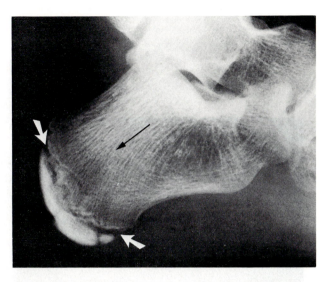

Figure 4-26. Calcaneal ossification. The physis (white arrows) allows posterior elongation of the calcaneus, indicated by the relative longitudinal arrangement of the trabecular bone between the physis and subtalar joint (black arrow). The secondary ossification center may be quite sclerotic.

single posterior spinal synchondroses serving as epiphyseal analogues (Fig. 4–25).

The tarsal and carpal bones form ossification centers that are structural modifications of the basic primary and secondary endochondral processes (Ogden, 1982a). Primary ossification of these small, nontubular bones is the same as the chondroepiphysis of a long bone. There is a pre-existent, extensive cartilage canal system with central initial ossification and centrifugal expansion. A primary bone collar does not form before this ossification. The calcaneus forms a specific cartilaginous growth center, the calcaneal apophysis, within which forms a secondary ossification center (Fig. 4–26). Other bones such as the talus and tarsal navicular may form secondary ossification centers that are often referred to as either a sesamoid or accessory ossification center (Fig. 4–27); however, with many of these purportedly accessory bones in the tarsus it is important to realize that, although there is apparent osseous separation on a radiograph, there is a single block of differentiating cartilage surrounding both ossification regions (Lawson et al., 1984).

Although secondary ossification centers are relatively common in the tarsal bones, they appear to be unusual in the carpus. The exception appears to be the cetaceans where multiple secondary ossification centers may be present (Fig. 4–28). These secondary ossification centers may be either small regions or may surround a considerable portion of the bone, almost like a shell. The purpose may be a method allowing rapid spherical enlargement.

Bipolar Physes

Each hemipelvis comprises three primary ossification centers, and several physes develop in each. The largest runs

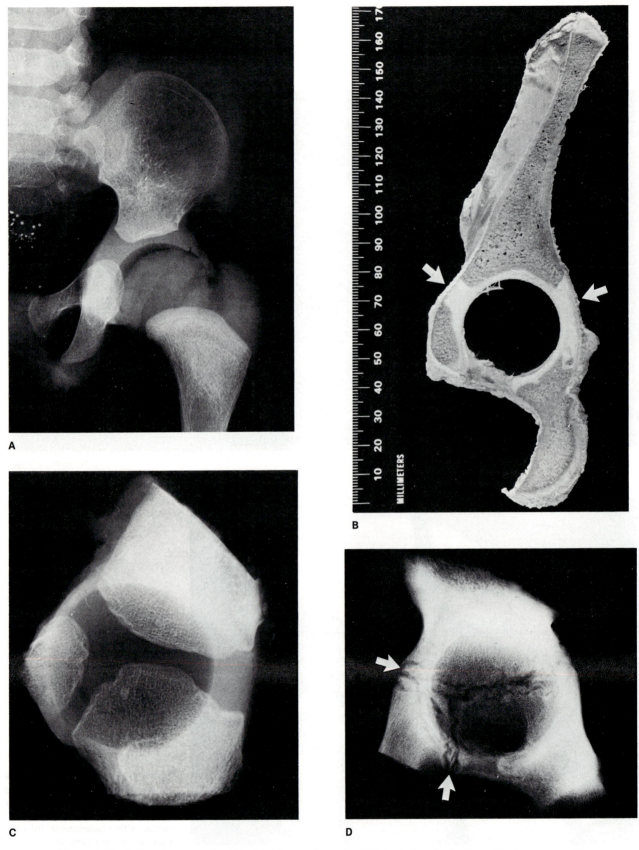

Figure 4–29. A. Roentgenograph of hip joint from a 3-month-old infant showing both cartilaginous as well as osseous components. **B.** Section through hip joint from a 5-year-old human showing portions of the triradiate cartilage (arrows). **C.** Roentgenogram of the acetabulum (round shadow) and triradiate cartilage in a 4-year-old. **D.** Roentgenogram of the acetabulum and triradiate cartilage in a 14-year-old human showing the secondary ossification centers (arrows) within the cartilage.

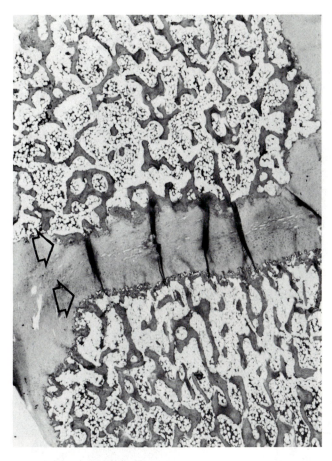

Figure 4-29. E. Bipolar growth zone from the triradiate cartilage.

along the iliac crest—the iliac apophysis. This structure is the major growth mechanism for the iliac bone. Like the greater trochanter, it is important to conceive that this is not just a traction apophysis since the attachments of the abdominal musculature are more than offset by the attachments of the gluteus maximus, tensor fascia lata, and iliac muscles, which must be considered as having a muscular (not weight-bearing) compression effect upon the physis. The cartilage of the iliac crest extends anteriorly to become the superior and inferior iliac spines. These latter two structures are more purely traction responsive to thigh musculature and better fit the criteria of an apophysis. The inferior spinous process becomes anatomically separate, whereas the superior one remains in continuity with the iliac crest.

The three primary ossification centers expand toward each other and form the triradiate cartilage at the hip joint (Fig. 4-29). This structure is composed of intersecting bipolar growth plates and is a unique situation that allows acetabular growth commensurate with enlargement of the femoral head.

The pubic rami centers meet at the midline to form a bipolar growth plate with intervening fibrocartilaginous tissue—the symphysis pubis. The pubic and ischial rami meet at the ischiopubic synchondrosis, a mass of cartilage continuous with the ischial tuberosity. The progressive ossification closing both regions create irregular appearances that may be misinterpreted as infection or tumor.

Apophysis

Physes have been arbitrarily divided into pressure (compressive) and traction (tensile) responsive structures, often on the basis of very simplistic interpretations of muscle actions. The latter have been classically referred to as apophyses. The histologic appearance of both types has been presumed the same; however, more recent studies demonstrate significant histologic differences, at least in the tibial tuberosity (Ogden et al., 1975; Ogden and Southwick, 1976; Ogden, 1984d).

The tibial tuberosity develops by a concomitant anterior outgrowth of the epiphyseal cartilage and a selected ingrowth of the fibrovascular tissue of the anterior zone of Ranvier. The hyaline cartilage outgrowth is progressively distally displaced anterior to the tibial metaphysis. About 4 to 6 months postnatally a discrete tibial tuberosity physis develops. This physis shows structural adaptations that specifically accommodate the large tensile stresses of the quadriceps mechanism through three distinct, adaptive regions: (1) a zone of endochondral bone formation, (2) a zone of membranous bone formation through fibrocartilaginous tissue, and (3) a zone of membranous bone formation through fibrous tissue (Fig. 4-30). The physis associated with the tibial tuberosity thus is histologically modified in a proximal-to-distal gradation of cellular adaptation to specific biomechanical demands in this region.

The tibial tuberosity begins secondary ossification between 7 and 9 years, usually as a distal focus (Fig. 4-31). This ossification focus progressively enlarges proximally and anteriorly while the main tibial ossification center concomitantly expands downward into the tuberosity. A section of epiphyseal cartilage remains between these two ossification centers until close to physeal maturity. The anterior chondro-osseous region at the site of patellar tendon attachment is a biomechanically susceptible region that may be acutely or chronically traumatized to create the Osgood-Schlatter lesion. Closure of the tuberosity physis occurs in a proximal-to-distal direction.

Similar structural (i.e., histologic) changes undoubtedly exist in other apophyses such as the lesser trochanter but certainly do not occur in the greater trochanter, which is misappropriately labeled an apophysis. Although there is some tensile force through the glutei, there are also major compressive forces directed through the vastus lateralis and external rotators, and so this structure is not purely responsive to tension. Thus, the cytoarchitecture of the greater trochanteric physis is similar to that of the capital femoral physis.

Short-Bone Patterns

In the smaller tubular (longitudinal) bones (phalanges, metacarpals, metatarsals), two planar physes and chondro-epiphyses initially form, but with subsequent skeletal

128

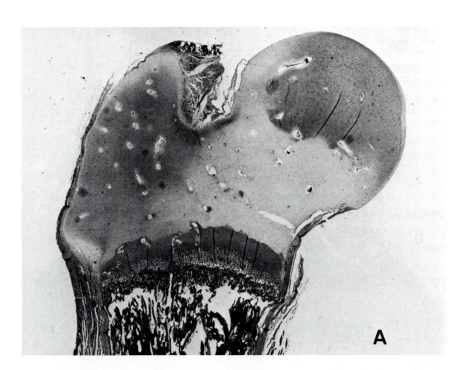

A

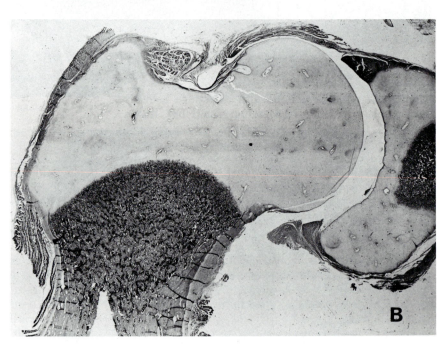

B

Figure 4-39. Sequential development of the proximal femur at **(A)** 5 prenatal months (× 7.50), **(B)** birth (× 2.25), **(C)** 3 years (× 2.25), and **(D)** 7 years (× 1.50) showing the evolution of the growth plate from a transverse structure into two relatively separate physes for the femoral head and trochanter.

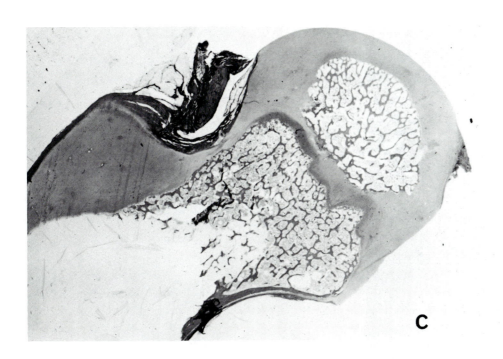

C

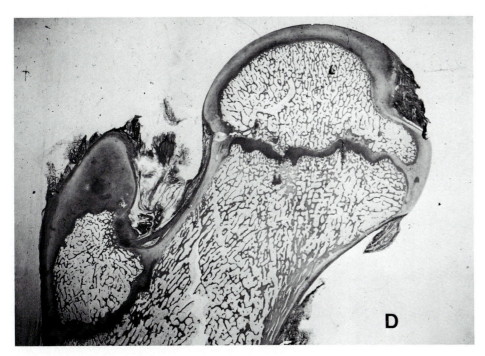

D

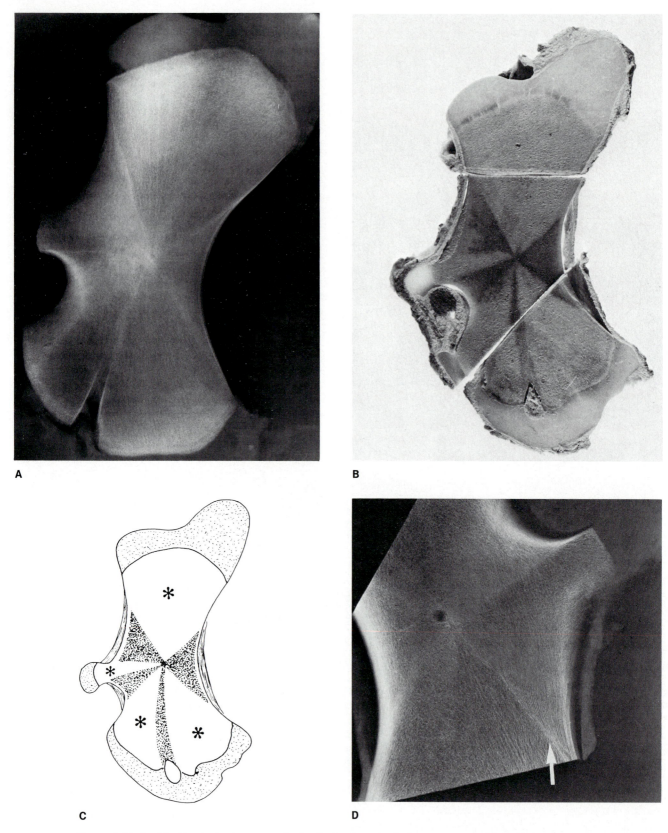

A

B

C

D

Figure 4-40. Ossification in the humerus of a leatherback turtle. **A.** Roentgenogram. **B.** Histologic section. **C.** Schematic showing endochondral (★) and periosteal (stippled) bone contributions evident in **A** and **B**. **D.** Roentgenogram of slab showing longitudinal layering (lamination) of periosteal bone (arrow).

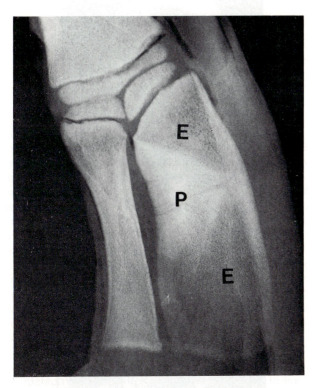

Figure 4-41. Roentgenograph of the humerus, radius, and ulna from a fetal narwhale. Note the eccentric periosteal bone (P) demarcated from the endochondral bone (E).

Endochondral Cone Concept

Developing bone enlarges by the aforementioned processes of endochondral and membranous bone formation, with the former ossification process creating a basic scaffold on which the latter ossification process is apposed and eventually remodeled to create the maturing diaphyseal cortex. This is a complex process in any mammal and may be disturbed at any stage by genetic alteration (e.g., skeletal dysplasia) or damage (e.g., trauma, infection, tumor) to the specific tissues responsible for each method of growth.

To understand these integrated growth mechanisms, it is best to look at appropriate animal models, since most vertebrates, especially mammals, appear to have similar patterns, and then derive simplified planar and solid geometric depictions (Felts and Spurrell, 1965, 1966; Oxnard and Yang, 1981). Elaborate remodeling and tubulation (medullary cavity formation) in children's bones mask many of the basic steps. Accordingly, animals without medullary cavity formation or extensive remodeling may serve as more appropriate, simplified schematic models of the more complex processes in terrestrial mammals. Marine mammals and one species of sea reptile, the leatherback turtle, readily demonstrate retained, juxtaposed patterns of endochondral and membranous bone forma-

tion without any of the modifications necessary for adaptation to a terrestrial or semiaquatic environment (Figs. 4–40 to 4–42). By extrapolating from these and other nonmammalian specimens, appropriate concepts of postnatal development and growth of the appendicular skeletal elements may be formulated.

The initial process of endochondral bone formation (primary ossification) leads to the formation (schematically) of two apposed structures that may be termed endochondral cones (Fig. 4–43). The apexes of these cones juxtapose at the prenatal site of the original primary ossification center formation and nutrient artery penetration of the original cartilaginous anlage. The bases of the cones, which are a composite of the epiphysis and physis, grow away from the juxtaposed apexes at variable rates. For example, the proximal humeral cone grows away four times as fast as the distal humeral cone in the human. These distances thus reflect the rates of longitudinal growth.

Concomitantly, the physis and epiphysis grow diametrically, thereby increasing the area of the base and width of the metaphysis and zone of Ranvier. The rates of longitudinal and latitudinal growth are closely integrated. At any point in time the exact distance of the periphery of the physis from the apex can be considered the vector of the longitudinal and latitudinal growth rates. Such a vector is really the contour of the metaphysis. Slow latitudinal enlargement versus rapid longitudinal enlargement causes a narrow elongated bone. In the radius or ulna, bones that are almost as long as the humerus, the proximal radial physis is small, with a cross-sectional area that may only be 10 to 20 percent of that of the proximal humeral physis. Again, such differences in latitudinal growth rates must reflect basic genetic control.

The surrounding bone collar concomitantly enlarges by membranous (periosteal) ossification to fill in the gaps produced by the endochondral cones (Eyre-Brook, 1984; Fell, 1932; Houghton and Dekel, 1979; Ogden et al. 1979; von Rohlig, 1966). This creates a cylindrical bone composed of endochondral trabecular (woven) bone and membranous trabecular (also woven) bone, with the latter being arranged in a laminated fashion similar to the growth rings of a tree and having more structural orientation than the underlying endochondral bone. In response to mechanical stresses in terrestrial mammals, this membranous woven bone is subsequently remodeled to create the more rigid cortical diaphyseal bone, characterized by haversian systems or osteons and termed lamellar bone (Oxnard, 1976; Oxnard and Yang, 1981).

Creation of the marrow cavity causes internal remodeling of both the endosteal (membranous) bone along the diaphysis and the secondary spongiosa (endochondral bone) of the metaphyseal–diaphyseal transition. This tubularization process also is responsive to the mechanical stresses to which the developing skeleton is subjected. In the child this area is filled with red (hematopoietic) marrow, whereas the mature skeleton eventually replaces much of this with fatty marrow.

In summary, growth in length occurs through the en-

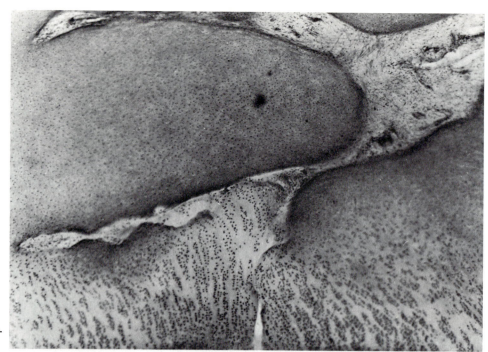

Figure 4-56. Discrete physeal circulation in a human.

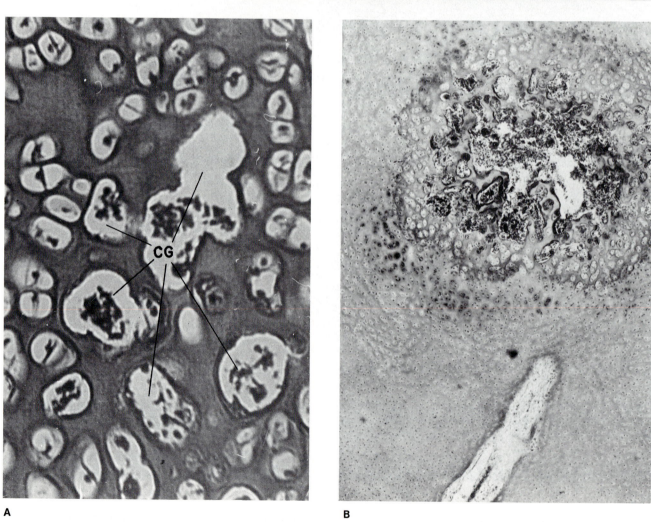

A

B

Figure 4-57. A. Canal capillary contribution to the initial formation of the secondary ossification center. There is cartilaginous hypertrophy around the capillary glomerulus (CG) ($\times$ 50). **B.** Later stage of early formation of the secondary ossification center with a contributing cartilage canal system coming toward the center.

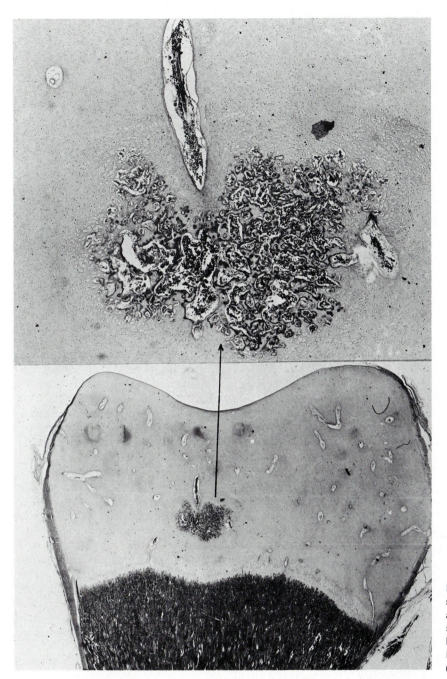

Figure 4–58. Distal femur of a human at birth showing the secondary ossification center and numerous canals, with one major canal system entering the ossification center. The hypertrophic cells radiate from this ossifying region creating a spherical growth plate (× 17, × 3.50).

ossification center. This site, defined as the preossification center, is probably genetically and biomechanically determined. The hypertrophic cells are in proximity to several cartilage canal systems. One or more of these canals will extend into this hypertrophic cell mass, but only after it has calcified and thus has become analogous to the calcified hypertrophic region of the physis. The ossification process then enlarges, with a zone of hypertrophic and calcified cartilage cells (a spherical physis) surrounding it. One or two vessels usually develop as the predominant blood supply (Figs. 4–57 and 4–58).

The continued centrifugal enlargement of the secondary ossification center is an extremely vascular-dependent process. When the normal rheology is disrupted, osteocyte death may occur rapidly. After recovery the damaged (dead) bone must be replaced by viable bone. The secondary ossification center bone was biomechanically responsive in its trabecular orientation; however, the rapidly formed new bone is not and is thus more susceptible to low-grade stress, especially at the interface of new and dead bone. This may lead to subchondral fracture, as in Legg-Perthes disease.

In smaller animals such as the mouse or rat the chondroepiphyses are never vascularized. The chondroepiphyseal cells hypertrophy and then calcify throughout the entire chondroepiphysis. One or more blood vessels then

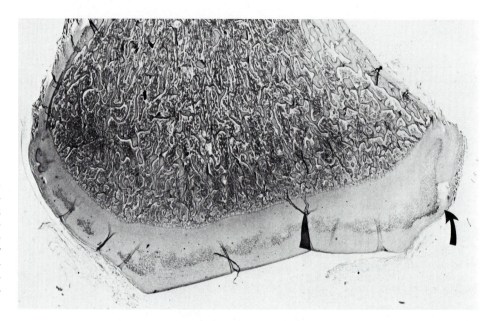

Figure 4–59. Hypertrophy and calcification throughout the nonvascularized chondroepiphysis in a platypus. Vascularization will subsequently ossify this entire region. The probable site of vascular penetration is indicated by the arrow where the hypertrophic cartilage is approaching the perichondrium.

invade from the perichondrium, forming bone in a peripheral to central (centripetal) direction, the opposite method of large mammals (Becks et al., 1948). This process leads to rapid replacement of the chondroepiphysis by an osseous epiphysis (Fig. 4–59) whereas the centrifugal process is a much slower chondro-osseous replacement.

Within the vascularized chondro-osseous epiphysis of large mammals, the spherical growth plate expands centrifugally, through rapid interstitial expansion as well as

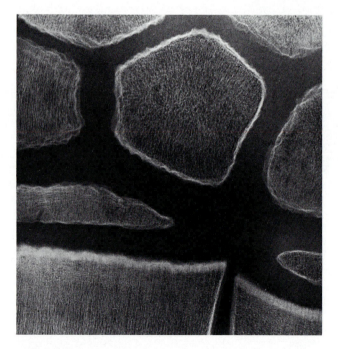

Figure 4–60. Progressive ossification in cetacean carpal bone exhibits spokelike or radial linear expansion in an animal that doesn't remodel.

radially directed longitudinal growth that corresponds to the metaphyseal ossification process (Fig. 4–60). Interstitial expansion of the spherical physis occurs virtually throughout the existence of the ossification center. During early formation of the ossification center, the margins are irregular and widely fenestrated. As the center expands, the outer surface contains more and more platelike bone and fewer fenestrations.

The enlargement of the secondary ossification center leads to juxtaposition of part of the spherical growth plate against the transverse (planar) growth plate, creating a variably bipolar growth zone. The epiphyseal contribution to the bipolar physis is eventually replaced by a subchondral bone plate, whereas the remainder of the spherical growth plate still may be found along the epiphyseal margins and the articular surface, thus allowing continued osseous expansion of the epiphysis commensurate with diametric expansion of the physis and metaphysis. Actual latitudinal expansion of the epiphysis occurs through the surrounding perichondrium, thus enlarging the cartilaginous model first.

Once the ossification center forms and enlarges, the epiphyseal circulatory pattern progressively changes. Several cartilage canal systems may contribute to the enlarging ossification center, thus creating variable anastomoses between canalicular systems that were previously endarterial. When the subchondral (cribriform) plate forms, small vessels cross this osseous plate and form vascular expansions that supply discrete regions of the physis.

The expanding, initially spheric secondary ossification center and surrounding physis eventually reach the various epiphyseal margins. At the articular surface the epiphyseal cartilage becomes divided from the articular cartilage by the tidemark (McKibbin and Holdsworth, 1967). At the periphery the perichondrium continues latitudinal growth of cartilage; however, near skeletal maturity (i.e., when physiologic epiphysiodesis commences)

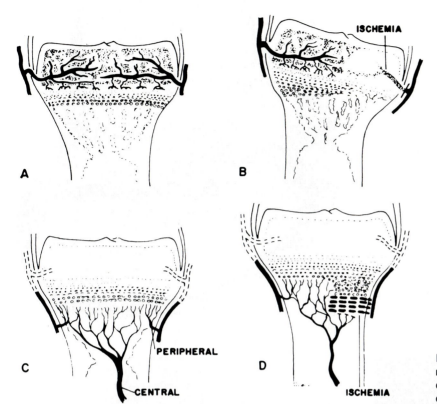

Figure 4-61. Schematic of the epiphyseal **(A)** and metaphyseal **(C)** circulatory systems; and the ischemic effects on each region **(B,D)**. See text for details.

the secondary ossification center reaches the periphery, and perichondrium becomes periosteum.

Vascular Disruption

The proximity of cells and vessels suggests that some germinal zone cells may originate from perivascular tissue. These epiphyseal vessels never penetrate between the cell columns so that the central zone of the physis is relatively avascular. This creates a gradient of oxygen tension that undoubtedly plays a role in cellular differentiation (Mooar et al., 1982). There are no anastomoses between these small arteries after they cross the subchondral osseous plate. Thus, they are effectively end-arterial to the particular segment of the physis that they supply.

When a region of the epiphyseal vasculature is compromised either temporarily or permanently, the zones of growth and transformation associated with these vessels cannot undergo appropriate cell division and maturation (Bucholz and Ogden, 1978; Catterall et al., 1982; Ogden, 1974b, 1981c, 1982d; Trueta, 1968). The unaffected regions of the physis continue longitudinal growth, resulting in the affected region being left behind (Figs. 4–61 and 4–62). The growth rate of the cells directly adjacent to the infarcted area will be more mechanically compromised than cells further away. If the involved area is peripherally located, an angular deformity may result.

Since vascular disruptions may be transient, the physis has a certain amount of recovery capacity; however, when restoration of circulation occurs, the cells that are most responsive are those encircling the physis in and adjacent to the zone of Ranvier. The more centrally lo-

cated cells are more likely to be permanently damaged and unable to recover. The result may be the formation of a conical appearance to the physis and epiphyseal ossification center as the cells at the periphery grow latitudinally and try to grow longitudinally, with the latter being mechanically restricted by the central growth impairment (Fig. 4–62).

The metaphyseal circulation is derived from two sources—the nutrient artery, which supplies the central region, and the perichondrial arteries, which supply the peripheral regions (Fig. 4–61). The terminal portions of both systems form a series of loops that penetrate between the trabeculae to reach the most mature cells of the zone of hypertrophy. The venular side of the loop enlarges to form a sinusoid (several adjacent venules may contribute to a sinusoid). The rheology imposed by the capillary loop and the sinusoids is one of the important factors rendering this area particularly susceptible to bacterial localization and subsequent osteomyelitis. Another factor is neovascularity, with temporary absence of the perivascular reticuloendothelial cells.

Interruption of the metaphyseal circulation has no direct effect upon chondrogenesis and sequential cartilaginous maturation within the physis; however, the transformation of cartilage to bone is blocked. This causes widening of the affected region as more cartilage is added to the cell columns, but none is replaced by bone (Fig. 4–61). When the metaphyseal circulation is reestablished, the widened, already calcified region is rapidly penetrated and ossified, returning the physis to its normal width.

Following a growth plate or metaphyseal fracture there

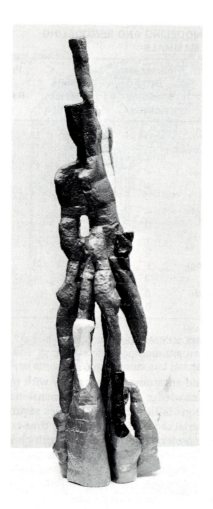

Figure 5-7. A model of more complex osteons in the femur of a dog. The variation in cross-sectional areas of different parts of the same osteon is evident, with the enlargement occurring gradually. The abrupt horizontal step cuts indicate anastomoses with other (unmodeled) systems. Lesser niches and bulges characterize the external contour. A blind osteon is seen at the right. *(From Cohen and Harris, 1958, with permission.)*

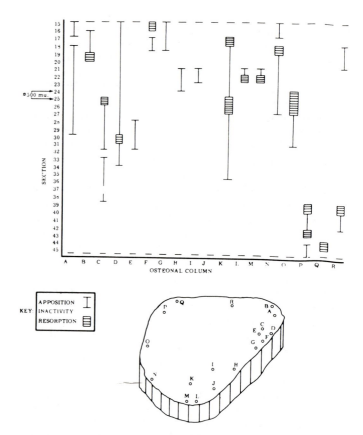

Figure 5-8. Spatial activity map from the left fibula of a dog. The oblique section at the bottom represents an average midsection on which active osteons are identified by capital letters. Activity is generally peripheral. Osteon activity, as determined from 30 sections, 100 μ thick, obtained from a 1.5-cm-long segment of fibula, is shown at the top. Most active osteons show intermittent apposition and resorption. *(From Enneking et al., 1972, with permission.)*

areas where the canal is uninvested by lamallae. Throughout the central portion of the cortex, however, concentric lamellae are invariably present (except around larger resorption spaces), but the internal structure of the canal may vary strikingly, with mature or partly formed osteons alternating with resorption spaces.

In other words, if a single canal were traced through the bone beginning at the periosteal surface, it might initially appear to be a longitudinally directed vessel in the circumferential lamellae. As it progressed deeper into the bone, concentric lamellae would be seen, some appearing to be primary osteons formed during growth. Further along, it would assume the appearance of a secondary osteon, with the stage of development changing every 0.1 to 1.0 mm or more. Large resorption spaces, mature osteons, and partly formed haversian systems would be encountered along its course, often repeatedly, with comparable changes in canal diameter and in overall osteon diameter,

which might be more than 25 to 30 times as great at one site compared with the next. Near the endosteum, about 1 cm from its periosteal origin, it might again lose its concentric lamellae before joining the vascular network in the medullary canal. Along most of its course, it would communicate frequently with other osteons, either through Volkmann's canals, direct anastomoses, or division into two or more descendents.

It must not be assumed that the aforementioned descriptive anatomy of an osteon indicates the direction of blood flow, which almost invariably is from the endosteal to the periosteal surface. The nutrient artery enters the medullary cavity through the nutrient canal, which characteristically points away from the faster-growing end of the bone, as in the femur where the vessels enter in a recurrent direction. Once within the medullary canal, the nutrient artery divides into branches that supply two separate vascular systems—the marrow sinusoids, which primarily drain into the nutrient vein, and the cortical capillaries, which drain into overlying periosteal plexuses (Fig. 5–10). Cortical capillaries are simple endothelial tu-

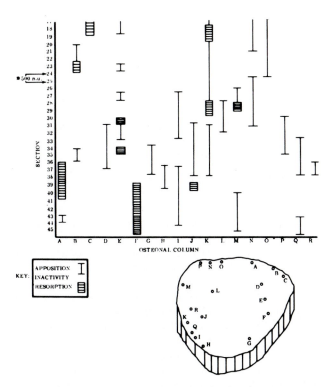

Figure 5-9. Spatial activity map from an identical site in the right fibula of the dog depicted in Figure 5-8. *(From Enneking et al., 1972, with permission.)*

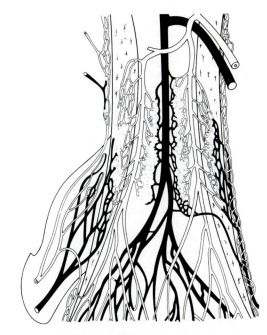

Figure 5-10. Diagram of the blood supply of a long bone—arteries, unshaded; veins, shaded. The nutrient arteries supply blood to the cortex with venous drainage into the periosteal system. The nutrient arteries also supply the medullary sinusoids, which drain primarily into the nutrient vein. The periosteal arteries supply the periosteum with little or no contribution to the cortex except in limited areas such as the linea aspera of the femur. *(Adapted from Warwick and Williams, 1973, with permission.)*

bules of unusually large diameter (15 to 30 μ), similar to sinusoids; they travel through the primary and secondary (haversian) canals of the cortex. The marrow sinusoids not only drain into the nutrient vein but also through metaphyseal veins, emissary veins that penetrate the cortex, or veins that accompany nutrient capillaries through the cortex. Although veins draining the sinusoidal system may accompany the cortical capillaries, there is no connection between the two systems. Blood flow through the cortex is brisk, so an isotope label in the nutrient artery appears in the periosteal vessels almost immediately; in contrast, the rate of flow through the marrow sinusoids is much more sluggish, with a prolonged delay before the isotope appears in the nutrient vein. The vessels in the cortex generally radiate in an oblique, radial direction from the site of the primary ossification center. Therefore, the direction of osteonal drift from endosteum to periosteum would be expected to vary in different parts of the bone.

On three-dimensional analysis, direct continuity of interstitial lamellae with osteons or with circumferential lamellae can be demonstrated; this usually occurs at sites of anastomosis between two osteons. Interstitial lamellae, therefore, rather than being isolated segments cut off from the mainstream of activity, are continuous with osteons and can be viewed as their extensions. For this reason, an isotope or other label given intravenously will appear almost as rapidly in the interstitial zones as in the intact osteons.

Trabecular Bone

General Features. Throughout the skeleton, trabecular bone exists as a three-dimensional lattice of bony plates and columns. The trabeculae are continuous with the endosteal surface of the cortex, but the number present and their extent vary with the location. Few trabeculae are found in the diaphysis, but in the metaphysis of a long bone and in short or round bones they usually fill the entire space inside the cortex.

Current knowledge of trabecular bone has in large part been acquired from studies on the spine and iliac crest, with less information available for long bones even though they contain over 50 percent of all the trabecular bone found in the skeleton. Detailed analyses of selected bones, together with observations on the morphology of cancellous bone throughout the body, suggest a pattern or organization that applies to all trabecular bone. Similar to cortical bone, trabecular bone provides support for transmitting applied loads; the trabeculae are oriented to provide maximum strength while using a minimum of material. Clark et al. (1975) produced direct evidence of this relationship using strain gauges in the calcaneus of sheep; during the stance phase of normal locomotion, the direction of principal strain remained fairly constant, and it coincided with that of the trabeculae.

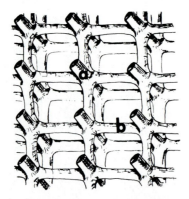

Figure 5–11. The idealized architectural pattern of trabecular bone includes both vertical (a) and transverse (b) trabeculae, which intersect at common points. In most locations, one plane of trabeculae (either horizontal or vertical) will be expanded into plates, which may be solid or fenestrated. *(From Arnold et al., 1966, with permission.)*

Idealized Architectural Pattern. On a microscopic level, the lamellar pattern and material composition of trabecular bone appear identical to those of cortical bone; but obvious structural differences are present, such as the degree of porosity and the number of haversian systems. The basic architectural model for cancellous bone includes sheets or plates of compact bone that are oriented either horizontally or vertically and are interconnected by rod-shaped supports running perpendicular to the plates (Fig. 5–11).* The plates do not form uninterrupted layers in all locations. When they contain large fenestrations they correspond to rods. The thickness of the plates, however, is more uniform, measuring between 100 and 200 μ (possibly because osteocytes more than 150 μ from the nearest bone surface lack adequate nutrition to survive). The plates may contain numerous holes (fenestrations) lined up with similar holes in adjacent plates, forming ill-defined cylinders that pass in a perpendicular direction through a series of plates.

In animals, the ideal trabecular pattern of parallel plates and regularly spaced transverse supports occurs throughout large areas of certain bones, or it may involve an entire bone; in humans, uninterrupted zones do not occur, and the trabecular orientation varies from area to area within the same bone. An accurate description of trabecular architecture, therefore, must include the three-dimensional changes encountered in different parts of the bone under discussion. Johnson (1966) has identified at least three patterns of trabecular plates: one pattern occurs in the proximal humerus where equally spaced plates of the same caliber exist; a second type occurs in the vertebrae where slightly curved plates extend between the cortical end plates; and the third pattern occurs in the femur where a mixture of smaller, evenly spaced plates, as in the humerus, and coarser, more widely spaced plates form a trajectorial system.

In the literature, detailed analyses of the trabecular pattern have been described for a number of human bones, including the proximal femur, the patella where five different areas have been characterized (Raux et al., 1975), and the vertebrae, which will be described in greater detail as representative of trabecular bone.

Normal Vertebrae. The cortical end plates (the laminae terminali), which transmit compressive forces from the intervertebral disk to the trabeculae, are composed of thin, solid plates of lamellar bone. The cortical walls of the vertebral body form a horseshoe-shaped cylinder (the open end faces posteriorly) flared outward above and below. The inner surface of the cortex contains concentric laminae, and the outer two thirds contain small, longitudinal haversian systems. The cortex is thickest centrally (up to 1 mm thick) and thins to 0.3 mm in areas toward the end plates. The external casement of cortical bone, though thin, not only interacts with trabeculae to transmit mechanical forces, but it can carry much of the load itself; if all the trabeculae are removed from a lumbar vertebra, the cortical shell can carry over 50 percent of the normal peak strength.

The organization of trabeculae within each vertebral body includes two general patterns, each located in different parts of the bone. One pattern can be found near each end plate (the end zones), and one occurs centrally (the central zone). Each end zone includes about one fourth of the total vertebral height, and the central zone includes half.

On sagittal section, the end zones contain regularly spaced longitudinal and transverse trabeculae at right angles to each other forming a grid of small squares (Fig. 5–12). The transverse trabeculae run parallel to the laminae terminali from the anterior to the posterior cortex (on frontal section they join the lateral cortices). The distance between them increases toward the center of the vertebra. The longitudinal trabeculae form less well defined rows; they arise from the laminae terminali and diverge slightly toward the center of the body.

On cross-section, a fairly uniform pattern of round holes (or cells) is seen in the end zones (Fig. 5–13). The transverse trabeculae can be considered to be fenestrated plates that when viewed on cross-section through the vertebra appear as a monotonous layer of round holes. Each transverse trabecula forms a separate fenestrated plate connected to adjacent plates by perpendicular (longitudinal or vertical) trabeculae arising from the "corner" of each hole. The holes in each plate generally line up with those in adjacent plates, forming vertical cylinders that may be unaltered for as much as 1 cm.

The central zone, unlike the end zones, is nonuniform. The basivertebral vein exits posteriorly through a

---

*In the past, it was commonly thought that the primary structural units in cancellous bone were thin interconnecting rods as in a wrought iron fence or grille; in fact, the derivation of the word cancelli actually means lattice. The appearance of trabeculae as thin strips in microscopic sections of cancellous bone explains the origin of this concept. A cut through a sheet of material appears as a line (strip of bone) in a two-dimensional section. Rods appear as isolated circles or ovals, except for those sectioned longitudinally, which occur much less frequently (Elias, 1971).

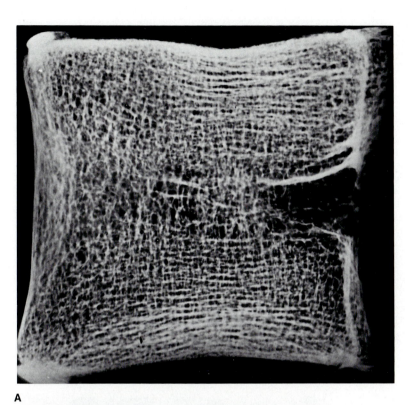

A

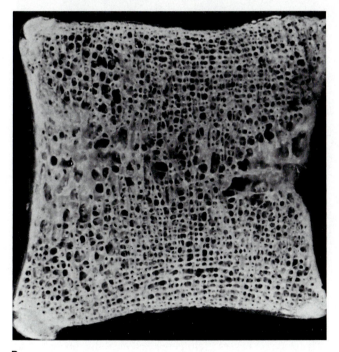

B

Figure 5–12. A. High resolution x-ray of a 1-cm–thick midsagittal slab of the first lumbar vertebral centrum of a 20-year-old female. The posterior cortex with its centrally placed foramen of basivertebral vein is on the right. The anterior cortex on the left forms the base of a fuzzy triangle composed of vertical plates whose apex lies almost at the center of the centrum. The horizontal lines beneath and more or less parallel to the terminal plates of the ends represent the fenestrated plates, which extend approximately one fifth of the length of the vertebra from each end and represent the end zones. **B.** Photograph of cleaned 2-mm–thick section from the surface of bone slab revealing the platelike structures surrounding the basivertebral vein on the right and the platelike structures on the left, which form the fuzzy triangle. The fenestrated plates of the end zones are seen as continuous, long, transverse trabeculae in this view. *(From Arnold, 1970, with permission.)*

channel that, on sagittal section, begins in the center of the body where two smaller cylinders running anterolaterally merge and extends to a large foramen in the posterior cortex. The walls of this channel are formed by moderately thick-walled plates of lamellar bone. Anteriorly, the central zone contains a triangle of vertically oriented plates that appear as homogeneous densities on x-ray; the vertical trabeculae from the end zones join these

plates. Centrally and posteriorly, the vertical trabeculae pass through the central zone to join those from the other end (except in the midline where they impinge on the basivertebral channel). On cross-section, the central zone contains a series of ovoid holes with their long axes perpendicular to the adjacent cortex; these are larger about the periphery (Fig. 5–14). The septa between the larger and many of the smaller holes in the peripheral zone are ac-

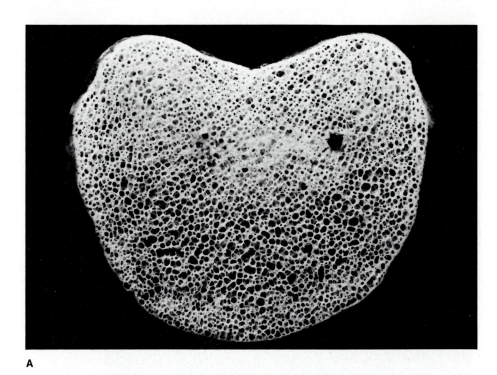

A

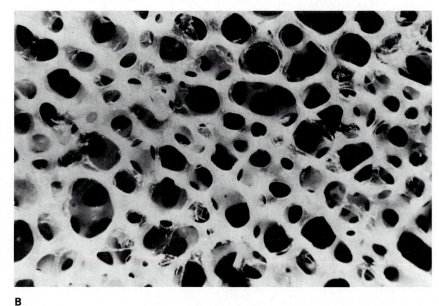

Figure 5-13. A. Cross-section of vertebra through the central portion of the end zone. Note that the round cells are somewhat smaller centrally where they are close to the lamina terminalis and progressively increase in size toward the periphery. Transverse trabeculae, as seen in Fig. 5-12, are inconspicuous since they form the walls of the cells. **B.** Cross-section of the end zone of a young individual immediately beneath the lamina terminalis revealing the circular holes in the delicate fenestrated plate and the deeper-placed underlying plates, which are barely visible in the depth of the section. *(From Arnold, 1970, with permission.)*

B

tually smooth vertical plates containing very few perforations. The plates enclose vertical cylinders that are continuous with the vertical holes in the end zones.

Composite Structure of Bone. Upon careful examination of a complete cross-section of a long bone, a variety of architectural patterns can be seen. These represent an accumulation of residual growth zones that have been rearranged and relocated during growth and altered by remodeling. Although the specific details in a given location vary between bones and between different areas in the same bone, the underlying principles apply to all bones. The basic processes include metaphyseal-diaphyseal alterations to accommodate for growth, and drift to accommodate for the normal curvature present along the long axis of the shaft. The composite result of these changes leaves a stratified cortex, with each stratum composed of a distinct kind of bone tissue, which in effect is the unaltered residual of a previous stage (Enlow, 1963).

Metaphyseal-Diaphyseal Modeling. Because bone is a hard, rigid material, it cannot increase its mass nor change

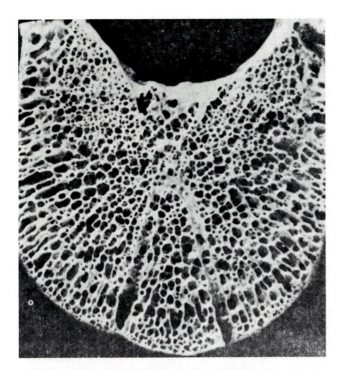

Figure 5-14. Cross-section through the central zone of the second lumbar vertebra from a 20-year-old individual. The edge of the basivertebral foramen is seen above, and its bifurcation within the center and branches running anterior-laterally are apparent. The large elliptical cells around the outer one third of the specimen, anteriorly and laterally, form the peripheral zone. The walls of these cells are formed by solid plates that run vertically. The walls of the smaller cells centrally are formed by transverse trabeculae. *(From Arnold, 1970, with permission.)*

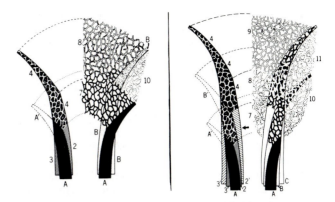

Figure 5-15. Formation of cortical zones. Three successive growth stages are shown on the right side of each diagram. The manner in which a stratified cortex, which is composed of multiple zones, is produced during growth and remodeling is schematized on the left. As stage A grows in length, the metaphysis is reduced in diameter so that A' is removed as the cortex grows in an inward direction by endosteal deposition and periosteal resorption. Since this endosteal growth proceeds into medullary cancellous bone (7), a convoluted, whorled, irregular pattern of compacted bone is produced (4). Inner circumferential lamellae, in the absence of cancellous bone, are laid down at surface 2. Reversal in direction of growth has produced a zone of outer circumferential lamellae at 3 as the midshaft now increases in diameter. With continued increase in size, B' becomes reduced during inward growth, and compacted cancellous bone (4) is progressively formed in the changing metaphysis. Additional zones of inner and outer circumferential lamellae (2' and 3') are subsequently deposited. Note that a middle zone of compacted cancellous bone has now become enclosed by endosteal and periosteal zones of circumferential lamellae (arrow). Medullary areas previously containing cancellous bone have been relocated toward the diaphysis because of increased longitudinal growth of the bone, and the cancellous trabeculae have been removed (7 and 8). Endosteal deposition in such regions, therefore, is in the form of flat circumferential layers. Cancellous bone formerly located in areas 10 and 11 no longer exists because of metaphyseal reduction in those regions. *(From Enlow, 1963, with permission.)*

its shape by interstitial expansion as do soft tissues (epiphyseal cartilage grows by interstitial expansion, but metaphyseal bone is laid down by apposition). The physical constraints imposed by its rigidity limit the mechanisms by which bone can increase in size; these include surface apposition of new bone and surface resorption of old bone. During growth, continual changes are necessary to maintain the normal shape of a bone. This requires new bone formation in some areas and resorption in others as the metaphysis advances longitudinally by epiphyseal growth while its trailing edge progressively decreases in diameter to that of the diaphysis (Fig. 5–15). The resultant effect leaves a multitude of architectural patterns in different parts of the diaphyseal cortex, and these areas are altered in turn by internal remodeling with haversian system formation.

As a bone grows in length, it also slowly increases in diameter, and various regions relocate into new positions. The bone tissue present in a given region does not move in a linear direction but remains at the same level as part of the new cortex; any area where the new bone does not overlap the old, however, is resorbed.

The contour of the existing surface acts as a template to determine the architectural pattern of the bone that is

subsequently deposited. If the surface is relatively flat, the new bone will be composed of flat sheets of lamellae. If the surface is irregular and convoluted, the new bone will contain corresponding convolutions, but the cancellous bone will have been converted into compact bone by lamellar deposition within the spaces; this type of bone is characteristically found in the cortex of the proximal and distal thirds of a long bone. Compacted cancellous bone generally has a coarse grain and results from inward relocation of the metaphyseal cortex into areas containing medullary bone. A fine grain occurs when the fine cancellous trabeculae produced at the epiphyseal plate become compacted into cortical bone without first being replaced by coarse trabeculae. Much of the compact bone in the diaphysis of a long bone, especially in the proximal and distal thirds, is of endosteal origin, deposited during metaphyseal reduction as its diameter decreases toward

TABLE 5-3 METABOLIC BONE SURFACES (m²)

	Mass (g)	Total Cell Surface		Total Cancellous Plate Surface		Total Cortex Canal Surface	
		Osteocyte Surface	Lacunar-Canalicular Surface*	Cancellous (g)	Cancellous Surface	Cortex (g)	Haversian + Volkmann Surface
Femur	400	4.8–9.6 (7.2)	96	130	1.1	270	0.2 + 0.02
Total skeleton	5000	60–120 (90)	1200	1000	9	4000	3.2 + 0.32

*Lacunar-canalicular surface after Robinson (1964) (adjusted upward for the larger total skeletal mass used).
(From Johnson, 1966, with permission.)

abolic units," represents an organizational unit of metabolic activity that remains after a remodeling unit has completed its task.*

The magnitude of surface available for mineral homeostasis is infinitely larger than that available for remodeling activity. Remodeling occurs on trabecular and endosteal surfaces as well as along vascular channels within bone, whereas mineral exchange takes place in the lacunae and canaliculae in addition to the larger spaces. The total surface theoretically available consists of a series of tenfold increments (Table 5–3). The least surface is in Volkmann's canals; haversian canals have ten times as much surface; cancellous bone adds a threefold increase (cancellous bone has 35 times as much free surface area per gram of bone as cortical bone, but there is less cancellous bone in the total skeleton, so overall there is about ten times as much cancellous as free cortical surface); lacunar surface is ten times larger; and canalicular surface adds another tenfold increase.

Theoretically, a separate bone fluid compartment exists between the lining cell syncytium and the underlying bone substance (Fig. 5–17). If true, insufficient fluid is present to obtain direct proof, but indirect evidence supports the existence of such a compartment. The syncytium acts as a barrier between the extracellular fluid of the body and the extracellular fluid in bone, and it also serves as a communications network within bone, a position of unique advantage for the rapid control of plasma-bone interchange. Electron micrograph studies of the surface osteocytes that envelop all spaces large enough to contain vascular channels show that the cells do not form tight junctions with each other as do similar lining cells in the bowel or kidney. In fact, definite channels or pores have been identified between adjacent cells. These spaces may have a crucial role in calcium and phosphorus regulation. In contrast, the junctions between osteocytes

within bone (beneath the surface osteocytes) are tight junctions, usually found in the canaliculi. The distance between a canaliculus and its vascular channel does not usually exceed 80 to 100 μ and diffusion through the canalicular system is extremely rapid, as seen in tracer studies. This system regulates mineral homeostasis and will be discussed in greater detail in Chapter 10.

Haversian Systems (Osteons or Basic Multicellular Units)

Structurally, the skeleton is maintained through the activity of basic multicellular (remodeling) units (BMUs) located on free bone surfaces and along the vascular channels. Remodeling events on these surfaces appear to have similar life cycles in both trabecular bone and cortical bone. The haversian systems found in cortical bone are the end result of previously active remodeling units. Structurally, a haversian system is an elongated cylinder 100 to 300 μ in diameter and several millimeters or more in length containing 0.05 to 0.1 mm³ of lamellar bone. In long bones, they run parallel to the long axis of the bone

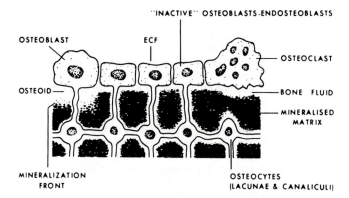

Figure 5-17. Schematic representation of the lacunar-canalicular system within bone and its relationship to the extracellular fluid. A layer of inactive osteoblasts lines all of the larger surfaces in bone, separating the extracellular fluid (ECF) from bone fluid. The borders of adjacent cells are loosely approximated rather than tightly sealed, permitting the extracellular transfer of water and of ions between the two fluid compartments. *(From Jaworski, 1976, with permission.)*

---

*These packets or groups of cells are known by several different names including basic multicellular units, basic (or bone) metabolic (or metabolizing) units, and bone remodeling units, all of which are symbolized by the letters BMU. To differentiate between the two major phases in the life cycle of these units, Rasmussen and Bordier (1974) have suggested that the term "bone remodeling unit" be used during the remodeling phase and "bone metabolic unit" once remodeling has been completed.

and appear round or oval shaped on transverse section. Their architecture and cellular relationships are best studied in longitudinal sections where the cylinder will be seen to have a blunt end that contains osteoclasts (the cutting cone) (Fig. 5–18). A short distance along the canal, active new bone formation is apparent over a length about seven times greater than the length of the cutting cone.

The configuration of remodeling units on endosteal and trabecular surfaces differs from the cylindrical shape of a haversian system, even though the cycle of activation-resorption-formation is the same. On these surfaces, the remodeling unit is flat as if an active osteon from cortical bone had been slit longitudinally and the cylinder unfolded to form a flat sheet of cells. A completed unit is 60 to 80 μ thick with a surface area of 0.5 to 1.0 mm^2.

Initiation of the remodeling cycle begins with activation of precursor (osteoprogenitor) cells in a localized area of bone. The stimulus produces mitotic division in the precursor cells. A batch of osteoclasts is produced first, and these cells resorb bone for about 1 month. After resorption subsides, the reversal phase lasts about 1 week, when a batch of new osteoblasts appears, and over a 3-month period lays down about the same amount of bone as was previously resorbed. Each BMU turns over approximately 0.05 to 0.1 mm^3 of bone during its active life. Once the cycle has been completed, cellular activity returns to its resting state, leaving the remaining osteoblasts as inactive lining cells (surface osteocytes).

Morphologically, the new bone made by a remodeling unit can be differentiated from adjacent bone by a cement (reversal) line, which remains as permanent evidence of previous activity (Fig. 5–19); the cement line forms at the outer limit of bone resorption just before new bone deposition and indicates the extent of resorption. Because of the method of bone formation, the new unit of bone is to some extent an independent entity since it does not communicate with adjacent bone across cement lines; its shape varies with its location; in cortical bone it is a haversian system (osteon), and in trabecular bone it is an irregular patch of bone, similar to a shingle on a roof and identifiable by its cement line (a remodeling unit in trabecular bone is flat, as if an osteon were slit longitudinally and unfolded).

The level of remodeling activity within a whole bone is equal to the sum of activity in all of its separate remodeling units. Secondary osteon development begins at about 1 year of age in the linea aspera and at about 6 years in the phalanges of the hand, but it then continues throughout life, so an increasing number of osteons and interstitial fragments develop with age. Conditions associated with an increased rate of remodeling activity, such as Paget's disease can be identified by the mosaic pattern of cement lines.

Activation. A remodeling unit must be activated before resorption can begin, and for this reason, methods to control the activation of new BMUs hold interest as the key to control of bone remodeling. Parathyroid hormone (PTH) is the most potent agent known to stimulate new foci of remodeling activity; the administration of PTH is followed by an increase in the number of osteoclasts present in bone, and continued administration produces a marked increase in total remodeling activity. The mechanism of PTH action appears to be as an activator of pluripotential precursor cells, leading to the elaboration of a batch of osteoclasts, which resorbs a packet of bone; when resorption is complete, the osteoclasts disappear, followed by the appearance of new osteoblasts that lay down an equivalent amount of bone to that previously resorbed. Recently developed monoclonal antibody techniques indicate that osteoclasts do not arise from monocytes or tissue-fixed macrophages but from previously unidentifiable mononuclear forms (Horton et al., 1985).

Bone formation appears to be inhibited initially, but it increases in 2 to 3 days, probably because of a coupling factor in bone that is released during the process of resorption (Baylink et al., 1982). Conversely, parathyroidectomy retards or prevents disuse osteoporosis. Calcium ions and 1,25-(OH)$_2$D$_3$ have also been found to activate precursor cells. Growth hormone, thyroxine, and physical stress stimulate activation, but their role is less well defined. In contrast, calcitonin, estrogen, and adrenocortical steroids inhibit activation.

Resorption. It is now generally acknowledged that bone resorption precedes formation and that this function is carried out by osteoclasts; even so, the possibility remains that surface osteocytes (or single-nucleated rather than multinucleate osteoclasts) may be able to resorb bone. In cortical bone, a resorption cavity results from the tunneling action of a cutting cone traveling along a vascular canal in line with, but slightly oblique to, the long axis of the bone. The sequence of events can be recognized most clearly in longitudinal sections that have been fortuitously cut through developing osteons (Fig. 5–20). The cutting cone is a broad, cone-shaped osteoclastic front about 150 μ long; as it advances, it leaves an elongated resorption cavity. Johnson (1964) has calculated that the cone contains approximately six osteoclasts in the plane of the section (in cross section about 12 osteoclasts are needed to make a cavity). Although the resorption cavity progresses in a longitudinal direction, the individual osteoclasts may resorb bone in a radial direction, with successive generations of cells accounting for the longitudinal advance of the cutting cone through bone (Johnson, 1964). This is not yet known with certainty, but it would be comparable to bone formation where the osteoblasts lay down new bone in a radial direction.

The life span of an osteoclast is uncertain because they are formed from mononuclear cells and require a steady supply of new nuclei that are continuously incorporated and shed. The nuclei are probably derived from proliferating cells in the area (Parfitt, 1984). An osteoclast advances approximately 2 to 4 μ per hour or 50 to 100 μ per day, and during a 24-hour period, it can resorb a cavity 100 to 300 μ in diameter containing 200,000 μ^3 of bone. This amount of bone is about three times its volume and contains three to six osteocytes (seven to ten generations of osteoblasts are needed to fill in the same amount). The resorption cavity itself advances longitudinally about 50

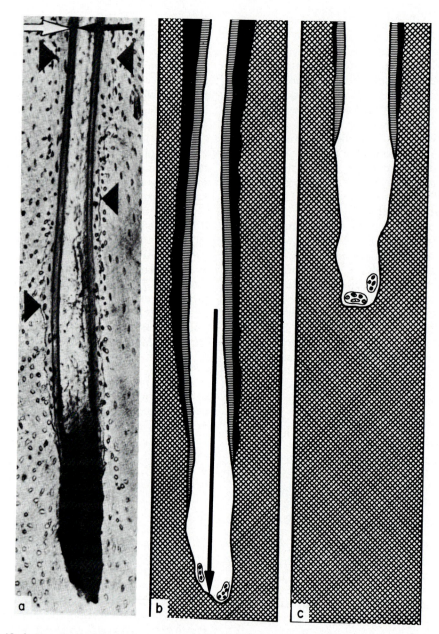

Figure 5–18. A. Longitudinal ground section, stained superficially with methylene blue, of the diaphysis of the radius of an adult dog (×90). The formation of an osteon involves a succession of events that is easily read: A tunnel is being bored downward and osteogenesis follows in the wake of bone destruction. Here a black arrow indicates the inner aspect of the preosseous layer, a white arrow indicates the demarcation line, and the indexes indicate the cementing line. The uniform thickness of the preosseous layer proves that the saw has cut the bone exactly all along the axis of the canal. **B.** The histologic picture is reproduced schematically. The preosseous layer is striated, the new bone is black, and the old bone is cross-hatched. Osteoclasts are in action at the blind end of the tunnel. This animal had received an injection of tetracycline 17 days before sacrifice. Examination of the section in ultraviolet light makes it possible to draw what the histologic picture would have been on the day of labeling. Said drawing is **C.** If it is superimposed on the schematic illustration in the middle, one sees at a glance the length of the tunnel that has been bored in 17 days. The linear rate of osteoclastic bone destruction (length of the arrow) and of bone formation (width of the black layer) in the field under study are thus visualized (Dhem, 1967). *(From Lacroix, 1971, with permission.)*

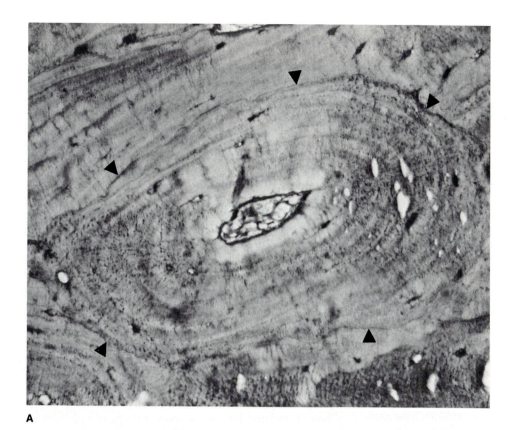

A

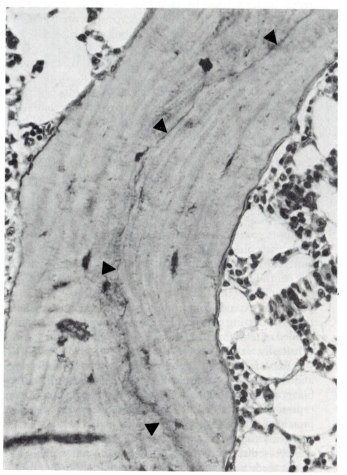

B

Figure 5–19. A. Cortical bone. The cement line (arrows) indicates the peripheral margin of the BMU (osteon); it acts as a barrier separating the physiologic function of the BMU from that of the surrounding bone (about ×350). **B.** In trabecular bone, a cement line indicates the margin of a BMU, but instead of a cylinder, the BMU borders an open surface. Undecalcified bone, 4-μ section (about ×350). *(Courtesy of Dr. Roland Baron.)*

of cellular activity and includes both the resorption phase (σ_r) and the formation phase (σ_f); it begins with initiation of a new remodeling center (BMU) and ends with eventual completion of the bone formation phase. The total remodeling period (σ) in children is 2 to 3 months, but it increases in duration with age, lasting 4 to 5 months in adults. It can exceed 13 years in osteomalacia. An increase in σ indicates that the individual cell performs less work than normal. For instance, a decrease in the rate of bone formation by osteoblasts (a decrease in the appositional rate) prolongs the duration of the formation phase (σ_f).

A change in the rate of activation of new BMU (μ) initially affects resorption activity, with formation inevitably changing later after osteoblasts have replaced osteoclasts in the normal remodeling cycle. Once a steady state has again been reached, the number of active BMU per unit of bone will be different from the number present initially, so the turnover rate (at the tissue level) will be permanently altered (Fig. 5–25, top). For instance, estrogen has been found to depress BMU activation. Therefore, re-

sorption will be decreased first, and biopsy analysis during this period will show a decrease in bone resorption and no change in bone formation. In time, formation will also decrease, so analysis after a period of time equal to one life span shows that estrogen permanently decreases both resorption and formation.

Changes in the remodeling period (σ) cause transient, but not permanent alterations of the turnover rate (Fig. 5–25, bottom). Sigma is longer than normal in some disease states and it can be lengthened by certain drugs, but it is questionable whether it is ever shorter than normal. If it takes longer for each BMU to complete its cycle but the rate of activation of new foci does not change, the total number of active foci will be increased. Once a complete cycle has occurred, however, the turnover rate will return to its previous level, regardless of the magnitude of change in the life span.

It is apparent that accurate results cannot be obtained from repeat bone biopsies, whether in humans or in animals, if performed sooner than one BMU life span (σ).

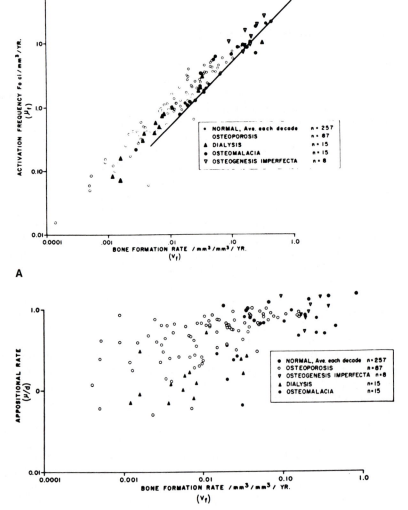

Figure 5-25. A. Relationship between the tissue-level bone formation rate and the BMU activation rate in a variety of conditions. An extremely high correlation exists between the two. **B.** Relationship between the bone formation rate and the appositional rate. No predictable relationship exists between the two. *(From Villanueva and Frost, 1970, with permission.)*

Therefore, σ is the shortest permissible interval between two biopsies, and to make certain a steady state has been reached, it must be calculated before obtaining a repeat biopsy.

Cellular-, Tissue-, and Organ-Level Remodeling. The physiologic behavior of the skeleton is dependent on remodeling activity at three basic levels of organization—cellular, tissue, and organ. Bone contains cells that together with extracellular matrix form bone tissue. The tissue, in turn, is part of a functional organ, a bone. Although activity at the various levels is interdependent, physiologic behavior may differ between the cell, tissue, and organ levels so that activity at one level cannot be inferred from that at any other (Fig. 5–26). Therefore, information obtained from measurements of bone remodeling must be viewed from the appropriate perspective, depending upon the level of organization to which it applies. The disease osteogenesis imperfecta illustrates these differences. The appositional rate in osteogenesis imperfecta has been reported to be either normal or decreased (σ is normal or prolonged), indicating that individual osteoblasts produce either a normal amount or a decreased amount of lamellar bone per day; i.e., cellular-level bone formation is normal or subnormal. Studies of these osteogenesis imperfecta cells in culture would be expected to show a similar level of activity. Such information, however, bears no relation to activity at the tissue level where bone formation and resorption are markedly increased; in fact, they may reach levels more than three to four times normal. This increase in tissue-level bone formation and resorption results from a marked increase in the number of active bone-remodeling units. Obviously, remodeling activity at the tissue level cannot be predicted from knowledge of activity at the cellular level. Likewise, information from cellular- or tissue-level activity does not predict activity at the organ level; these patients have a severe decrease in the amount of total bone present in their skeletons, as indicated by thin cortices and narrow diaphyses. In effect, the increased amount of new bone formation at the tissue level (three times normal) appears to balance the deficit in total skeletal bone (assuming it to be about one third of normal), so the total amount of new bone formed per patient may be close to normal. Consequently, studies that measure organ-level activity such as urinary hydroxyproline or kinetic tracers may yield normal results.

The Triple-Surface System (also see the section, "The Triple Envelope System"). One additional variable must be considered in measurements of bone remodeling, that of the triple-surface system (periosteal, intracortical, and endosteal surfaces are envelopes). The cells in these envelopes form a complex group of subsystems in which the behavior of the osteoblasts and osteoclasts in one envelope is distinctive from that in the others. Each envelope shows a typical pattern of changes with age. The periosteal envelope increases in size throughout the period of growth, and it continues to increase slowly throughout adult life. The haversian envelope shows the fewest changes with age. The endosteal envelope includes the en-

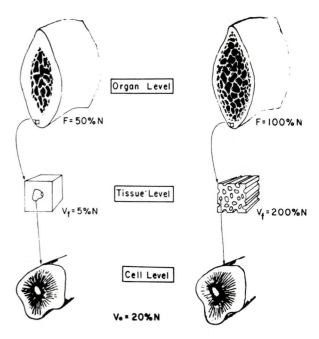

Figure 5-26. Diagram of cellular-, tissue-, and organ-level remodeling in two different conditions (right and left). Two actively forming osteons representing cellular-level bone formation are shown at the bottom, each making bone only 20 percent as fast as normal (V_o). The cellular level does not reflect activity at the tissue level, which can be even lower as on the left where there is only one active bone-forming site instead of the normal four (per cubic millimeter of cortex), so that tissue-level bone formation (V_f) is only 5 percent of normal. In contrast, on the right there are 40 such centers in 1 mm³ of bone so that 200 percent of the normal amount of bone is being made. Similarly, tissue-level activity does not reflect organ-level activity, which varies with the total amount of bone tissue in the skeleton (top). An excess amount of bone is present on the left, which raises organ-level cortical bone formation to half of the normal; this can be seen in osteoporosis. Less bone than normal is present on the right, causing normal organ-level bone formation; this can be seen in osteogenesis imperfecta. *(From Frost, 1969, with permission.)*

dosteal wall of cortex, which progressively loses bone throughout most of adult life, resulting in slow enlargement of the medullary canal. In cancellous bone, the trabeculae are continuous with the endosteal wall of cortex, and functionally their behavior is similar, but the trabeculae have from 10 to 200 times more surface area than an equivalent amount of cortical bone, and this exposes them to a correspondingly greater amount of remodeling activity. The various analyses carried out on bone can be classified according to their effect on one or more envelopes.

Biopsy Site

Selection of Site. The type of specimen selected for analysis is of crucial importance since the results will be viewed as representative of events occurring throughout the skeleton as a whole. Therefore, the site of the biopsy

Rasmussen H, Bordier P: The Cellular Basis of Metabolic Bone Disease. Baltimore, Williams & Wilkins, 1974.

Raux P, Towsend PR, Miegel R, et al.: Trabecular architecture of the human patella. J Biomech 8:1, 1975.

Robinson RA: Observations regarding compartments for tracer calcium in the body. In Frost HM (ed): Bone Biodynamics. Boston, Little, Brown, 1964, p 423.

Schenk RK: Endosteal formation surface estimated by histological technique in iliac bone. In Jaworski ZFG (ed): Proceedings of the 1st Workshop on Bone Morphometry. Ottawa, University of Ottawa Press, 1976, p 185.

Schultz A, Delling G: Age related changes of new bone formation. In Jaworski ZFG (ed): Proceedings of the 1st Workshop on Bone Morphometry, Ottawa, University of Ottawa Press, 1976, p 189.

Takahashi H, Norimatsu H: The longitudinal and transverse rate of resorption of the haversian system in canine bone. In Jaworski ZFG (ed): Proceedings of the 1st Workshop on Bone Morphometry. Ottawa, University of Ottawa Press, 1976, p 143.

Urist MR, Mikulski AJ, Lietze A: Solubilized and unsolubilized bone morphogenic protein. Proc Natl Acad Sci USA 76:1828, 1979.

Villanueva AR: Methods of preparing and interpreting mineralized sections of bone. In Jaworski ZFG (ed): Proceedings of the 1st Workshop on Bone Morphometry, Ottawa, University of Ottawa Press, 1976, p 341.

Villanueva AR, Frost HM: Evaluation of factors determining the tissue-level Haversian bone formation rate in man. J Dent Res 49:836, 1970.

Vu Van Nguyen N, Jowsey J: A study of bone formation in dogs of different metabolic states using autoradiographic visualization of ^{45}Ca. Acta Orthop Scand 40:708, 1969.

Warwick R, Williams PL: Gray's Anatomy, 35th Brit. ed., Edinburgh, Churchill Livingstone, 1973.

Woods CG, Morgan DB, Patterson CR, Gossman HH: Measurement of osteoid in bone biopsy. J Pathol 95:441, 1968.

Chapter 6

Bone: Mineralization

H. Catherine W. Skinner

HISTORY
THE INORGANIC COMPONENT OF BONE
  Identification of the Minerals in Bone
  Studies on the Synthetic System CaO-P$_2$O$_5$-H$_2$O

MINERALIZATION
  Roles of collagen, mucopolysaccharides, cells
SYNTHETIC BONE, PROSTHETIC DEVICES,
  AND IMPLANTS

Bone tissue is an intimate mixture of cells, fibrillar organic molecules, and mineral. It is the presence of mineral that distinguishes bone from other normal tissues in the human body and bestows bifunctionality on the organs composed of bone tissue. The vertebrate skeleton, which has evolved over eons to permit the upright stance, the mobility, and dexterity unique to *Homo sapiens*, is most importantly the site of muscle attachment. Mineral is the stiffening agent essential to the formation and stability of bony structures. Bones enclose the marrow cavity, the site of blood production, and protect the spinal column and the brain. In addition, the mineral in the tissues is the conserved, locally available storehouse of the many chemical elements required in metabolism, the ultimate pool in homeostasis. The skeleton is composed of a variety of mineralized tissues that continually grow and remodel throughout the lifetime of an individual and is really a complicated composite material. The composition, distribution, and rate of turnover of the mineral in skeletal tissues play essential roles in the well-being and quality of life. Without mineral and appropriate mineral dynamics, the proper function of the skeleton is compromised.

This chapter will briefly summarize our present knowledge of the mineral in bone tissue and mention some of the contributions that mineral makes to skeletal tissues from the molecular to tissue and organ levels.

HISTORY

The adult human skeleton contains over 200 bones, each one composed of mineralized tissues and having a distinctive structure and shape. The external portions of all bones are composed of dense, compact, highly mineralized tissue known as cortical bone. The limbs or appendicular skeletal elements are tubular bones with a central marrow cavity. The skull, clavicle, and axial skeleton (the vertebrae) are flat bones that also contain marrow but in discontinuous internal areas defined by spicules of mineralized tissue called trabeculae. Trabeculae are also found in the flared ends (metaphyses and epiphyses) of long bones. The preferred orientation of these mineralized structures along lines of stress (Wolff's law) produce distinctive internal architecture: the arcades in the longitudinal cross section of the femur; the struts in human vertebrae that change, thickening with age (see Figs. 5–1, 5–11, and 5–12).

There are two pathways from mineralized tissues to mature, functioning bone organs. Some bones, notably the long bones, are preformed in cartilage. As early as 1631, Spigelius had distinguished bones formed from a mucous substance (cartilage) that "hardened into bone" from those made of intermembranous bone where an aggregate of cells produced mineralized bone tissue directly without a car-

Leonard and Scullin (1969) proposed an interesting source for the phosphorus needed in bone mineralization by calling upon the cycle of cell metabolism. Hydrolysis of ATP in the presence of calcium ions (Ca^{+2}) intracellularly could lead to the formation of a calcium phosphate complex and release of adenine and HPO_4. Adenine recombines with some of the HPO_4, forming adenosine monophosphate (AMP), and with more HPO_4 through adenosine diphosphate (ADP) to reform ATP. Cells, therefore, could control mineralization by modulating ATP production. The mechanism for extruding the calcium phosphate complex into the extracellular environment, as required for mineralization of the matrix in an orderly fashion typical of bone, has not been identified, but the vesicles previously mentioned may be important in some tissue systems.

Enzymes, perhaps induced by extracellular signals, may play important roles in mineralization. Alkaline phosphatase has been suggested as aiding the precipitation of mineral by providing phosphate (Solomons and Neuman, 1960). The pyrophosphatases may act by destroying inhibitors of mineralization (Fleisch and Neuman, 1961). Proteases specific for the removal of proteoglycans may create localities and sites for mineralization. Baylink and Wergedal, (1972) demonstrated that proteoglycans were lost precisely at the mineralization front preceding mineral formation. Osteoid contains a high level of chondroitin sulfate, which decreased (using radiolabeled sulfur on the proteoglycan) as the calcium content increased. It seems reasonable that the loss of the macromolecule signals mineralization.

Small calcium-chelating proteins have been found in mineralized tissues. They may be transport agents or act as local nucleating agents (Hauschka et al., 1975). Several role(s) have been identified for calcionectin and fibronectin, and they are important molecular species; however, these molecules are not confined to bone tissue.

It is quite possible that all of the aforementioned hypotheses for initiating or sustaining mineralization operate at some site or at some time during the generation or repair of normal bone tissue. It must be remembered that bone, as distinct from the dental tissues, enamel and dentine, is resorbed and redeposited many times over the lifetime of the individual. It is also true that bone tissue formation through the action of osteoblasts that first produce extracellular matrix and subsequently mineralize is not a symmetrical reversible process (Bordier and Rasmussen, 1974). Osteocytes may locally affect the amount of mineral in the matrix surrounding them (Belanger, 1969; Baylink and Wergedal, 1971), but osteoclasts are necessary to resorb the tissue and do so by destroying mineral and matrix together and effectively at the same time (Hancox, 1972; Hall, 1975). The cellular control that serves formation and resorption must be individualized and specifically respond to some, perhaps systemic level, requirements (homeostasis?). Hydroxyapatite located in and on the biomolecules must *pari passu* be involved in all the metabolic events. The presence of the mineral must dictate some of the cellular actions. The basic physical chemistry of the calcium phosphate species must be the foundation, the modulator, or both, of at least some of the biologic reactions that produce and maintain bone.

SYNTHETIC BONE, PROSTHETIC DEVICES, AND IMPLANTS

The significance of the mineral phase in the normal woven or lamellar tissues is perhaps best appreciated when we attempt to replace bone with substitute materials.

We know that whenever a foreign object or material is placed within the body there is often a characteristic tissue reaction. If the chemical composition of the material is nontoxic and nonreactive, the object may remain for extended periods and may become encapsulated, or sealed off from the biologic regime by fibrous (collagenous) tissue. When the material is a substitute for bone or joint, however, the many facets of bone and the bone system of growth development and repair become important and, if not too much of a pun, painfully obvious.

Substitution for a portion of a bone such as at small but highly biologically active sites, the alveolar crest, for example, is often mandated when disease is treated by surgical resection. An empty tooth socket or discontinuous alveolar ridge would create nonfunctional areas in a highly used portion of the anatomy—the oral cavity. From this dental or maxillofacial application to the insertion of total hip and knee prostheses, there are complicated functional and mechanical requirements for any device substituting for bone or bone organs. The strength and structure of these devices, so important to their usefulness, is a reflection of the presence of mineral in bone tissues.

Over the past 15 years there has been a remarkable proliferation in the variety and availability of prosthetic devices. As might be anticipated there has also been a plethora of studies on these devices to determine their clinical stability and benefit to the patient and especially to test and estimate their longevity in vivo. In many ways all the factors that are considered when attempting to produce an appropriately useful and stable implant emphasize the molecular and cellular as well as the functional characteristics of bone. Much useful information on bone tissues, their reactions, and remodeling have been obtained from studies undertaken to examine whether prosthetic devices are of optimum shape and constructed from appropriate materials.

Putting aside the mechanical problems of joint replacement, including the clinical restraints, let us focus on the materials chosen for implants. The criteria for using a particular material are, that it be strong and maintain strength under mechanical use (not be brittle) and in the biologic environment. The biologic environment, it has been found, is highly corrosive to metals, even stainless steel. The materials chosen must be nontoxic, tissue compatible, and virtually indestructable to stay in place for the duration of use and, it is hoped, the life of the individual. Alternatively, some implants are intended to be transient; therefore, the material should be resorbable, but continue to function while new bone tissue invades and restores the original structure.

In the early stages of research on implants, metal and ceramic devices were affixed to bone by polymethyl methacrylate (PMMA) cement. Biocompatibility difficulties arose as metal fragments were abraided from the devices, and some tissue necrosis resulted from the exothermic (heating) effect of the curing cement. Many materials and shapes were investigated. The use of porous implant materials facilitated the ingrowth of tissue and minimized the need for cements. Portions of the larger structural replacements (joints) were coated or were made with sintered exteriors simulating roughened surfaces, potentially to take advantage of the opportunity of bonding the device to the bone or soft tissues. The reactivity of bone and the surrounding soft tissues had to be taken into account in fashioning implant devices (Hood et al., 1983).

Over the past several years surface-active biomaterials such as hydroxyapatite ceramics and Bioglass have become the materials of choice, at least as the coating for many different prosthetic devices (Hench and Wilson, 1984). The materials are biocompatible and may aid early fixation of the larger metallic or ceramic devices (Ducheyne et al., 1980). The use of these materials highlights the information we have obtained from the synthetic studies on the mineral system.

From our previous discussion we might expect that hydroxyapatite ceramics would be biocompatible. They are also biodegradable. The glasses constructed for use with implants are composed of the same dominant elements as the mineral materials—CaO, P_2O_5—and contain in addition Na_2O and SiO_2.

Figure 6–7 delineates the chemical composition of the bioactive glasses that have been investigated as bioim-plant materials. A portion of the composition range expressed in the diagram has been shown to be useful: those that become involved in direct bonding to bone (A), those that have reacted relatively favorably by not being rejected but encapsulated by fibrous tissue (B), and those that dissolve (C) under biologic conditions, which means they are not useful but are also not harmful.

It has been shown that a bond between the implant core and a glass coating is essential for implant longevity. A bonding between the glass and the tissues prevents movement of the implant, inflamation, and scarring (fibrous tissue formation) that could ultimately destroy or cause rejection of the implant. The present objective in research for replacement bone and bone organs is to replicate as close as possible the composition and tissue characteristics of bone. For weight-bearing applications, bioglass materials may be used as a coating over a device mostly composed of specialty metals such as Vitallium. Bioglass-coated wires have also proved useful in orthodontic manipulation. If the coating shears off, biocompatible material remains in the healing wound. For nonweight-bearing situations porous hydroxyapatite, made in one case by treating natural coral ($CaCO_3$) samples with phosphate solutions, has been most successful (Holmes, 1979). Rapid bone regeneration within the channelways created during growth of these colonial sea creatures facilitated penetration (and fixation) of the bone cells and tissues. The result is physiologic in that the implant degrades as new bone tissues are put in place. The coral's inorganic architecture functions as the house for bone (re)generation. The hydroxyapatitic coralline material is satisfying the dual roles we mentioned at the outset of this chapter: the mineral provides structural support as well as compositional compatibility for homeostasis, contributing to the physical and chemical needs of functioning bone and bone tissues.

ACKNOWLEDGMENT

I am indebted to J. A. Albright for suggestions and for the opportunity to include the discussion of bone implants and synthetic bone in this revision. My thanks to A. W. Crompton, Department of Biology, Harvard University, for the space and time, so generously made available to compose the original version of this chapter. My gratefulness has not diminished in the intervening years.

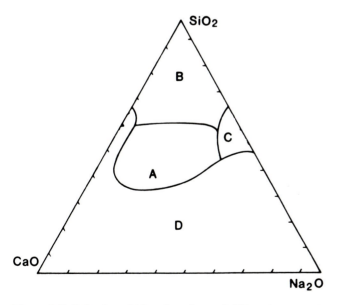

Figure 6-7. Behavior of bioactive glass of different compositions. Region A, bone bonding; B, fibrous tissue encapsulation; C, dissolution; D, non–glass-forming. All compositions have a constant 6 percent P_2O_5 by weight. *(From Hench and Wilson, Copyright © 1984 by AAAS, with permission.)*

REFERENCES

Anderson HC: Vesicles associated with calcification in the matrix of epiphyseal cartilage. J Cell Biol 41:59, 1969.

Armstrong W, Singer L: Composition and constitution of the mineral phase of bone. Clin Orthop 38:179, 1967.

Barzel ES (ed): Osteoporosis. New York, Grune & Stratton, 1970.

Bassett H: The phosphates of calcium. V. Revision of earlier space diagram. J Chem Soc 601:2949, 1958.

Baylink D, Wergedal J: Bone formation and resorbtion by osteocytes. In Nichols G. Wasserman RH (eds): Cellular Mechanisms for Calcium, Transfer and Homeostasis. New York, Academic Press, 1971, p 257.

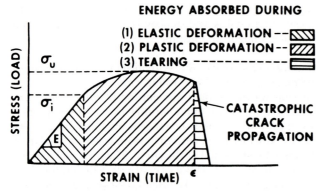

Figure 7–1. Idealized stress–strain (or load-time) curve in tensile impact showing energy absorbed during elastic, plastic, and tearing phases. σi = the proportional limit or yield point. σu = ultimate or maximum stress. E = modulus of elasticity or the slope of the straight line portion of the curve. u = total plastic deformation. (*From Saha and Hayes, J. Biomech 9:243–251, Pergamon Press, Ltd. 1976, with permission.*)

terial is unloaded, the curve will return to zero immediately with no residual deformation.

Viscoelastic properties can be detected by several types of mechanical tests. With rapid loading, the elastic properties assume increased importance relative to the viscous properties, which results in a steeper stress–strain curve and, therefore, a higher modulus of elasticity. A constant force, such as a dead weight, applied to a viscoelastic material usually causes an instantaneous deformation, but progressive deformation occurs slowly with time (creep). If a viscoelastic material is stretched and then maintained at a constant length, its resistance force will immediately rise to a maximum level and then decrease progressively with time (stress relaxation).

Fatigue. Fatigue studies measure the susceptibility of a material to failure from cyclical loading using a stress or a strain level below yield strength. Most materials have an endurance limit, a level of stress below which cyclical stress can continue indefinitely without failure.

Hardness. Hardness is the indentability of a material. An indentation is made under standard conditions and the defect is measured. Microhardness, rather than macrohardness, measurements are usually made on bone because of the multiple microscopic spaces (voids) present. These spaces will decrease the accuracy of the results when a larger indenter is used, as it is for macrohardness testing.

Units of Measurement

The terminology used in the literature has undergone a number of changes in recent years. In this chapter alone four different designations for strength have been quoted from articles published within the last 20 years. Fortunately, the results from one system can be changed to those of the other systems by using the proper conversion factors. Table 7–2 lists the currently recommended terms (SI units) used to describe bone, with conversion factors for other systems. In the United States the International System of Units (SI units), based on the metric system, is often used for scientific and medical purposes, but neither engineers nor technologists have yet made the transition to the metric system, nor has the general public.

Measurement Conditions

Studies can be performed on whole bones or on machined specimens, with each providing information that complements the other but at a different level of interest. To study fracture behavior and repair, or the response of bone to physical stress, or the effect of various treatment programs requires the testing of intact bones; either paired bones (one side treated and the other side untreated) from the same animal can be compared, or the bones can be grouped according to categories of treatment. Whole bones have usually been loaded in torsion or in bending; bone, however, does not have a uniform cylindrical shape, so the exact orientation is critical in bending tests, where even slight differences in rotation will effect the results. Axial loading in line with the forces sustained during normal activity is often preferable.

To characterize bone as a material requires the use of machined specimens. Although the overall size of the bone automatically limits specimen size, most studies have utilized samples having a cross-sectional area of 4 to 20 mm²,

TABLE 7–2. UNITS USED TO DESCRIBE THE MECHANICAL PROPERTIES OF BONE

Category	Term	Equivalent SI Unit	Other
Force	1 pound force (lb f)	4.448 Newton (N)	0.45359 kg f
	1 kilogram force (kg f)	9.807 Newton (N)	
	1 kilopond force	9.807 Newton (N)	
Stress	1 lb/in² (psi)	6894.8 N/m²	0.070307 kg/cm²
(pressure or strength)	1 kg/cm²		
	1 kip/in² (Ksi)		1000 lb/in²
	1 Pascal (Pa)	1 N/m²	
Energy (work)	1 Nm	1 Joule (J)	
	1 ft lb f	1.3558 J	
	1 in lb/in²	175.13 J/m²	
Torque (moment)	1 ft lb f	1.3559 Nm	0.13826 kgf m

which is usually large enough to include several Haversian systems. The resulting information represents the average properties of a material whose internal architecture changes continuously from one area to the next, and it includes countless spaces of varying size, from canaliculae to large resorption cavities, plus a variety of structural components, including primary osteons, and secondary osteons, with interstitial bone intertwined in patterns that defy accurate three-dimensional analysis. Because bone is a viscoelastic, anisotropic material that undergoes plastic deformation, its properties vary somewhat with the conditions of measurement. Variations due to viscoelasticity can be minimized by controlling the rate of loading and the moisture content at the time of study. The ultimate strength is directly proportional to the strain rate (Fig. 7–2). In contrast, toughness (ability to absorb energy prior to fracture) is greater at low than at high loading rates. Drying increases the breaking strength of bone, but it decreases the capacity for plastic deformation prior to fracture, resulting in decreased toughness. The degree of control needed over these factors during testing must be determined by the type of study. It is always preferable to closely simulate physiologic conditions, and it often is essential to do so, as when evaluating the properties of normal bone. The experimental conditions are not as critical for many studies, such as the comparison of two methods of internal fixation on paired bones. Due to the anisotropic nature of bone, specimen orientation must be controlled; for a complete evaluation of the physical properties, samples must be obtained from different directions along the bone.

Material Composition

Bone is a composite material that contains approximately two-thirds mineral (by weight) and one-third collagen. Although the details of this relationship are incompletely understood, the mineral component, when tested alone as an isolated material, primarily resists compression, while collagen resists tension. This can be appreciated by comparing demineralized bone (for instance, a specimen that has been demineralized during histologic processing), which is very flexible and resistant to fracture, to deproteinated bone, which is hard, rigid, and brittle (Fig. 7–3).

Bone mineral, similar to a ceramic material, is stronger in compression than in tension, and it is much more rigid than bone. It has a modulus of elasticity (E) as high as 114 giganewtons/m², whereas the modulus of bone itself is about 18 giganewtons/m². Collagen, on the other hand, offers almost no resistance to compression, but its tensile strength (per unit weight) is five times greater than bone, and it is over ten times as flexible (E = 1.2 giganewtons/m²) as bone. Both materials occupy an approximately equal volume in bone, as is evident when either the mineral or the collagen is removed leaving the other intact, or when the relative weight of either component is divided by its density (density = weight/volume).

In any case, bone has unusual properties in that its tensile strength (100 to 150 meganewtons/m²) is relatively high compared to its compressive strength (200 to 250 meganewtons/m²). Other brittle materials with a high mineral content, such as porcelain, have markedly greater strength in compression than tension. Bone has been compared to reinforced concrete, an analogy that may be inappropriate, since it has been calculated that the mineral, which has a higher elastic modulus (more rigid), would bear most of the load when subjected to a tensile force, whereas that borne by collagen would be minimal. Therefore, other analogies have been proposed to explain the material properties of bone (Halstead, 1974). Even so, the organic component is probably responsible for the ductile behavior of bone (Saha, 1977).

Bone has resemblances to fiberglass, which contains fine glass fibers embedded in an epoxy resin, giving it

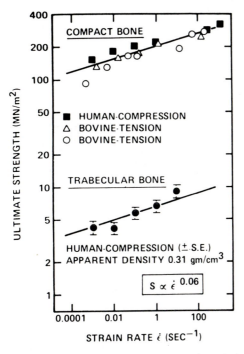

Figure 7-2. Influence of strain rate on the ultimate strength of compact and trabecular bone. *(From Carter and Hayes, 1976, with permission.)*

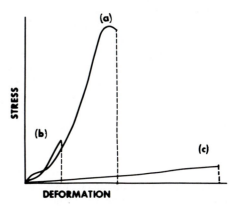

Figure 7-3. Typical stress deformation curves for the following types of bone specimens: **a.** Intact; **b.** Deproteinated; **c.** Demineralized. *(From Saha, J. Mat Sci 12, 1798–1806, 1977, with permission.)*

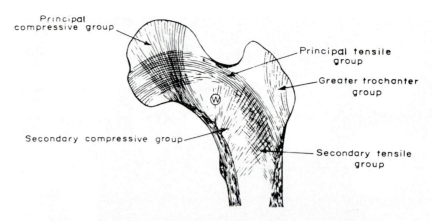

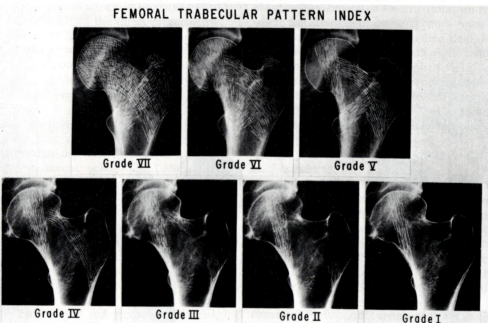

Figure 7–23. Top. The major groups of trabeculae normally present in the upper end of the femur. Ward's triangle (W) is a relatively clear area containing the fewest number of trabeculae. (*From Singh, 1970, with permission*). **Bottom:** Characteristic disappearance pattern of trabeculae in the proximal femur. (*From Singh, 1976, with permission.*)

lowed by the secondary tensile, the primary tensile, and eventually the primary compressive.

The disappearance pattern is predictable enough to use as a guide for judging the severity of demineralization in osteoporosis (Singh, 1970).

Pattern of Response. (This topic is discussed more fully in Chapter 8.) The flexibility of bone and its ability to withstand stress vary in different bones due to differences in shape and internal structure, yet a common pattern of response probably occurs in all bones, with the internal changes dependent on the type and magnitude of force applied. The development of bone hypertrophy is thought to require mechanical compression. With tension, bone appears to atrophy by periosteal resorption and intracortical osteolysis.

Compression. Chamay and Tschantz (1972) have identified three distinct "load zones" in an intact bone loaded repetitively in compression. This concept permits a coherent overview of the response of bone to repetitive forces. It should be viewed as an aid toward better comprehension of the subject, not as an impeccable technical description of the process. Depending on the magnitude of force applied, the three zones include: (1) the elastic load zone, in which bone responds as an elastic body; (2) the fatigue zone, in which repetitive stimulations progressively weaken the bone; and (3) the overload zone, in which a single stress produces plastic deformation.

ELASTIC LOAD ZONE. In the elastic load zone, the deformation (strain) is proportional to the force applied. For practical purposes, repetitive loading within the elastic zone does

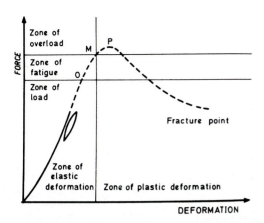

Figure 7-24. Repeated strain in the load zone produces a stable, closed hysteresis loop. (O) limit of the elastic zone, where neither a single nor multiple loading causes permanent deformation; (M) limit of the fatigue zone, where a single loading produces no visible deformation; (P) point of maximum (ultimate) stress. A single loading in the overload zone results in permanent deformation. *(From Chamay A: Mechanical and morphological aspects of experimental overload and fatigue in bone. J Biomech 3:266, 1970, with permission of Pergamon Press, Ltd.)*

not result in fatigue failure* (Fig. 7–24). The ultrastructural changes associated with strain cannot be adequately explained, since no permanent histologic differences have been detected; most likely, the deformation results from intramolecular elongation or from a minimal degree of slippage along cement lines and interlamellar planes, followed by recovery after load release. In any case, loads within the elastic zone stimulate slow adaptational changes in living bone, but the stimulus is much weaker than with higher loads. Maximal elastic compression in the ulna of a dog is approximately 6 to 8 kg/mm² (this would be more accurate if expressed in units of strain, not stress). Plastic lesions appear above this level.

FATIGUE ZONE. The fatigue zone is characterized by the absence of detectable histologic changes in a single loading, even though some permanent (plastic) deformation results (Fig. 7–25). Repetitive loading causes progressive plastic deformation, and prefailure slip lines appear in the compressed cortex (Fig. 7–26). Eventually, a fatigue fracture develops, with the fracture always situated in the middle of the area crossed by the slip lines.

OVERLOAD ZONE. Overload causes permanent (plastic) deformation with parallel prefailure slip lines obliquely oriented at an angle of about 30 degrees to the long axis of the diaphysis. These oblique lines begin as narrow lines,

---

*Dead bone may not have an endurance limit (a maximum level of stress below which cyclical loading can continue indefinitely without failure). Living bone, however, can adapt, so that, functionally, it probably has an endurance limit, allowing it to be loaded repetitively in long-term studies without evidence of fatigue.

which progressively enlarge and eventually form fissures; they may cross part or all of the cortex, as well as the larger trabeculae in cancellous bone, and they often cross small osteons without changing direction. Prefailure slip lines are due to shear with buckling or rupture of collagen fibers in the lamellae and disruption of the crystal pattern. As the force increases to its maximum (ultimate) level, internal failure accelerates and the bone offers decreasing resistance, so that at the time of fracture the force has decreased. The duration of the plastic phase varies, being shorter for dense cortical bone, which fractures closer to the ultimate force, and much longer in children, where a greater degree of deformation occurs prior to fracture.

HYPERTROPHY VERSUS FATIGUE FAILURE. Although the mechanism by which stress leads to hypertrophy of bone remains unknown, the process is markedly stimulated by the production of plastic slip lines; intermittent compression causes massive hypertrophy, presumably because of alternating shearing in the slip lines. Whatever the specific stimulus might be, whether electrical, mechanical, chemical, or enzymatic, the internal motion causes a mechanical–biologic irritation that maintains and continuously reactivates osteogenesis. Plastic slip lines, therefore, are associated with either bone hypertrophy or, if excessive, with fatigue failure. Whether a given stress will produce hypertrophy or fatigue fracture depends upon the magnitude of force, the frequency of loading, and the duration.

It must be kept in mind that a basic difference exists between the mechanisms that cause bone to adapt and those that initiate most clinical fractures. Bone adapts to stress by remodeling until the deformation is stabilized in the elastic zone. The bone is then capable of transmitting all the stored energy. During normal activity, the skeleton primarily resists compression forces, which constantly vary in magnitude, so that the major stimulus to remodeling is the degree of compression, together with the frequency and magnitude of its cyclical variation. In contrast, most clinical fractures result from bending forces or from torsion, and failure begins along lines of maximum tension (it seems appropriate that bone, which normally resists compression, is weaker in tension).

Tension. There appears to be a completely different mechanism of failure in tension than in compression. In a bone subjected to tension, slipping occurs along cement lines bordering osteons and interstitial lamellae. Scattered transverse cracks then appear through isolated substructures, permitting greater slippage; eventually, one of the cracks continues to propagate and a clinical fracture occurs (Fig. 7–27). As a result, the fracture surfaces may contain osteon remnants that have been "pulled out" of the bone, although in a rapidly propagating fracture, the surfaces may be relatively smooth. The optical properties and staining characteristics of bone change when plastic deformation begins, probably because of the multiple interfaces that have been produced at the ultrastructural level.

Several studies have reported that tension leads to

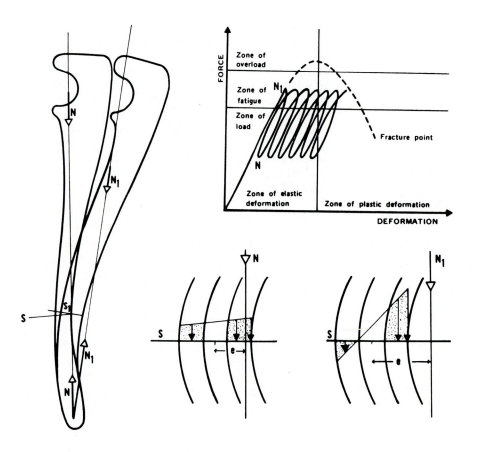

Figure 7-25. Distribution of the stresses and strains in the diaphysis. The diagram of force/deformation shows the fatigue effect. A slow bone deformation is observed, progressing to the plastic phase under the influence of repetitive mechanical stimulations. The hysteresis loops are not superimposable as they remain open. With minimal forces N, both cortices are under compression; whereas with maximal forces N_1, the convex cortex is in tension and concave cortex is in compression. *(From Chamay A, Tschantz P: Mechanical influences in bone remodeling. Experimental research on Wolff's law. J Biomech 5:173, 1972, with permission of Pergamon Press, Ltd.)*

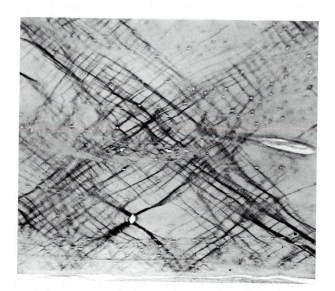

Figure 7-26. Zone of plastic deformation in a compressed cortex. Prefailure slip lines and microcracks are obliquely oriented, forming an angle of about 30 degrees with the long axis of the diaphysis (× 88 sagittal section). *(From Chamay, 1970, with permission.)*

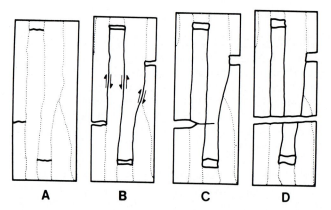

Figure 7-27. Diagram of suggested mechanism of yield in bone. **A.** Bone loaded in tension parallel to the long side of the page. Transverse cracks appear, which are stopped by discontinuities. Unbroken interfaces are indicated by dots. **B.** Shear (arrows) allows relative movement of parts of the tissue and the cracks open. **C.** A crack starts to travel across old interfaces. **D.** The bone breaks, apparently by brittle failure. *(From Wainwright et al., 1976, with permission.)*

bone resorption. Yet, in a physiologic or functional setting, tension does not produce bone resorption (see Chap. 8). This relationship is not clear at the present time and needs better elucidation.

REFERENCES

Ascenzi A, Bell GH: Bone as a mechanical engineering problem. In Bourne GH (ed): The Biochemistry and Physiology of Bone, Vol. 1 Structure. New York, Academic, p 311, 1972.

Ascenzi A, Bonucci E, Simkin A: An approach to the mechanical properties of single osteonic lamellae. J Biomech 6:227, 1973.

Atkinson PJ, Weatherell JA: Variation in the density of the femoral diaphysis with age. J Bone Joint Surg 49B:781, 1967.

Backman S: The proximal end of the femur. Acta Radiol Suppl 146, 1957.

Bassett CAL: Biophysical principles affecting bone structure. In Bourne GH (ed): The Biochemistry and Physiology of Bone. New York, Academic, p 1, 1971.

Bell GH, Dunbar O, Beck JS, Gibb A: Variations in strength of vertebrae with age and their relation to osteoporosis. Calcif Tissue Res 1:75, 1967.

Binderman I, Shimshoni Z, Somjen D: Biochemical pathways involved in the translation of physical stimulus into biological message. Calc Tiss Int 36:S-82–85, 1984.

Blaimont P: Contribution a l'etude biomechanique du femur humain. Acta Orthop Belg 34:665, 1968.

Blaimont P, Halleux P: Un paradoxe des contraintes osseuses. Acta Ortho Belg 38, Suppl I:63, 1972.

Burr DB, Martin RB, Schaffler MB, Radin EL: Bone remodeling in response to *in vivo* fatigue damage. J Biomech 18:189, 1985.

Burstein AH, Currey JD, Frankel VH, Reilly DT: The ultimate properties of bone tissue: The effects of yielding. J Biomech 5:35, 1972.

Burstein AH, Frankel VH: The viscoelastic properties of some biological materials. Ann NY Acad Sci 146:158, 1968.

Burstein AH, Reilly DT, Martens M: Aging of bone tissue: Mechanical properties. J Bone Joint Surg 58A:82, 1976.

Carter DR: Mechanical loading histories and cortical bone remodeling. Calc Tiss Int 36:S-19–24, 1984.

Carter DR, Caler WE: Cycle-dependent and time-dependent bone fracture with repeated loading. Trans of the ASME 105:166, 1983.

Carter DR, Hayes WC: Bone compressive strength: The influence of density and strain rate. Science 194:1174, 1976.

Carter DR, Hayes WC, Schurman DJ: Fatigue life of compact bone–II. Effects of microstructure and density. J Biomech 9:211, 1976.

Carter DR, Caler WE, Spengler DM, Frankel VH: Fatigue behavior of adult cortical bone: The influence of mean strain and strain range. Acta Orthop Scand 52:481, 1981.

Chamay A: Mechanical and morphological aspects of experimental overload and fatigue in bone. J Biomech 3:263, 1970.

Chamay A, Tschantz P: Mechanical influences in bone remodeling. Experimental research on Wolff's law. J Biomech 5:173, 1972.

Chen IIH, Saha S: A model of streaming potentials in osteons based on charge fluid flow between the haversian canal and lacuna. Advances in Bioengineering (ed. by N.A. Langrana), ASME (in press), 1985.

Clark EA, Goodship AE, Lanyon LE: Locomotor bone strain as the stimulus for bone's mechanical adaptability. J Physiol 245:57P, 1975.

Currey JD: The mechanical consequences of variation in the mineral content of bone. J Biomech 2:1, 1969.

Currey JD: The mechanical properties of bone. Clin Orthop 73:210, 1970.

Currey JD: Tensile yield in bone. Calcif Tissue Res 15:173, 1974.

Currey JD: What is bone for? Property–Function relationships in bone. In Cowin SC (ed): Mechanical Properties of Bone, AMD-Vol 45. ASME, NY, 1981, pp 13–26.

Davidovitch Z, Shanfeld JL, Montgomery PC, et al.: Biochemical mediators of the effects of mechanical forces and electric currents on mineralized tissues. Calc Tiss Int 36:S-86–97, 1984.

Doyle F, Brown J, La Chance C: Relation between bone mass and muscle weight. Lancet 1:391, 1970.

Eriksson C: Electrical Properties of Bone. In Bourne GH (ed): The Biochemistry and Physiology of Bone, Vol. IV. New York, Academic, 1976, p 330.

Evans FG: Mechanical Properties of Bone. Springfield, Ill, Chas. C Thomas, 1973.

Frost HM: The presence of microcracks in vivo in bone. Henry Ford Hosp Med Bull 8:25, 1960.

Frost HM: An Introduction to Biomechanics. Springfield, Ill, Chas. C Thomas, 1963.

Frost HM: The Bone Dynamics in Osteoporosis and Osteomalacia. Springfield, Ill, Chas. C Thomas, 1966.

Gibb A: Appendix. Calcif Tissue Res 1:83, 1967.

Goodship AE, Lanyon LE, McFie H: Functional adaptation of bone to increased stress. J Bone Joint Surg 61A:539, 1979.

Goldhaber P: Remodeling of bone in tissue culture. J Dent Res 45:490, 1966.

Halstead LB: Vertebrate hard tissues. London, Wykeham, 1974.

Hasegawa S, Sato S, Saito S, et al.: Mechanical stretching increases the number of cultured bone cells synthesizing DNA and alters their pattern of protein synthesis. Calc Tiss Int 37:431, 1985.

Inman VT: Functional aspects of the abductor muscles of the hip. Bone Joint Surg 29A:607, 1947.

Jendrucko RJ, Hyman WA, Newell PH Jr, Chakraborty BK: Theoretical evidence for the generation of high pressure in bone cells. J Biomech 9:87, 1976.

Johnson LC: The kinetics of skeletal remodeling. In Structural Organization of the Skeleton. Birth Defects Original Article Series. New York, National Foundation, p 66, 1966.

Johnson MW: Behavior of fluid in stressed bone and cellular stimulation. Calc Tiss Int 36:S-72–76, 1984.

Justus R, Luft JH: A mechanical hypothesis for bone remodelling induced by mechanical stress. Calcif Tissue Res 5:222, 1970.

Kayser CH, Heusner A: Étude comparative du métabolisme energétique dans la série animale. J Physiol Paris 56:489, 1964.

Keller TS, Lovin JD, Spengler DM, Carter DR: Fatigue of immature baboon cortical bone. J Biomech 18:297, 1985.

Kimura T, Amtmann E: Distribution of mechanical robustness in the human femoral shaft. J Biomech 17:41, 1984.

Kummer BFK: Biomechanics of bone: Mechanical properties, functional structure, functional adaptation. In Fung YC, Perrone N, Anliker M (eds): Biomechanics. Its foundations and objectives. Engelwood Cliffs, NJ, 1972, p 237.

Lakes R, Saha S: Long-term torsional creep in compact bone. J Biomech Eng 102:178, 1980.

Martin RB: Collagen fiber orientation in osteonal bone: Measurement technique and mechanical significance. Ortho Trans 9:302, 1985.

Mather S: Observations on the effects of static and impact loading on the human femur. J Biomech 1:331, 1968.

Mayer DC, Ashman RB, Cowin SC, Van Buskirk WC: Radial variations in the elastic properties of bovine cortical bone. Trans Ortho Res Soc 8:284, 1983.

McElhaney JH: Dynamic response of bone and muscle tissue. J Appl Physiol 21:1231–1236, 1966.

Meickle MC, Reynolds JJ, Sellers A, Dingle JT: Rabbit cranial sutures in vitro. A new experimental model for studying the response of fibrous joints to mechanical stress. Calc Tiss Int 28:137, 1979.

Meikle MC, Sellers A, Reynolds JJ: Effect of tensile mechanical stress on the synthesis of metalloproteinases of rabbit coronal sutures in vitro. Calc Tiss Int 30:77, 1980.

Moyle DD, Bowden RW: Fracture of human femoral bone. J Biomech 17:203, 1984.

Munro M, Piekarski K: The microstructure of cortical bone. Microstructural Science 3B:941, 1975.

Munro M, Piekarski K: Stress-induced radial pressure gradients in liquid-filled multiple concentric cylinders. J Applied Mechanics 99(2):218, 1977.

O'Conner JA, Lanyon LE, MacFie H: The influence of strain rate on adaptive bone remodelling. J Biomech 15:767, 1982.

Pal S, Saha S: Effect of deformation rate on the flexural fracture behavior of long bones. Med Biol Eng Comput 22:251, 1984.

Piekarski K: Mechanically enhanced perfusion of bone. In Cowin SC (ed): Mechanical Properties of Bone, AMD-Vol 45. Am Soc Mech Eng, 1981, pp 185–91.

Pollack SR, Petrov N, Salzstein R, et al.: An anatomical model for streaming potentials in osteons. J Biomech 17:627, 1984a.

Pollack SR, Salzstein R, Pienkowski D: The electric double layer in bone and its influence on stress-generated potentials. Calc Tiss Int 36:S-77–81, 1984b.

Reilly DT, Burstein AH: The mechanical properties of cortical bone. J Bone Joint Surg 56A:1001, 1974.

Rodan GA, Bourret LA, Harvey A, Mensi T: Cyclic AMP and cyclic GMP: mediators of the mechanical effects on bone remodeling. Science 189:467, 1975.

Rubin CT, Lanyon LE: Regulation of bone formation by applied dynamic loads. J Bone Joint Surg 66A:397, 1984.

Rydell N: Forces acting on the femoral head prosthesis. Acta Ortho Scand Suppl 88, p 1, 1966.

Saha S: Longitudinal shear properties of human compact bone and its constituents, and the associated failure mechanisms. J Materials Sci 12:1798, 1977.

Saha S: The dynamic strength of bone and its relevance. In Ghista KN (ed): Osteoarthromechanics. New York, McGraw-Hill, pp 1–43, 1982.

Saha S, Hayes WC: Tensile impact properties of human compact bone. J Biomech 9:243, 1976.

Sedlin EA: A rheologic model for cortical bone. A study of the properties of human femoral samples. Acta Orthop Scand Suppl 83, 1965.

Singh M: Changes in trabecular pattern of the upper end of the femur as an index of osteoporosis. J Bone Joint Surg 52A:457, 1970.

Singh M: Femoral trabecular pattern index for grading osteoporosis. In Jaworsky ZFG (ed): Proceedings of the 1st Workshop on Bone Morphometry. Ottawa, University of Ottawa Press, p 86, 1976.

Smith AH, Pace N: Differential component and organ size relationship among whales. Environ Physiol 1:122, 1971.

Somjen D, Binderman I, Berger E, Harell A: Bone remodeling induced by physical stress is prostaglandin E_2-mediated. Biochem Biophys Acta 627:91, 1980.

Stanwyck TS, Fischer R, Pope M, Seligson D: Studies on prestress in bone. Biorheology 19:301, 1982.

Szilágyi M, Kovács AB, Pálfalvi I: Relationship between the ash content and microscopic hardness of swine bones. Acta Vet Acad Scient Hungaricae 28:455, 1980.

Townsend PR, Rose RM, Radin EL: Buckling studies of single human trabeculae. J Biomech 8:199, 1975.

Wainwright SA, Biggs WD, Currey JD, Gosline JM: Mechanical Design in Organisms. New York, Wiley, 1976.

Weaver JK: The microscopic hardness of bone. J Bone Joint Surg 48A:273, 1966.

Wood JL: Dynamic response of human cranial bone. J Biomech 4:1, 1971.

Wright TM, Hayes WC: Fracture mechanics parameters for compact bone—Effects of density and specimen thickness. J Biomech 10:419, 1977.

Yeh C-K, Rodan GA: Tensile forces enhance prostaglandin E synthesis in osteoblastic cells grown on collagen ribbons. Calc Tiss Int 36:S-67–71, 1984

Chapter 8

Mechanical Determinants of Skeletal Architecture:
Bone Modeling

H. M. Frost

In trying to understand his skeleton's biomechanics, man sought a predetermined master blueprint utilizing knowledge gained from making machines such as cranes. But mature skeletons develop in another way and only lately have we been able to perceive the mechanism. Both design and construction divide into two phases. First, in the uterus a miniature, preformed skeletal model arises that follows a predetermined master blueprint drawn from evolutionary experience accumulated since paleozoic times. Second, each tissue of that model is endowed with special action principles that determine its responses. As the model grows to adult size it is used with increasing vigor, and it continuously adapts its postnatal architecture to that usage. The engineering behind such a finished machine will remain an enigma until one knows its principles of action and the factors they respond to.

In the sixteenth century, both Vesalius and Galileo suspected the shape of bones might be related to the loads they supported. Nearly 300 years later Wolff proposed that bones could alter their internal architecture in response to changes in load.

Now known as Wolff's Law, that statement, while relevant, cannot predict the specific architectural change caused by a change in mechanical usage. Improved methods of investigation and better understanding of musculoskeletal tissues led to the formulation of principles that can predict skeletal architectural features from mechanical factors. This chapter presents concepts that are useful in understanding skeletal biomechanics and related clinical effects.

THE INTERMEDIARY ORGANIZATION OF THE SKELETON

General Remarks

Numerous organs, such as the kidney (Berliner, 1971), brain, liver, lung, pancreas, gonads, gut, thyroid, and skin, have an intermediary organization (IO). The basic scheme looks like this:

Organ Level
  Intermediary Organization
    Cell Level

All IOs contain the internal machinery that makes organs work, and specific principles of action govern the responses of that machinery to challenge. The skeleton also has an IO, and people such as Gegenbaur (1867), Koelliker (1873), and Virchow (1850) knew many of its histological signatures before 1870. However, it remained unsuspected as an operational entity before 1962–1966 (Frost, 1964, 1966), it took a further decade to perceive its larger design and, due in part to some controversy (Frost, 1981), it began to gain acceptance as such only after 1980 and its first brief descriptions appeared in 1982–1983 (Frost, 1982, 1983a, 1983b). Consequently the handful of investigators who studied it after 1966 learned much that others remained unaware of or misunderstood, and while spectacular advances have occurred in the clinical, cellu-

lar, and molecular–biologic aspects of skeletal pathophysiology, the skeletal IO still remains an enigma to most clinicians and investigators. Yet it directly underlies skeletal architectural adaptations to mechanical usage as well as many clinically apparent effects. The complex skeletal IO has at least three levels of organization and each has special multicellular entities that provide particular functions and other properties (Parfitt, 1979; Courpron, 1981; Jaworski, 1981; Courpron et al., 1982). The overall plan follows this scheme:

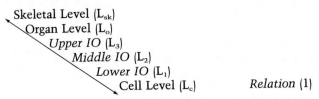

Skeletal Level (L_{sk})
  Organ Level (L_o)
    Upper IO (L_3)
      Middle IO (L_2)
        Lower IO (L_1)
          Cell Level (L_c)   *Relation* (1)

Each level in that organizational ladder has properties peculiar to its own operational entities and space–time domain, and each entity forms an organized association with lower levels. Many functions arising at a particular level lack exact analogs at other levels, either above or below. As examples, articulated skeletons can jump, as over fences, but isolated bones at the L_o-level, haversian systems at the L_2-level and cells at the L_c-level cannot jump; they merely go along for the ride. Or, only L_2-level entities produce osteoid seams; no lower or higher level ones can do so. Such transformations in functions and other properties accompany changes in organizational levels in all biological systems, not just in the skeleton (Mayr, 1961). Table 8–1 lists a few features peculiar to each IO domain.

TABLE 8-1. EXAMPLES OF SKELETAL PHENOMENA (ACCORDING TO LEVEL OF ORGANIZATION)

Biologic Domain	Structures	Activities	Morbid States
L_{sk}	Articulated skeleton	Motion Work	Limb alignment
			Short stature
L_o	Intact bone	Growth Modeling Remodeling	Osteopenia Osteosclerosis Fragility
L_3	Envelopes Spongiosa Epiphyses	Modeling Remodeling Growth in length	Thin cortex Sparse spongiosa Low turnover
L_2	Trabeculum	Osteoid formation	Osteomalacic bone
	Osteon	Resorption drift	Incompetent drift
	Circumferential lamellae	Formation drift	Rachitic cartilage
L_1	Hyaline cartilage Lamellar bone	Formation of new tissue	Mineralization defect Abnormal matrix
	Fibrous tissue	Resorption	Lack of resorption
L_c	Cell	Metabolism	Slowed metabolism

The Basic Common Plan (L_1 Level)

While middle IO level entities provide the direct origins of functions known as growth, modeling, remodeling, homeostasis, repair, and the regional acceleratory phenomenon (RAP) (Frost, 1981, 1983a) they all stem from associations of L_1-level units that have a common basic plan. In general terms, external factors regulate all IO units.

In more specific terms, all L_1-level units can undergo extrinsic regulation by systemic agents such as hormones, drugs, and mechanical effects, as well as by local factors in the unit's immediate surroundings. Circulating systemic agents reach most such units via their own capillaries. Continued skeletal health requires the continual production of new L_2-level units, although on different time scales for different tissues and kinds of units. No new unit can begin until its precursor cells produce new daughter cells, some of which differentiate into specialized cells such as osteoblasts, chondroblasts, or fibroblasts. Factors inherent in the unit organize those cells and their capillaries into microscopically recognizeable entities. Specialized cell activities then occur, perhaps to form intercellular materials such as bone, cartilage or fibrous tissue, or perhaps to resorb them. (Fig. 8–1). Intercellular materials become inherent parts of the units. If "X" signifies other important factors, not yet recognized, then a simple notation suggested elsewhere (Frost, 1983b) can encode the above phenomena. Let $f(S_k)$ signify "a function of the skeleton" or the unit's net effect or output; then:

$$f(S_k) = (S:L):\overrightarrow{(C:P:D:O:A:M:X)} \qquad \textit{Relation (2)}$$

The arrow above the right hand brackets means the activities within them occur in the given sequence and after characteristic time delays at each step. A colon means that the first factor acts on or interacts with the other factor. The following is a list of the above "factors" or "terms." They appear repeatedly in this chapter, and "X" will be understood in subsequent relations:

A = *Activities* of differentiated effector cells (exs: osteoclast, osteoblast)

C = *Capillary* supplying any multicellular IO unit

D = *Differentiation* or specialization of newly produced cells

L = *Local* or environmental source of regulation

M = *Materials*, solid, made by "A" (exs: lamellar bone, hyaline cartilage, ligament)

O = *Organization* of the various IO elements into a functional unit

P = *Precursor* cell proliferation that makes new daughter cells

S = *Systemic* or extrinsic source of regulation such as a hormone or mechanical load

X = The unnamed or unknown but still important to the IO

The common L_1-level plan can create elementary structures such as dentine or lamellar bone, elementary activities such as resorption or formation, and elementary morbid states such as poorly mineralized osteoid, defective collagen, or lethargic cell-level resorption. The plan

does so by varying the kinds, numbers, activities, and organization of its cells, and its intercellular materials, or by varying its pathways of regulation. As for those pathways, IO units have additional properties shown by the following "programmed" state equation:

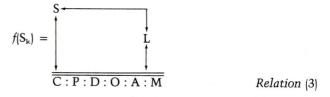

$$f(S_k) = \qquad \textit{Relation (3)}$$

External regulating agents, (S and L), will always lie above the double horizontal "bus" (as in a computer), while the intrinsic parts of the unit lie below. The bus represents the communication channel provided by the unit's intrinsic or intercellular space. In principle any term could communicate with or act directly on any other, and under some circumstances could bypass or change the sequences in Relation (2). If a message represented by "S" enters the system through another term in that relation, such as "M," then the latter becomes a gate that imposes its special properties on the unit's behavior. Such gating occurs widely in life.

Activities of the Intermediary Organization

Three activities of the IO are of concern: growth, remodeling, and modeling (Jee et al., 1963; Frost, 1972, 1973a, 1973b; Kimmel et al., 1981; Jee, 1983). Growth determines size, modeling the growing architecture, and remodeling the turnover and maintenance of the resulting skeletal structures. We will describe them next, noting that the clinical evidence of all three has its origins in L_2-level units that combine various L_1-level units.

Growth means those increases in cells and intercellular materials that increase the size of the organism, for example the embryo to the man. Growth occurs independently of the external architecture of tissues and organs, and its determinants and effects reveal two different classes of architectural phenomena. Cell proliferation causes growth, and directly so: no proliferation, then no growth. However, there are two different classes of proliferation. The growth-related class increases the total number of cells and the size of a tissue or organ. Growth hormone and somatomedin control it; it stops at maturity (Fig. 8–1C), and it enables most bone modeling. A second class of proliferation occurs throughout life, and it replaces previously made but exhausted or dead cells without changing an organ's size or its total number of cells (Fig. 8–1E). Throughout life it helps to maintain the functional competence of established tissues such as the blood, connective tissue, endothelia and epithelia, it enables wound and fracture healing and it also supports bone remodeling.

Inherent organizing properties, represented by the "0" term in Relation (2), act independently of extrinsic influences and determine the intrinsic architecture of the L_1 level elements of a tissue. These elements can be seen microscopically at about 1200 ×, as in Figure 8–1A

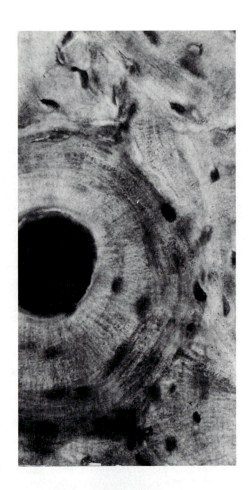

G

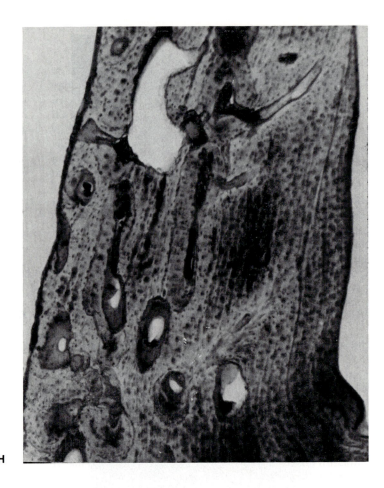

H

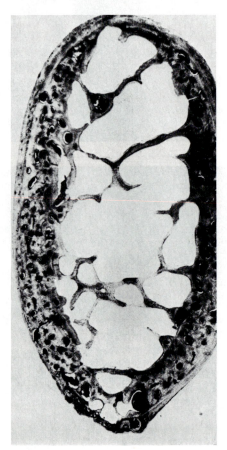

I

Figure 8-1. *(cont.)* **G,H,I.** More photomicrographs of undecalcified, basic fuchsin stained sections of human bone. **G.** Cross section of compacta at approx. 150× showing part of a secondary osteon surrounded by interstitial lamellae, both made of lamellar bone as in top row middle, but L_2-level "L" factors imposed different forms on them during their deposition. **H.** Cross section of fibular cortex of a boy with familial vitamin D resistant rickets, marrow to left, periosteum to the right, haversian canals lined with thick osteoid seams within. This L_3 domain structure associates both modeling and remodeling activities, the former representing drifts on the periosteal and cortical-endosteal envelopes, the latter appearing as packets of turnover on the haversian envelope. The section also illustrates two morbid states, one the L_2-domain-origin abnormally thick and slowly mineralizing osteoid seams, the other the L_c-domain-origin dark blurs of incompletely mineralized bone or halos around many osteocytes. About 30× (case referred by Dr. B. Frame). **I.** A rib at approx. 5× of a young woman who had active thyrotoxicosis. This represents a cross section through an L_{sk} domain structure, an organ.

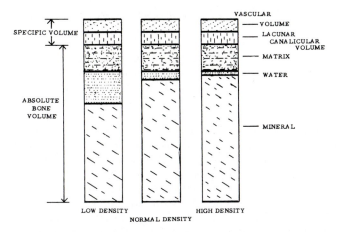

Figure 8-2. Excluding the marrow cavity, the bulk volume of lamellar bone sums several fractions, the organic, mineral, and fluid volumes or phases. The vascular spaces shown in Figure 8-1 G and H, plus the lacunae and canaliculae form one part of the fluid volume, and both combined equal about 9 percent of the total bone volume that is filled by cells and extracellular fluid. This volume fraction remains constant as young bone ages. The organic matrix occupies a second fraction, and the mineral deposits the remaining fraction. A volume of interstitial fluid lies within the matrix but outside the lacunae and canaliculae, and as the mineral deposits increase the interstitial water is displaced and decreases. Thus young, low density bone has a larger interstitial fluid volume than old, high density bone. The interstitial fluid is partly mobile so it can flow under pressure gradients caused by bone strain.

(Frost, 1963), in response to local stimuli that seem inherent in the woven bone itself (Frost, 1972). When deformed or strained, dry lamellar bone generates microvolt range piezoelectric potentials on its surfaces, and fresh wet bone develops millivolt range streaming potentials that derive from the flow of its fluid phase. Mineral deposits begin to appear in newly formed bone matrix about a week after its formation and take a year or more to become complete. In the process the mineral displaces equal volumes of water from the matrix without affecting the amount of matrix per unit volume of bone. Thus, young bone has less mineral and more water per unit volume than old bone so it is less stiff, but both have similar amounts of organic matrix. Lamellar bone also has a nerve supply in its vascular channels, endosteum and periosteum.

Bone Modeling

Modeling occurs primarily during growth (Weinmann and Sicher, 1955), and it is detectable grossly. The writer coined the term circa 1966 to distinguish the activity from growth and from remodeling (Frost, 1972, 1973b). Some earlier observers such as Lacroix (1951) and McLean and Urist (1960) suspected that modeling and remodeling differed but it required new investigative techniques and analytical insights to prove and explain it (Frost, 1969, 1978; Melsen and Mosekilde, 1981). Two different forms of bone modeling, micromodeling and macromodeling, may be distinguished by differing determinants and effects. In lamellar

bone, the former causes the preferred fiber orientation (in the 0.01 mm to 0.1 mm domain) of newly forming bone to parallel the local compression or tension strains. Its causes remain virtually unstudied but could represent smaller strains than those that control the macromodeling process. This chapter will say nothing further about micromodeling.

Macromodeling sculpts or models the visible architecture of growing bones, except for cartilage effects, including cross and longitudinal shapes, periosteal and marrow cavity diameters, and cortical thickness (Enlow, 1963; Rubin, 1964; Frost, 1973b). Modeling can correct post fracture deformities in children but not in adults, and it determines how much compacta a child accumulates (Enlow, 1963; Rubin, 1964). (Semimicroscopic analogs of modeling on trabeculae and on the haversian envelope, in adults as well as in children, do not concern this chapter but they do account for some of Wolff's anatomic observations.)

Two kinds of L_2-level entities cause bone modeling: the osteoclastic or resorption drift, and the osteoblastic or formation drift (Enlow, 1963; Frost, 1973b). During normal growth those drifts account for all bone surface alterations, except for chondral effects. While the cells causing growth and modeling of cartilage and fibrous tissue lie inside these tissues, the cells that model bone lie only on "free" surfaces, and these surfaces adjoin soft tissues. Figures 8-1 and 8-3 illustrate examples of that phenomenon. The difference may help explain some of the principles that govern the growth and modeling of bone, cartilage, teeth, and fibrous tissues.

The Resorption Drift. Organized groups of short-lived osteoclasts progressively plane away an affected bone surface, as in Figure 8-3, often in waves rather than continuously, particularly after infancy. A special capillary system supplies each resorption drift. Jaworski (1980), Jee (1977), Owen (1970), Simmons (1979), and Walker (1975) have shown that osteoclast precursor cells probably represent mononuclear cells circulating in the blood, themselves likely the daughters of progenitor cells in the marrow tissue at large rather than locally (Bonnucci, 1981; Tonna, 1981).

In L_2 space–time (i.e., over domains ≈ 0.1 mm, and a month) each resorption drift occurs alone, without accompanying or associated bone formation, but it must be initiated by precursor cell activity. The process includes a mechanical load applied to the bone resulting in deformation (strain), which creates a signal (see discussion of the Bone Modeling Signal, later in this chapter) that crosses the local environment at the bone's cortical–endosteal or periosteal surfaces to reach the cells in the drift unit. More concisely:

load → bone → strain → bone surface signal → precursor cells → rest of the IO unit → resorption drift.

So for mechanical as opposed to other mechanisms that control bone modeling, the bone itself becomes the

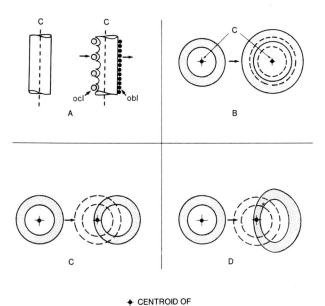

◆ CENTROID OF
ORIGINAL SECTION

Figure 8-3. A. Osteoclasts on the left of this diaphyseal segment erode the underlying surface, moving it in tissue space, to the right. Osteoblasts build up the surface on the right, moving it also to the right. When combined those two drifts move the entire bone to the right relative to the original center line or centroid (C). **B.** When periosteal formation drifts and endosteal resorption drifts distribute equally around the circumference of a cross section then it expands symmetrically without moving the centroid. **C.** But if the drifts occur only along one diameter of the cross section then the diaphysis moves as a unit in the same direction. **D.** Combining those two phenomena can enlarge the section, move it to the right and create noncircular cross sections.

primary gate, and the space between the bone and the cells on its surfaces acts as a secondary gate. Thereby those terms can impose their special properties on the response of the whole drift unit to the mechanical load. Parenthetically, differences in composition, cells, and organization of the varied skeletal materials (e.g., lamellar bone, tendon, hyaline cartilage, dentin) probably cause some of their different responses to identical mechanical factors.

The Formation Drift. Organized groups of short-lived osteoblasts progressively build up an affected bone surface with accumulating thicknesses of new bone, named circumferential lamellae, as in Figure 8–3, and also often in waves, each of which deposits a smooth arrest line, as in Figure 8–4 (Weinmann and Sicher, 1955; Putschar, 1960). A capillary system supplies each formation drift and its osteoblasts derive from local precursor cell division as noted by Owen (1970), Jee and Kimmel (1977), and Tonna (1981).

In L_2 space-time each formation drift occurs alone without any associated resorption, but it responds to the same mechanical regulation as the resorption drift. (No systematic studies of L_1-domain drift phenomena have been published, but those phenomena may prove rather

complex.) Its "A" cells (osteoblasts) make new intercellular bone matrix.

Drift Systems. At the organ level, drifts occur in organized collections on the periosteal and cortical–endosteal surfaces of an intact bone such as a femur or a radius, and the surface drift patterns prove highly stereotyped among all normal individuals of a given species (Enlow, 1963). While drifts determine the amount of compacta in a given bone by the mechanisms shown in Figure 8–3, the amount of spongiosa depends primarily on longitudinal growth mechanisms, not on cortical bone modeling (Enlow, 1963).

Lamellar bone modeling occurs most rapidly during infancy, slows in the adolescent, and stops for practical purposes at skeletal maturity (Frost, 1973b), so modeling depends upon the growth-related class of cellular proliferation (whereas micromodeling, a maintenance function, can occur throughout life). If precursor cell activity stops, then after about two weeks in a rat and a month in a child, all modeling will stop too. Modeling occurs in all growing vertebrates. It can reactivate in adults in some diseases, for example acromegaly, Paget's disease of bone, Ribbing's disease, chronic osteomyelitis, and malunion (Jaffe, 1972; Aegerter, 1975; Anderson, 1977). Its activity in adults never approaches that seen during growth, especially during infancy. As an aside, histologic evidence reveals two types of formation drifts, according to the magnitude of the activating stimulus. The physiologic stimuli of concern here typically cause new circumferential lamellae to deposit on periosteal and cortical endosteal surfaces, as in Figures 8–3 and 8–4, but pathologically large stimuli can evoke woven bone deposition that is eventually replaced by lamellar bone via the bone remodeling mechanism. Little is known about the matter at present.

In a child, correction of a typical long bone malunion during subsequent growth combines the effects of two kinds of skeletal modeling, described by Karaharju et al. (1976). Bone modeling tends to restore a normal configuration to the diaphysis and metaphysis, while chondral modeling tends to restore normal alignment and direction of growth of the regional epiphyseal plates, epiphyses, and articular cartilage. Each form of modeling follows different action principles. We consider those that govern bone modeling next, in the process changing the focus of attention from what constitute the intraskeletal mechanisms of present concern, to the principles of action that govern why and how they respond and affect organ and skeletal level structure.

MECHANICAL DETERMINANTS OF LAMELLAR BONE MODELING

Background
Since Wolff's time, two assumptions about the mechanical determinants of bone modeling have become generally accepted (Frost, 1983). First, the mechanical loads applied to a growing bone can affect its subsequent architecture. Second, the architectural change produced by a change in bone loading usually improves the bone's ability to carry

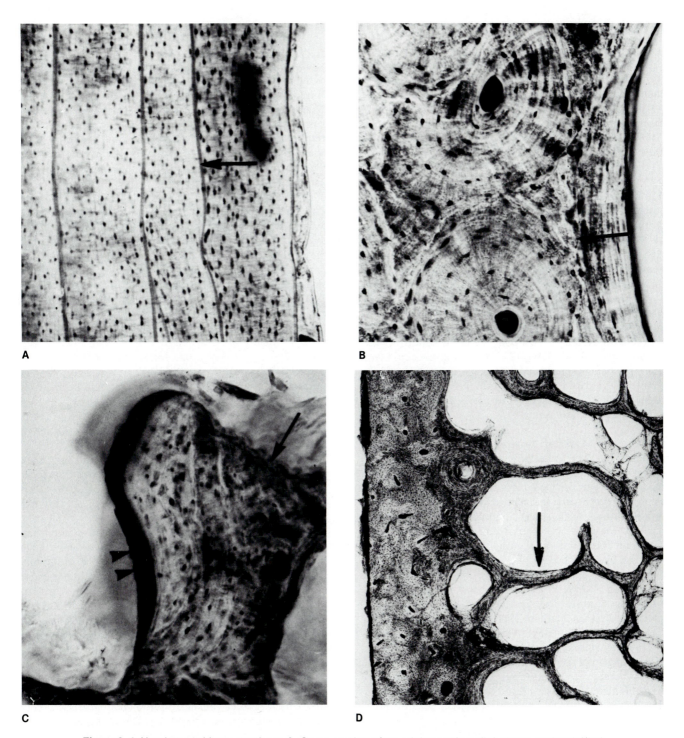

Figure 8-4. Hand-ground bone sections. **A.** Cross section of an adolescent's radial cortex, undecalcified, basic fuchsin, periosteum to right. The three dark, smooth vertical bands are special cement lines, named arrest lines, where a new formation drift arose on the circumferential lamellae deposited by an earlier, completed drift. Thus four separate formation drifts have left a record or signature of their birth, activity, and passing. Direction of surface motion caused by those drifts: to the right. The dark spots are osteocytes (approx. 50×.) **B.** Cross section, (approx. about 150×) cortical-endosteal surface of adult human rib, marrow cavity to the right, basic fuchsin stained. Note the scalloped contours of the cement lines (reversal lines) bordering the bone adjoining the marrow space. These represent signatures of previous remodeling (turnover) phenomena, and they have removed all traces of the original circumferential lamellae that once formed this part of the compacta, for before it was remodelled it looked like the section to the left. **C.** An ARF remodeling process on a trabeculum from human spongiosa, with the R phase above (long arrow), and the F phase to the left (short arrows). Undecalcified, basic fuchsin (approx. 300×). **D.** Cross section of adult human femoral metaphysis, periosteum to left, marrow and spongiosa to the right. L_3-level modeling phenomena have created the naked eye architectural features of both compacta and spongiosa from the same L_1-domain "bricks" or building material, lamellar bone.

the new loads, so the architectural adaptations evoked by loads that threaten structural competence reduce rather than accentuate that threat.

Until recently, the specific principles that underlie those assumptions remained elusive. Enlow (1963), Evans (1957), Putschar (1960), and Weinmann and Sicher (1955) have summarized some of the ideas considered in the past: (1) direct genetic control of each structural feature; (2) direct control of local growth by juxtaosseous tissues; (3) stimulation of formation by compressive stress and resorption by tensile stress; and (4) when applied to teeth, stimulation of resorption by compression and formation by tension. Epker (1965, 1982), Frost (1973b), and Lanyon (1982) have shown that these principles do not apply universally, although some of them have merit in special situations.

Provisional Bone Modeling Laws

The author has proposed nine axioms that can predict certain specific responses of a bone's architecture to its mechanical usage (Frost, 1964, 1973, 1983) and one could term them provisional bone modeling laws. They work only as a collective entity for if one examines the play of any one of them without considering the others, some apparent inconsistencies can appear.

The Growth–Modeling Axiom. As described earlier, bone modeling sculpts lamellar bone architecture primarily during growth (chondral effects excepted). To influence modeling, the underlying drifts, including their initiation, kind, location, surface extent, speed, and ultimate magnitude (Frost 1973b), must be controlled. Modeling does not sum the activities of unorganized effector ("A") cells alone, for modeling stops without the continual backup provided by the other terms in Relation (2).

The Strain Axiom. Mechanically controlled bone modeling relates more directly to strain than to the corresponding stresses (Lanyon, 1966; Liskova, 1971; Pauwels, 1973; Frost, 1973b, 1983). A load on any structure produces a deformation (strain), not only of its gross dimensions, but also of the intermolecular bonds in the material. Those bonds resist deformation with an elastic force termed stress. When the strain becomes constant or fixed, the internal stresses equal but oppose the external load. Thus *strain* means any deformation, *stress* the resisting internal force, and a *load* the external force that causes both (Popov, 1952; Jensen and Chenoweth, 1975). Strain can be measured directly, but stress must be inferred.

Materials like steel or glass retain a reasonably constant stress–strain proportionality over their safe loading ranges and over time so one can define their useful strength as either a strain or a stress. In a structure, one can predict stress more easily than strain because Young's modulus (stiffness) and viscoelastic properties (Jensen and Chenoweth, 1975) must be considered in order to predict strain. Accordingly, engineers choose to focus on stress rather than strain, and that habit carries over to most analyses of bone mechanics. Indeed, some analysts thought the distinction trivial. But like other living, growing struc-

tural materials such as wood, chitin, tendon and cartilage, living bone converts strain into signals that control modeling (Fukada, 1957; Frost, 1973b, 1983; Eriksson, 1974; Chakkalakal, 1981), whereas the associated stresses relate indirectly and variably to those strains and signals. For example, new bone is less mineralized and thus more compliant than old bone, so it deforms (strains) more under the same load (and stress), and it models more readily too (Frost, 1973b; Curry et al., 1975; Burstein et al., 1976).

The Minimum Effective Strain (MES). A negative feedback controls strain, keeping it within the limits needed to maintain the integrity or stability of the system, and the system's design sets those limits. Strain beyond those limits generates an error signal that makes the system change itself in a way that reduces both the error and its signal. One could diagram those relationships thus:

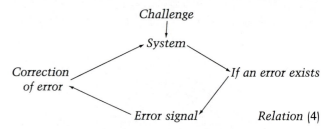

$$\text{Relation (4)}$$

All feedback systems require some minimum error signal to make them respond. Smaller signals represent trivia that do not threaten their integrity (Frost, 1983). This principle applies to the factors that control all soft and hard tissue modeling.

For bone, tension or compression strains smaller than some minimum effective strain (MES) do not evoke adaptive bone modeling, but larger strains do. The MES probably represents a range, below which strains do not cause modeling, above which they regularly do, and in between which they do increasingly. Currently, in vivo strain data place the lower MES limit at about 0.0008 unit tension or compression strain (or 800 microstrain), and its upper limit at about 0.002 unit strain (or 2000 microstrain). Accordingly, loads causing less strain than the MES represent trivial loads, while all larger loads are nontrivial.

Figure 8–5 shows a tentative graph of those phenomena, which predict that adaptive modeling arises where and when bone strains exceed the MES (qualified of course by the other modeling axioms). During normal usage strain in a biomechanically adapted bone seldom exceeds the lower MES limit. The MES property itself does not specify the nature of that adaptive modeling but other axioms do.

The Dynamic Strain Axiom. Bone modeling responds to dynamic or changing strain, not to constant strain, at least in any presently obvious way (Frost, 1973b, 1982).

The Strain–Averaging Axiom. The modeling system averages repeated nontrivial strains to produce an architecture that fits a history of its usage rather than occasional large strains (Frost, 1973b, 1982). How that averaging occurs is unknown but stochastic notions seem reasonable

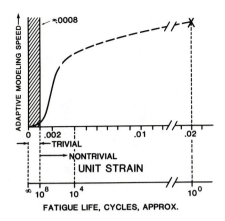

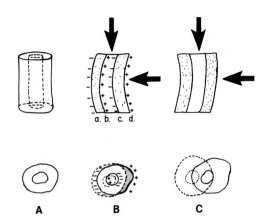

Figure 8-5. This graph shows the tentative snape of the MES curve according to information available in 1984. Dynamic, repeated strains are assumed and increase to the right while the amount of modeling they evoke increases on the vertical axis. The shaded vertical bar represents strains below the MES, and thus trivial. Between 0.0008 and 0.002 unit strain, modeling responds and seems to increase sharply, and then less sharply above that. Bone breaks at about .025 unit strain. It appears that the subMES strain range represents a small fraction of the total strain at which bone breaks under a single load.

Figure 8-6. A. An unstrained diaphseal segment or free body. **B.** It now carries two load components, as in life: a vertical uniaxial compression end-load, and a side or direct flexural load causing flexure with the concavity pointing toward the right (surfaces b and d). The + signs indicate formation drifts and the − signs resorption drifts. The drift pattern moves the diaphysis towards the reader's right (lower middle insert), to create the longitudinal shape shown in C. **C.** The end-load now generates a cantilever-origin flexure that opposes the direct flexural load.

(Frost, 1964). The relative roles and possible interactions of strain rate, frequency, magnitude, and range in this system also remain unknown, but investigators have begun to study them (Lanyon, 1982).

The Flexure–Drift Axiom. Whether uniaxial strains can control bone modeling still remains unclear but substantial evidence indicates that dynamic flexure does (Frost, 1982). That perception formed the first breakthrough in understanding how bone modeling responds to mechanical usage (Frost, 1964). In effect, repeated, nontrivial flexural strains evoke drifts that move all affected bone surfaces in the concave-tending direction, as shown in Figure 8–6. The converse applies to convex-tending flexure. Accordingly, dynamic flexure causes concave-tending bone surfaces to add bone, and convex-tending surfaces to erode. The surface distribution of flexural strains determines the type and location of drifts, and, therefore, the bone's final cross sectional and longitudinal shape.

The flexure–drift response of growing bone to compression end-loads plus side-loads, causes the bone to adopt a shape that neutralizes or limits excessive flexure, including buckling. This response is called the "flexural neutralization" (Frost, 1964) mechanism (Fig. 8–7). Flexural neutralization also limits the shearing strains and stresses that accompany flexure. One can minimize flexural strain by enlarging the cross section, by reshaping the diaphysis, or by reducing or reorienting loads or moments, or by a combination.

Drift-Barriers. Drifts do not arise on any bone surface covered by cartilage (Frost, 1973b, 1982). Such surfaces obey chondral modeling laws. They include articular cartilage, epiphyseal and apophyseal plates, and the cartilage

layer interposed between bone and attachments of tendon, ligament, or fascia. Bone beneath a cartilage covering always copies the separately controlled chondral contour. The bone-drift–barrier property of cartilage makes it a closed gate that blocks bone-strain–generated stimuli from local bone modeling units. Other drift barriers include a dead bone surface, a bone surface covered by dead soft tis-

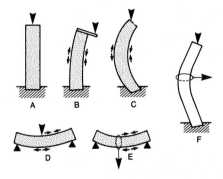

Figure 8-7. Loading and flexural terminology. **A.** A uniaxial compression end-load causes equal strains and stresses at all points along the column. **B.** An eccentric load generates a cantilever-origin flexure. **C.** The cantilever-origin flexure accentuates the original curvature. Both tend to make the column buckle under end-loads. In both **B** and **C**, the compression strain and stress on the concave-tending surface (right) exceeds any tension strain on the convex-tending surface (left). **D.** A direct flexural load on the beam also causes flexure. **E.** A tension load on the beam produces the same response as a compression load. **F.** The analogous real-life situation. A large end load on a curved column accentuates its curve by the cantilever effect, while another direct side load opposes that accentuation, thereby reducing or limiting the flexural moments and strains. Note that F could represent a longitudinal section of one cortex of a bone, or a whole bone.

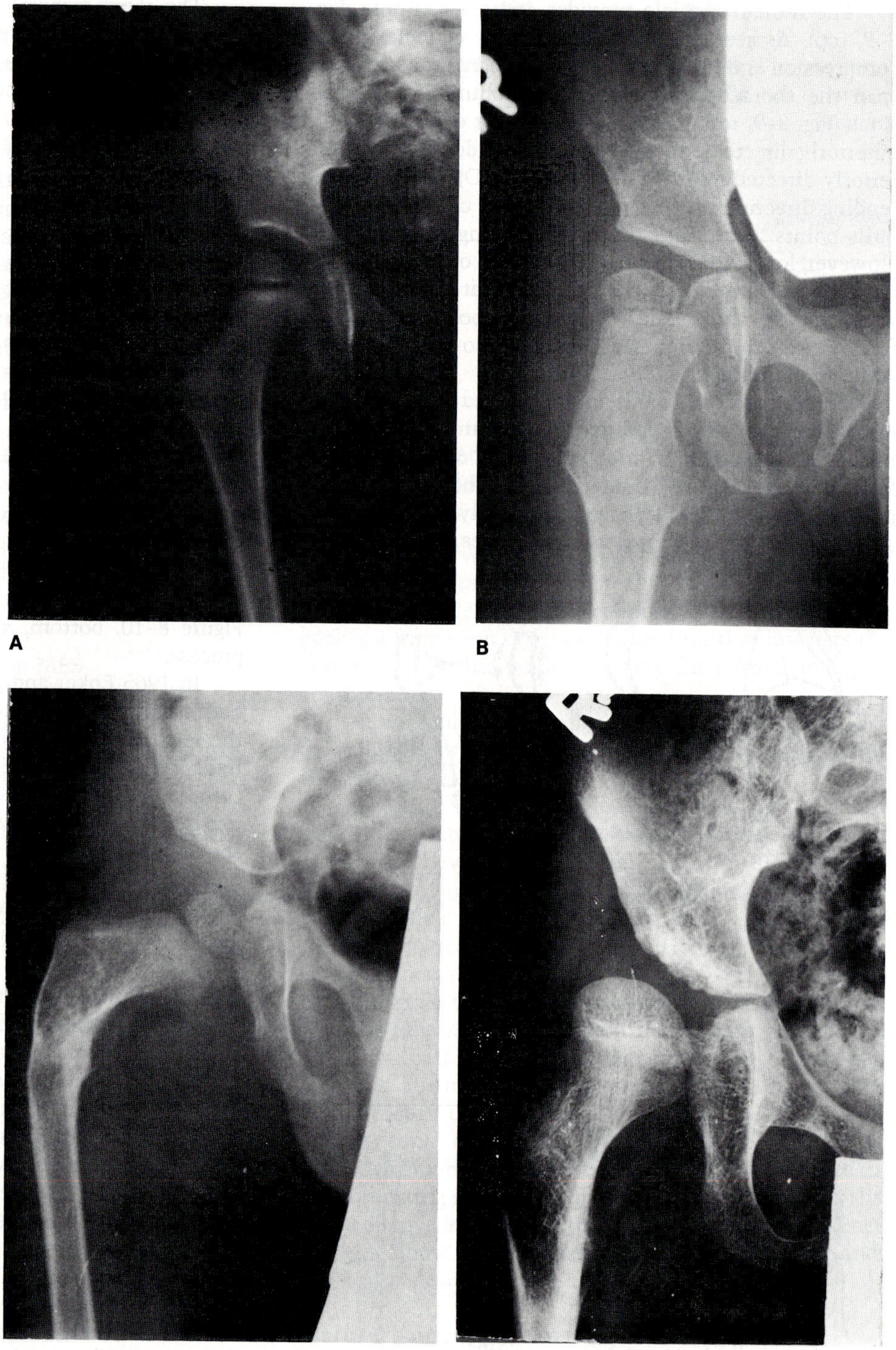

Figure 8-10. A. AP x-ray of the hip of a child with muscular dystrophy. A mild coxa valga exists (compare to Fig. 8-11A), associated with small outside diameters of the neck and femoral shaft, thin cortices and a horizontal alignment of the capital epiphyseal plate. **B.** Coxa valga in a young patient with spasticity; femoral torsion also exists but does not change the argument in the text. **C.** Coxa vara after osteotomy of the femur in a patient with amyotonia congenita. The load resultant across this hip represented mostly body weight that aligned purely vertically, resulting in subluxation. The purpose of the osteotomy was to shorten the bone, to tilt the pelvis in order to better cover the head, to reduce vertical muscle pull, and to increase the resting length of the short external rotators. The varus position created abnormal flexure during walking (Fig. 8-9, lower half). **D.** Three years later the original shape has been restored, due in part to bone modeling during subsequent growth, and in part to chondral modeling. The medial cortex has become much thicker than the lateral.

medial cortex the periosteal formation drift must exceed any endosteal resorption drift. This phenomenon occurs regularly in malunions (Fig. 8-10D).

Modeling of Young or Recently Fractured Bone

As a material, bone has about 40 percent greater compliance in children than in adults, according to Currey and Butler (1975). The metaphyseal compacta has greater compliance than the diaphyseal compacta, and a recently frac-tured bone has greater compliance than an unfractured bone. In each of those situations the more recently deposited or more rapidly turning over bone has more water and less mineral, and thus greater compliance because the mineral content provides most of a bone's mechanical stiffness. Under equal unit loads and unit stresses, therefore, such bone strains more, so it should model more readily, as in fact it does. This at least partly explains the more rapid modeling in infants, and in recently malunited bones, as well as the lack of effective modeling in the stiffer bone of normal adults. An increased sensitivity of children's cells to various stimuli, when compared to adults, may also play a role, as well as the potentiating effects of the regional acceleratory phenomenon (RAP) evoked by most fractures (see Discussion section, later in this chapter), plus other factors not mentioned.

Neuromotor Effects

In Wolff's and Koch's times most analysts believed the major loads on bones came from body weight. They were also stress-oriented rather than strain-oriented, and lacking insight into skeletal dynamics, they tended to look for predetermined master blueprints of skeletal architecture. Consequently, they studied the architecture of mature bone and considered only the stresses generated by body weight alone. More realistic analyses of in vivo loading, begun by M. Janssen in 1920 and pursued by Vernon Inman and his associates in the 1940s (Inman, 1947), revealed that even in weight bearing bones and their associated joints muscle forces produce the largest loads which, during strenuous activities, can exceed body weight more than five-fold, and regularly more than two-fold. In fact, in normal people the maximum strains generated in the femur by simply standing are less than a third of the MES (Koch, 1917). Assuming that mechanical control of growing bone architecture depends in part on dynamic

bone strain, and that greater strains evoke greater modeling, then muscle forces must influence modeling more than body weight alone.

Accordingly, bone architecture should be closely related to the demands of muscle anatomy and nontrivial usage (Frost, 1973b). "Muscle anatomy" includes the lines of action of muscles, their points of attachment to bones, and the nature of those attachments, whether concentrated at a tendon attachment or diffusely spread over a broad surface, as by the fleshy origins of the vasti, brachialis, iliacus and scapular muscles. "Muscle Usage" includes strength plus muscle coordination (which affects the loads carried by bones), so the central nervous system also affects growing bone architecture (Frost, 1972, 1973b, 1982). Several examples of neuromotor effects on bone modeling and architecture during growth follow.

Coxa Valga. The time-averaged resultant of loads transferred across a normal hip parallels the major trabecular orientation within the femoral neck and head, forming a line between the calcar femorale and the third lumbar vertebra, as in Figure 8–11, left. That resultant sums two components: a major vertical component that sums body weight plus vertical adductor, hamstring, iliopsoas and abductor muscle forces, and a medially directed minor horizontal component that sums transverse obturator, hip abductor, and proximal adductor muscle forces. (Most ex-

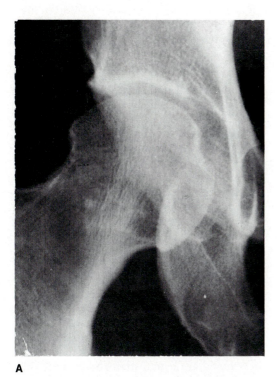

A

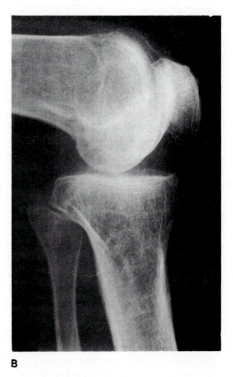

B

Figure 8–11. A. AP x-ray of a normal adult hip, showing the thick calcar and inferior neck, and the oblique group of vertical trabeculae that parallel the time-averaged load resultant across the hip joint and proximal femur. **B.** Lateral x-ray of the knee of an adult who developed postpolio hamstring paralysis in childhood but retained good quadriceps power. The change in muscle force caused the anterior concavity of the upper tibia. (See text discussion).

tant analyses of this situation omitted the nevertheless important adductor and obturator loads.) The normal neck–shaft angle and the thick femoral calcar represent responses to that resultant by two modeling modalities: bone modeling on the inferior–medial neck and calcar, and chondral modeling on the cartilage-covered capital epiphyseal plate, superior neck, and greater trochanter.

If the vertical component should increase relative to the horizontal component, then a normal neck–shaft angle represents a flexural error and the exaggerated loads will cause medially facing concave-tending flexure in the inferior femoral neck and calcar, as in the femoral diaphysis in Figure 8–9. During growth this can evoke formation drifts on the periosteal surface of the calcar and inferior neck, and resorption drifts on their cortical-endosteal surfaces, a combination that moves the neck and calcar medially relative to the femoral head to produce a coxa valga, as in Figure 8–10.

The loading imbalance described above occurs most often in two different clinical circumstances, the paretic and the spastic.

In the paretic hip that develops early in life, as in early-onset muscular dystrophy or poliomyelitis, the vertical load due to body weight does not change but all muscle forces decrease, including the medial component, so the resultant force orients more vertically and a coxa valga develops, accompanied by a decrease in cortical thickness and a decrease in the outside diameter of the calcar and femoral neck (Fig. 8–10, top left). In contrast, when paresis develops near the end of growth the bone is less compliant, so the strain produced by similar loads decreases. In that case the neck–shaft angle will not change, because mechanically induced architectural adaptations occur only when typical peak strains equal or exceed the MES.

In the spastic hip the central nervous system disorder alters the pattern of muscle contraction. This causes a weakened horizontal component with a normal or even accentuated vertical component. The total loads on the hip may approximate normal but again their resultant aligns more vertically. A coxa valga arises but now the thickness of the calcar and the outside diameter of the femoral neck remain normal (Fig. 8–10, top right).

The Paralyzed Hamstrings. Figure 8–10, right, shows a lateral knee x-ray of a man who developed a postpolio hamstring paralysis during childhood but retained good quadriceps function. During the stance and thrust phases of walking both hamstrings and quadriceps normally contract, so their direct flexural components on the upper tibia tend to neutralize or cancel out. But with paralyzed hamstrings, the quadriceps cause unneutralized, anteriorly facing, convex-tending flexure of the proximal tibia (exactly the same as a posteriorly facing, concave-tending flexure). The flexure-drift axiom requires such a cortex to drift posteriorly until the added cantilever-origin flexural force caused by the vertical load on the now inwaisted cortex becomes large enough to neutralize the anteriorly directed component of quadriceps pull via the patellar ligament.

Predictably, the opposite configuration can occur when quadriceps paralysis occurs early in life, but the hamstrings remain.

To repeat, such structural adaptations do not occur when the altered neuromotor function arises near or after maturity, partly because the growth-related precursor cell proliferation no longer occurs, partly because the material of adult bone becomes stiffer than that of a child so it strains less under equal loads, partly because the abnormally patterned loads usually are too small to cause strains equal to or above the MES, and possibly for other reasons too.

Total Paralysis from Birth. The lower limbs of a child paralyzed below the T 12 level by a myelomeningocele provide a natural experiment for bone growth and development in the absence of nontrivial loads. In Figure 8–12, left, the normal "S" shaped curve of the tibia is absent, and the diameter of the diaphysis is reduced. This child did walk in braces so the tibia carried some uniaxial loads during growth. The architectural features indicate that other determinants of bone architecture exist beyond those described in this chapter. These determinants include an inherently determined plus hormonally controlled bone growth, modified by effects of the local juxtaosseous tissues, including cartilage, marrow, muscle and periosteum.

DISCUSSION

A Crane Analogy

This analogy can clarify some features of the foregoing material. Thus:

A hypothetical builder had to construct a large and complex articulated crane so he scaled up an old design of a smaller crane, copying its layout of girders, bearings, guy wires and ropes. Here we consider the girders, which he made in tubular form but in ignorance of the actual loads they would carry during the crane's intended use. Accordingly, he did not know how large to make them or how to shape them. However, he knew their material would fail in fatigue if repeatedly loaded beyond 5 percent of its ultimate strain, and that the material would gradually work harden (become stiffer) with use. He also had a plethora of strain guages and workmen, and equipment to add or remove material at any part of any girder, and plenty of time.

So he constructed the crane with slender girders and covered their inner and outer surfaces with strain guages monitored by workmen instructed to add new material wherever concave-tending flexural strains exceeded the 5 percent limit, and to remove material wherever convex-tending flexural strains exceeded that limit. He then tested the crane, at first with small loads and simple tasks, gradually progressing to the intensive usage required by the purchaser. At the completion of testing he laid off the workmen, disconnected the monitoring system, and turned the crane over to the buyer.

257

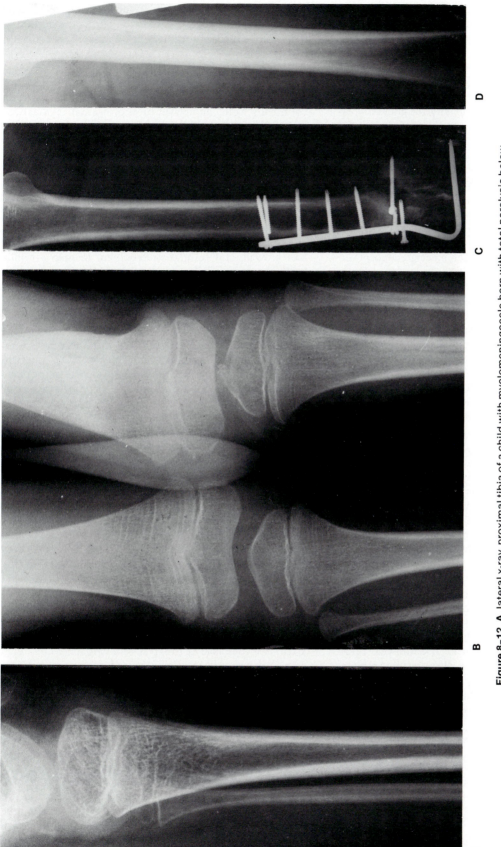

Figure 8–12. A. lateral x-ray, proximal tibia of a child with myelomeningocele born with total paralysis below the hips. The patient did some walking in braces. The normal overall curves of the tibia are absent, and both the tibia and fibula have nearly circular cross sections. **B.** Multiple transverse arrest lines due to earlier abuse of vitamin preparations are present in the distal femoral metaphysis on the reader's left. A recently healed fracture of the other femur evoked a concomitant RAP, and the resulting increase in local bone turnover eradicated all radiographic evidence of the transverse arrest lines. **C** and **D.** The femur on the reader's left sustained a supracondylar fracture that remains ununited in spite of several operations. The associated RAP has expanded both the periosteal and endosteal diameters and thinned the cortex, thereby also reducing radiographic bone density.

Given those game rules, the shape and strength of each girder would fit its major loads and tasks perfectly, but not its minor ones, and the crane would provide a satisfactory service life.

Substitute lamellar bone for girders, the fetal skeletal for the older and smaller design, aging for work hardening, the strain-induced signals for strain guages, the MES for the 5 percent limit, growth and activity for gradually escalating usage, bone drifts for the work force and equipment, and skeletal maturity for laying off the workmen. And there is the essence of modeling in growing human bones. Clearly, a laboratory analysis of such a crane could show a meaningful fit between its loads, functions, shapes, and strengths only for major loads, only for some time-averaged history of its typical usage rather than for some momentary act, and only if the flexural axiom was taken into account.*

One word can characterize such a design concept: *elegant.*

Sigma for Modeling

All biologic systems from macromolecules to societies have "natural" time periods or lead times that define how long their transient responses to a challenge will last, and when their steady state responses will appear. Transients always arise first and steady states afterwards. For bone remodeling that lead time has become known as sigma (Frost, 1973a,c). Modeling also has that property, for after a major change in loading the modeling system needs time to respond [time represented by the horizontal arrow in Relation (2)]. That period increases during growth from a month or less in an infant to longer than the remaining life span by age 15 to 18 years. Hence an infant can completely correct a major bone deformity during subsequent growth but a 12 or 15-year-old cannot, so a fracture deformity permissible in the former requires intervention in the latter. Experimental studies must account for the real time value of this property of modeling.

The Relative Modeling Rate

In part the above differences reflect age-related differences in the absolute speeds (i.e., in mm/year) at which tissues can model. Here the infant excels. But in part that difference pertains to the relative modeling rate, for example the time an absolute diaphyseal drift of 4 mm/year takes to move the bone surfaces the full diameter of the bone. Because bone diameter increases during growth, a 4 mm drift is a greater fraction of an infant's bone diameter than an adolescent's. Consequently, the relative modeling rate declines steadily during growth, and the potential total rate falls steeply in adolescence as the potential absolute rate also declines.

Thus, bone modeling is a game of active growth played by the young. It can correct a deformity or achieve a desired structural change only if sufficient modeling time remains before skeletal maturation closes the curtain on that stage. One cannot study it effectively in adult animals.

The Regional Acceleratory Phenomenon (RAP)

First described in 1979 (Frost, 1979, 1981), this phenomenon constitutes an acceleration of normal regional soft and hard tissue vital processes in response to major noxious regional stimuli. Those stimuli include trauma, particularly fractures and surgical procedures that strip, osteotomize or drill holes in bone, as well as burns, infections, crushing injuries, and acute paralyses. The greater the stimulus the greater the RAP. The accelerated processes include both primary and secondary bone healing (Schenk, 1978), fibrous tissue, bone and cartilage growth and modeling, bone remodeling (see Figure 8–12, middle), hair growth, and cellular metabolism. In man a typical RAP, say after a Colles' fracture, lasts 3 to 5 months but after major trauma or paralysis it can persist over 2 years. A RAP usually dominates other influences on those processes, including endocrine, nutritional, and mechanical stimuli.

The RAP normally evoked by a fracture also accelerates its healing, making it a desirable "SOS" phenomenon. An ineffective RAP following fracture can cause a delayed union or nonunion in spite of proper treatment. In that regard, all currently successful treatments of nonunions evoke a new RAP (Schenk, 1978; Takahashi, 1982). A RAP can increase regional longitudinal bone growth, for example, after long bone fractures, sudden paralysis, juvenile rheumatoid arthritis (Kelley et al., 1981), or in the presence of a juxtaarticular osteoid osteoma. A RAP can accelerate corrective modeling of bony malunions in children and it can also accelerate the increase in periosteal diameter, especially in children, but also in adults, (Fig. 8–12, right). Comparison of a previously fractured bone to the contralateral unfractured bone reveals larger periosteal and endosteal diameters in the fractured bone. The more protracted the healing or the more numerous the operations that led to union, the greater the final difference.

RAP effects have perturbed most experimental animal studies of mechanical effects on the growth and modeling of skeletal tissues. Many of the changes currently attributed to disuse or to stress-relieving hardware, relate at least in part to RAP effects instead, as some recent studies have shown (Todd et al., 1972; High et al., 1981a,b; Churches and Howlett, 1982).

The Bone Modeling Signal: A Hypothesis

Numerous facts suggest how bone can amplify strain and then use it to control the biologic modeling processes.

Before the work of Fukada and Yasuda (1957) no known mechanism could transduce a mechanical load on a bone into a biologic message that could control modeling. Their work suggested that the microvolt-range piezoelectric signals arising on dry bone strained in flexure might constitute that signal (Becker, 1964). But Chakkalakal and Johnson (1981) and Eriksson (1974) found that strained, fresh, wet bone develops millivolt-range stream-

---

*There lies part of the reason that analyses of stress–strength distributions in various human bones under unrealistic loads have produced a lot of data but, at least so far, no predictive design-meaningful principles of action for bone architecture.

ing potentials and other effects from the flow of electrolyte solution in its fluid space. If bone modeling responds to an electrical voltage, it should obey the signal produced by streaming potentials, for it is much larger than the piezoelectric signal.

In that respect, the present modeling laws imply certain properties of any signal that controls modeling in response to mechanical usage (Frost, 1980). First, the signal should arise if, when, and where supraMES strain occurs. Second, under flexure it should have two properties or signs, one on concave-tending surfaces that selects formation drifts, the other on convex-tending surfaces that selects resorption drifts. Third, it should arise during changing rather than constant strain; and fourth, greater strains should evoke larger signals.

The interstitial fluid in bone can flow under internal pressure gradients via canaliculae, lacunae, and vascular channels but the mineralized matrix cannot. A momentary 0.002 unit compression strain decreases a bone's bulk volume by approximately 0.2 percent (we ignore Poisson's ratio here), and it can create a pressure in the bone of 300 to 800 psi that makes its interstitial electrolyte solution flow. Normally the interstitial fluid occupies less than 3 percent of the bulk bone volume and most bulk compression should occur in the spaces that contain the fluid, so its fractional volume change will be 15 to 30 times larger than the fractional volume change of the bulk bone, in effect producing mechanical strain amplification. The flow of electrolyte through very small spaces produces a voltage named a streaming potential (Eriksson, 1974). The presence of an electrical charge on the walls of those spaces would momentarily change the proportions of anions and cations in the fluid emerging from the bone. Both effects, the streaming potentials and the ionic imbalance, would transduce bulk strain into phenomena that cells can readily respond to. Changing strain can cause that flow but a fixed strain cannot. Furthermore, flexural strain gradients within the bone cause corresponding internal pressure gradients that would force flow in one direction relative to concave-tending flexure, so the direction of flow should match the direction of flexure. Because recently formed bone is more compliant and because it has a larger interstitial fluid volume than old bone, equal unit loads and stresses would produce larger strains, larger flows, and thus larger signals in young compared to old bone.

Nonmechanical Regulation of Bone Modeling

Bone modeling determines the shape of a bone, but it primarily affects compacta rather than spongiosa. Even so, it can create a bone of inappropriate configuration, and with too little or too much compacta. The modeling process primarily fits the bony skeleton to its mechanical usage, including architectural adaptations to muscles and to longitudinal bone growth, whether or not growth is accelerated or retarded. The forces generated during normal activity have the greatest effect on bone modeling, while growth of bone and of muscle has a less direct secondary effect.

Experimental studies and naturally occurring diseases provide information on the influence of nonmechanical factors. When a genetic error in its cells impairs the functions of the IO an IO-intrinsic disease arises (Fig. 8–13). Although the resulting bony architecture may not adversely affect function, as in osteopoikilosis, it may become inappropriate for the demands on it, as in osteogenesis imperfecta (Frost, 1981), and even if external regulation is normal. When intrinsic function of the IO remains normal but its extrinsic regulation malfunctions, an IO-extrinsic disease results, for an intrinsically normal IO faithfully follows even flawed extrinsic instructions. An infrequent but diverse third disease category represents combinations of the first two. Some IO-intrinsic diseases are osteogenesis imperfecta, pycnodysostosis, osteopetrosis, hyperphosphatasia, and Paget's disease. IO-extrinsic diseases include all acquired childhood osteopenias—biliary stenosis, Gaucher's, malnutrition, juvenile rheumatoid arthritis, corticosteroid-induced, Turner's; myopathies, paralyses; Marfan's Syndrome; Caffey's disease; femoral and tibial torsions; coxa valga; Ehrenfried's disease; fluorosis; lead intoxication; and acromegaly.

There is little evidence that the pediatric endocrinopathies; metabolic, nutritional, and biochemical disorders; or systemic infections and intoxications have major direct effects on bone modeling. For instance, the bones of a child with advanced muscular dystrophy or with a myelomeningocele appear markedly osteopenic relative to the bones of healthy children of comparable age and stature, but biomechanically they are appropriate for a level of activity that has been profoundly reduced by paralysed muscles during growth.

In addition, the osteopenia seen in biliary stenosis probably reflects the reduced physical activities of the sick child, more than a direct nutritional effect on bone modeling.

Further Architectural Determinants

While excessive flexure is one determinant of bone architecture, it fails to explain the architecture of the trivially loaded cranial vault, of the nasal or ethmoid bones, of the tibia in a totally paralyzed leg (see Fig. 8–12), or of the anterior femoral concavity above the adult knee (see Fig. 8–10). Clearly, other determinants exist. SubMES strains over long time periods, constant strains, or juxtaosseous soft tissues might also affect bone modeling and architecture. If so, the underlying principles await formulation. The basic plan of the IO entities predicts that such phenomena could occur and their state equation might look like this, where $f(M)$ represents the net modeling effect:

$$f(M) = \quad \begin{array}{c} S \longrightarrow \\ \qquad\qquad \downarrow \\ \Big\vert \longrightarrow L \\ \overline{\overline{C : P : D : O : A : M}} \longrightarrow \end{array} \qquad \textit{Relation (5)}$$

Here the "L" term might represent dura or galea for the skull, or subepithelial tissue for the ethmoid, and the endocrine control for growth ("S") could gate through that

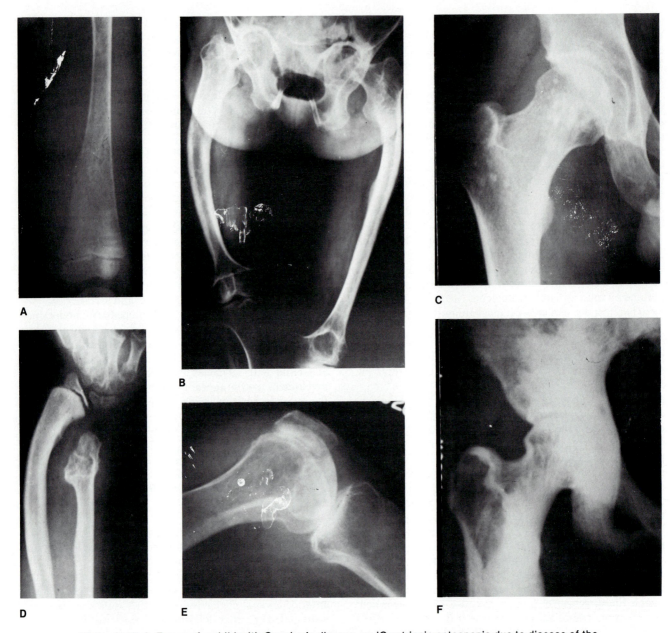

Figure 8-13. A. Femur of a child with Gaucher's disease, an IO-extrinsic osteopenia due to disease of the adjoining marrow tissue. The cortical-endosteal and trabecular envelopes are affected. An "L" gated phenomenon. **B.** Woman with osteogenesis imperfecta, and IO-intrinsic modeling disease with normal BMU-based remodeling. **C.** Osteopoikilosis, and IO-intrinsic disorder that causes no disability and apparently affects only the trabecular envelope. **D.** Multiple, hereditary exostoses or Ehrenfried's disease is an IO-extrinsic disease with abnormal architectural demands made by local chondral and fibrous tissue structures. **E.** Lateral x-ray of a knee with chronic synovial hypertrophy present for years. Under IO-extrinsic control, modeling of the anterior femoral cortex produced a recess to accommodate the synovia (an "L" effect). **F.** Osteopetrosis, an IO-intrinsic disorder of both bone modeling and remodeling due to a proven cell-level (L_c-domain) disorder: functionally incompetent osteoclasts.

"L" to affect the cell proliferation ("P" activity) that is essential to all bone growth, modeling, and remodeling.

To reiterate, bone architecture has multiple determinants and mechanical control represents only one of them.

The Influence of the Marrow Cavity
Varied evidence suggests that something about the marrow cavity, whether it be its tissue, varying pulse pressure,

temperature, or something else, inherently weights the net cortical–endosteal and trabecular bone modeling and remodeling processes in favor of net bone loss. A negative bone balance on trabecular and cortical–endosteal surfaces appears first in the fetus and it persists throughout life. That marrow-gated influence could modify simultaneously acting mechanical modeling activities (funneling agents through different gates at the same time often occurs in the IO). Since other evidence suggests that mechanical usage can restrain the tendency to net endosteal bone loss, the increased endosteal bone loss that follows prolonged deloading of an adult bone may reflect the removal of that usage-induced restraint. Two studies by Jaworski and Uhthoff strongly support the idea (Uhthoff and Jaworski, 1978; Jaworski et al., 1980).

Accordingly, retaining the bone deposits in one's skeletal bank may require regular activity to produce frequent and sufficiently large strains (or possibly other effects, as on bone blood flow) to restrain the inherent tendency to net loss on the endosteal envelopes. A usage-induced restraint may also apply to the bone adjacent to loadbearing endoprostheses, meaning that to make the bone supporting them last longer one should not only not overuse them, but should not underuse them either.

The Role of Microdamage

Under a single load, fresh adult bone breaks at approximately 0.015 to 0.03 unit strain and an infant's bone at 0.04 or more (Currey, 1975; Burstein, 1976). Also, the fatigue life of fresh adult bone relates closely to cyclic strain (Carter, 1981; Carter and Caler, 1981). With a unit strain of 0.004 (which is about five times larger than the lower MES limit but five or more times smaller than the ultimate strain of mature bone, as suggested in Figure 8–5) the fatigue life of bone can be only a few tens of thousands of cycles, or much less than 2 month's usage (Carter, 1981; Carter and Caler, 1981). When contrasted to the unquestionably superior fatigue life of healthy living bones, such facts suggest that fatigue failure became a major threat during skeletal evolution, and failure under single overloads a lesser threat. Consequently the MES limits probably fit the needs of the former better than those of the latter (Carter, 1981).

Microscopic physical damage in healthy living bone occurs under normal usage and it most likely represents a fatigue phenomenon. The writer discovered it in 1960 (Frost, 1960, 1981), others have verified it (Arnold et al., 1966; Radin and Tolkoff, 1970; Todd et al., 1972; Freeman et al., 1974; Watson, 1975) and Figure 8–14 shows some examples. The bone remodeling process repairs that microdamage during the period when its effects on the integrity of the intact bone remain mechanically trivial (Frost, 1966, 1973a). Accordingly, in preventing gross fatigue failure ("spontaneous" or stress fracture) bone modeling and remodeling appear to collaborate. The former minimizes the development of new microdamage foci by adjusting bone size and shape in a way that keeps typical strains below a certain threshold, the MES. The second repairs the microdamage before it threatens the structural integrity of the intact bone. The following list suggests general design guidelines for structural tissues:

1. Designed primarily to sustain cyclic loading-deloading
2. The primary objective: protection from fatigue failure under cyclic normal loads
3. A secondary objective: protection from failure under single large normal loads

4. A tertiary objective: protection from failure under catastrophic overloads.
5. Strain magnitude or range is the most important phenomenon in all three forms of failure
6. Macromodeling of structural *organs* during growth specifically limits their typical strains and thus fatigue-induced microdamage, by controlling their shape and size, and thus their bulk strength and stiffness
7. Micromodeling of structural *tissues* specifically minimizes their typical strains and thus fatigue-induced microdamage, by controlling their preferred grain orientations

While older thought emphasized ultimate strength and stress, newer thought increasingly emphasizes fatigue and strain.

Biomechanical Competence of Fracture Callus

The primary healing phase of a fracture includes the elaboration and mineralization of callus made of unoriented woven bone and cartilage. Standard texts describe the accompanying cellular and biochemical processes that are of little concern here but they omit something of considerable clinical importance. Callus needs 5 to 12 weeks to mature (attain biomechanical competence). If loaded before that it will deform plastically, allowing malposition, angulation, rotation or overriding. But if loading resumes only after maturation, and gradually, the callus will have become sufficiently rigid to escape plastic deformation. It then undergoes piecemeal internal replacement by correctly oriented lamellar bone via the BMU-based remodeling process. After 2 years or so the callus will have been completely replaced by functionally competent lamellar bone and its contour will fit the needs of its typical mechanical usage. Those processes represent the secondary phase of fracture healing.

Hence, "biomechanical competence": *The ability of a tissue to model and remodel in response to overstrain and microdamage.* If an inadequate RAP develops during fracture healing it can delay both union and the development of biomechanical competence in spite of technically adequate primary treatment. Most if not all successful methods of treating nonunions, including various forms of electrical stimulation, also evoke a new RAP that accelerates the local healing, remodeling, and modeling processes.

The term also applies to uninjured structural tissues. Thus a bone or tendon too weak to endure normal usage without straining at or above the level of its MES will ultimately fail due to progressively increasing burdens of microdamage. Equally, when abnormally sluggish microdamage repair mechanisms cannot repair microdamage as fast as it develops, a fatigue failure must occur eventually. Osseous examples of such biomechanical incompetence occur in osteogenesis imperfecta (an IO-intrinsic modeling disorder), many osteomalacias and many osteoporoses (most of them IO-extrinsic remodeling disorders).

Load-Bearing Endoprostheses

In several respects the above material bears on the design of load-bearing skeletal endoprostheses. The designs have

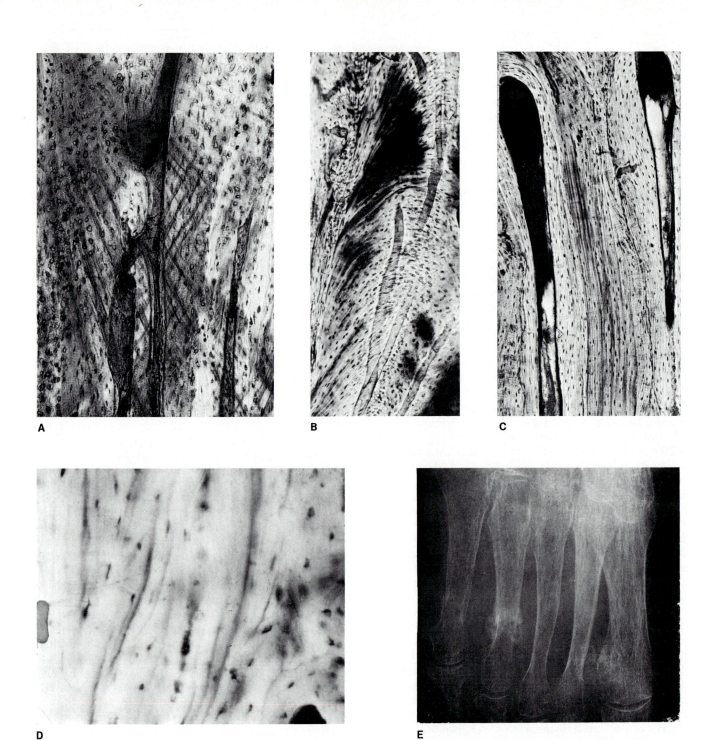

A

B

C

D

E

Figure 8–14. Except for the x-ray at bottom right, these are photomicrographs of undecalcified, basic fuchsin stained longitudinal human bone sections. **A.** Sample from a bone longitudinally sheared with a compression end-load. The intersecting oblique dark lines represent prefailure shear planes, an early kind of microdamage causing defects in the bone substance large enough to admit the stain molecules but too small to see with the light microscope. **B.** Analogous prefailure planes arising in vivo in the tibia of a youngster with Blount's disease. Note that they parallel the grain. Specimen obtained at corrective osteotomy. **C.** Further prefailure planes in a bowed femur of an adolescent who came to corrective osteotomy for a varus related to vitamin D resistant rickets. **D.** Cross section of a rib of a patient with asthma on long-duration steroid treatment. Bulk sample stained in basic fuchsin for 4 months before sectioning. The vertical lines are true microscopic cracks in the bone, almost certainly due to fatigue and in this case visible in the light microscope. The prolonged staining period before sectioning the tissue ensured that the stained cracks were not sectioning artifacts. **E.** A healing metatarsal stress fracture in an osteoporotic woman receiving corticosteroids for a chronic medical problem. Here microdamage accumulated faster than the steroid-depressed remodeling process could repair it, leading ultimately to a complete failure that evoked the perfectly competent primary bone healing process, a process far more resistant to depression by corticosteroids than the remodeling process.

improved to the point that most failures now occur in the host bone rather than in the implants, and they relate to fatigue phenomena rather than to loading beyond the ultimate strength of the bone. Our present understanding of bone modeling and remodeling suggests certain design criteria that must be satisfied if an endoprosthesis is to have a satisfactory service life, and violations probably underlie the above failures.

First, to prevent fatigue failure of bone the loads on an implant should not cause typical bone strains parallel to the grain that equal or exceed the MES nor that exceed about half that magnitude across the grain. Second, the corresponding bone shearing strains should nowhere exceed limits of approximately half the MES in tension or compression. Third, the bone accepting an implant's load should remain alive so its microdamage repair mechanism(s) can function, because some microdamage will always occur. Fourth, to neutralize any nontrivial internal bursting loads, either the bone cortex must be inwaisted or be able to inwaist by appropriate modeling, or the implant's geometry must substitute for that function. Among other things, no endosteal or periosteal drift barriers should exist, and one must recognize that adult bone can only model very slowly.

Impact
Loading rates and peak loading phenomena associated with impact have important effects on bone and cartilage healing, modeling, and maintenance. The chapter on fibrous tissue (see Chap. 14) modeling discusses these effects.

Summary
The following are biomechanical rules of thumb for normal lamellar bone:

1. Strain rather than stress most directly controls modeling. The structure's shape, stiffness, and the loads it carries determine its strains
2. Macromodeling determines the cross section size and shape, the longitudinal shape, and the location in tissue space, of growing bony diaphyses and metaphyses, excepting chondral effects
3. Local dynamic and repeated flexural bone strains can control that macromodeling
4. The size and shape of a bone reflect the magnitudes and orientations of the typical dynamic loads it carried during its growth, and those loads are applied primarily by muscle, and under the control of the CNS
5. Micromodeling aligns the preferred grain of lamellar bone during its deposition, to make it parallel the typical local tension or compression strains
6. The callus that heals a complete fracture in man normally requires 6 to 12 weeks to attain the biomechanical competence it needs to become replaced by lamellar bone and properly contoured to sustain normal usage
7. To occur in significant amounts, bone modeling requires general body growth to occur too
8. A RAP accelerates all of the processes listed above

REFERENCES

Aegerter E, Kirkpatrick JA Jr: Orthopaedic Diseases, 4th ed. Philadelphia, Saunders, 1975.

Albright JA: Bone: Physical properties. In Albright JA and Brand RA (eds): The Scientific Basis of Orthopaedics. New York, Appleton-Century-Crofts, 1979, pp 135–183.

Anderson WAD, Kissane JM: Pathology, 7th ed. St. Louis, C.V. Mosby, 1977.

Arnold JS, Bartley MH, Tont SA, Jenkins DP: Skeletal changes in aging and disease. Clin Orthop 49:17–38, 1966.

Becker RO, Bassett CA, Bachman CH: Bioelectric factors controlling bone structure. In Frost HM (ed): Bone Biodynamics. Boston, Little, Brown, 1964, pp 209–232.

Berliner RW: Outline of renal physiology. In Strauss MB, and Welt LG (eds): Diseases of Kidney. Boston, Little, Brown, 1971, pp 31–85.

Bonnucci E: New knowledge on the origin, function and fate of osteoclasts. Clin Ortho Rel Res 158:252–269, 1981.

Burstein AH, Reilly DT, Martens M: Aging of bone tissue: Mechanical properties. J Bone Joint Surg 58A:82–86, 1976.

Carter DR: The relationship between in vivo strains and cortical bone remodeling. CRC Critical Reviews in Biomechanical Engineering, 8:1–28, 1981.

Carter DR, Caler WE: Uniaxial fatigue of human cortical bone. The influence of tissue physical characteristics. J Biomech 14:461–470, 1981.

Chakkalakal DA, Johnson MW: Electrical properties of compact bone. Clin Orthop Rel Res 161:133–145, 1981.

Churches AE, Howlett CR: Functional adaptation of bone in response to sinusoidally varying controlled compressive loading of the ovine metacarpus. Clin Orthop Rel Res 168:265–280, 1982.

Courpron P: Bone tissue mechanisms underlying osteoporoses. Ortho Clin N Amer 12:513–545, 1981.

Courpron P, Lepine PM, Meunier PJ: Analyse Par l'Histomorphométrie osseuse des Mécanismes de L'Ostéopénie du Spongieux Iliaque Humain. Francheville, Hôpital A. Charial, 1982.

Currey JD, Butler G: The mechanical properties of bone in children. J Bone Joint Surg 57A:810–814, 1975.

Enlow DH: The Principles of Bone Remodeling. Springfield, Ill, Chas. C Thomas, 1963.

Epker BN, Frost HM: Correlation of patterns of bone resorption and formation with physical behavior of loaded bone. J Dent Res 44:33–42, 1965.

Epker BN, O'Ryan F: Determinants of Class II dentofacial morphology. I. A biomechanical theory. In McNamara JA Jr, Carlson DS, and Ribbens KA (eds): The Effect of Surgical Intervention on Craniofacial Growth. Ann Arbor, Univ. of Michigan, 1982, pp 169–206.

Eriksson C: Streaming potentials and other water dependent effects in mineralized tissues. Ann NY Acad Sci 1974, 238–321.

Evans FG: Stress and Strain in Bone. Springfield, Ill, Chas. C Thomas, 1957.

Frost HM: Presence of microscopic cracks in vivo in bone. Henry Ford Hosp Med Bull 8:25–35, 1960.

Frost HM: Bone Remodeling Dynamics. Springfield, Ill, Chas. C Thomas, 1963.

Frost HM: The Laws of Bone Structure. Springfield, Ill, Chas. C Thomas, 1964.

Frost HM: Mathematical Elements of Lamellar Bone Remodelling. Springfield, Ill., Chas. C Thomas, 1964.

Frost HM: Bone Dynamics in Osteoporosis and Osteomalacia. Springfield, Ill., Chas. C Thomas, 1966.

Frost HM: Tetracycline based histological analysis of bone remodeling. Calc Tiss Res 3:211–237, 1969.

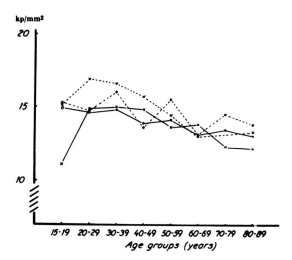

Figure 9-6. Changes in the ultimate tensile strength of cortical specimens with age; ○ = males, × = females; femur, solid lines; humerus, broken lines. *(From Lindahl and Lindgren, 1967b, with permission.)*

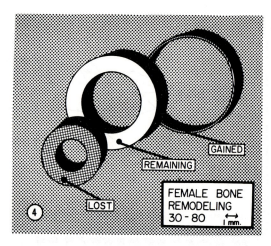

Figure 9-8. Adult female bone remodeling in second metacarpal showing washer of bone lost at endosteal surface over a 5-decade period (shaded), thin collar of bone gained at subperiosteal surface (black), and tube of bone remaining at age 80 (shown in white). For some bones, such as femur, subperiosteal apposition may actually exceed area of bone lost in endosteal resorption. *(From Garn, 1970, with permission.)*

Cortical Bone

To obtain comparative information on the life-long behavior of tubular bone, the measurements made on growing bone must not be confused by the effects of epiphyseal growth; for this purpose, cross-section analyses of the middiaphysis have been found to be a reliable source of information (Fig. 9–8). Relatively simple measurements can be made from x-rays using a technique that permits large-scale studies of populations (Fig. 9–9). The results demonstrate clear differences in the behavior of bone among the three envelopes (Fig. 9–10).

Periosteal Envelope. At the periosteal surface, bone deposition proceeds unidirectionally throughout life, with a slow, steady increase in bone diameter once growth is complete. The rate of expansion is much greater in grow-

ing bone, but the subperiosteal diameter continues to increase at all ages (except in areas of metaphyseal modeling adjacent to the advancing epiphyseal plates); the direction is rarely reversed, even in disease states that cause a reduction in total skeletal mass. The same pattern of expansion has been noted in rib, vertebra, and skull, as well as in the femur and metacarpal.

The reason the periosteal diameter of bone continues to enlarge throughout life is not known, but it can be assumed that bone hypertrophies in response to the stresses placed upon it; hence, mechanically, progressive expansion would be expected. The stresses in a cylinder, such as the diaphysis, are greatest on its surface; therefore, the

Figure 9-7. Schematic diagram showing the pattern of bone formation rates in various bones of the dog skeleton. The rate in the middiaphysis of the tibia equals one. The numbers represent the mean and standard error of the ratio between the respective bone and the tibia middiaphysis in 21 dogs. The rates in the proximal epiphysis and metaphysis of any bone can be determined by multiplying the rate in its diaphysis by the numbers at the proximal end of the isolated drawing of a long bone (these numbers represent the mean and standard error from five long bones in eight dogs). *(From Marotti, 1976, with permission.)*

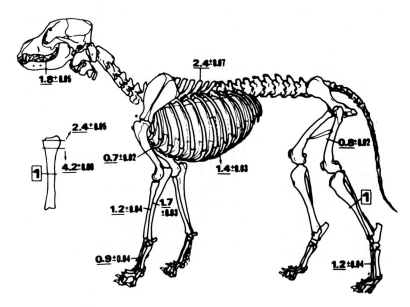

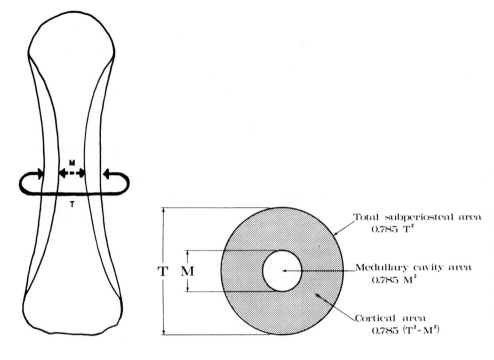

Figure 9–9. Left. Diagrammatic representation of tubular bone showing midshaft measurements of T, total subperiosteal diameter and M, medullary cavity width. Using 0.05-mm readout Helios caliper and expressing cortex (C) as T–M, measurement accuracy is maximized. **Right.** Diagram illustrating total subperiosteal area, medullary area, and cortical area as derived from T and M. *(From Garn, 1970, with permission.)*

Total subperiosteal area
$0.785 \ T^2$

Medullary cavity area
$0.785 \ M^2$

Cortical area
$0.785 \ (T^2 - M^2)$

stimulus to new bone formation is maximum at the periphery and minimum at the endosteum.

Haversian (Intracortical) Envelope. The least number of age-related changes occur in the intracortical envelope (as determined by changes in cortical porosity). Porosity refers to the percentage of cortical bone occupied by spaces (haversian canals, Volkmann canals, resorption spaces, actively forming (closing) osteons, and osteocyte lacunae). Normally, the canals and osteocyte lacunae are relatively unimportant in determining porosity, since they only occupy about 15 percent of the total space, while resorption spaces, and to some extent newly forming osteons, make a much larger contribution (osteocyte lacunae provide a larger percentage of the total surface area, which explains their importance in calcium homeostasis, but when considering the capacity of a bone to provide structural support, porosity and not surface area is the relevant parameter). For example, a typical resorption cavity has a cross-sectional area of about 0.035 sq mm, while that for a haversian canal equals 0.0006 sq mm. Thus, large changes in cortical porosity usually result from an increase or decrease in the number of resorption spaces, rather than alterations in the smaller spaces.

The number of resorption spaces and actively forming osteons is greatest during the growth period, and together with the overall metabolic activity in bone, it decreases with maturity. Porosity then remains relatively stable throughout life; after 50 years of age, it may actually decrease somewhat due to occlusion of increasing numbers of osteons (micropetrosis) and osteocyte lacunae (during this period the cortex is becoming progressively thinner due to endosteal erosion). The lack of major changes in cortical porosity partly explains why the physical properties of cortical specimens remain relatively stable with age, while the bone as a whole steadily decreases in strength (cortical bone in patients with the diagnosis of osteoporosis usually shows cortical thinning, rather than true porosis). In the femur, the most severe loss of cortical bone occurs along the neutral axis, with preservation of bone in the areas of maximum stress (Blaimont, 1968); a similar pattern probably occurs in other bones as well. Resorption spaces often develop on the endosteal side of the cortex during aging, and these coalesce to enlarge the marrow canal. Haversian canal diameter changes very little with aging, nor does it vary much from bone to bone, but at all ages osteon diameter is greater near the endosteum than near the periosteum.

The fact that cortical porosity remains relatively stable during the normal aging process does not mean that true "osteoporosis" never occurs, since it often accompanies various disease states such as thyrotoxicosis. Paget's disease, hyperparathyroidism, and disuse osteoporosis, which undoubtedly is the most common cause. Early in its course intracortical porosity is transient and can be reversed by removal of the inciting stimulus, but cortical thinning due to endosteal resorption appears irreversible. Intracortical porosis can often be recognized on x-ray by a mottled or moth-eaten appearance, as commonly seen after a fracture. During this period, mineral turnover, as measured kinetically in patients with severe paralytic disorders such as paraplegia, increases for 6 to 12 months and then decreases, as does the x-ray appearance of porosis, leaving a cortex that is thinner but not porotic. The bone behaves as if the loss of muscle activity establishes a new threshold, which necessitates an extended transient phase before reaching a new steady state. This sequence becomes significant during investigative stud-

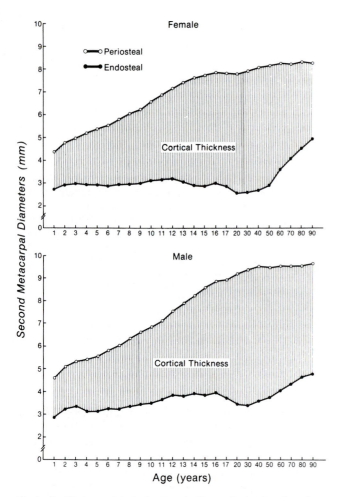

Figure 9–10. Age-related changes in the periosteal and endosteal diameters of the second metacarpal for white males and females in the United States. Maximum cortical bone is attained between 30 and 40 years of age. The figures were obtained by direct measurement of x-rays of the hand (*n* = 5086 for males and 6391 for females). (*From data of Garn et al., 1976.*)

ies, particularly when disuse atrophy may be a factor or when the study involves any change in physical activity; the detection of cortical porosity could easily be interpreted as an end stage, rather than as a temporary phenomenon unless the phase of remodeling activity is accurately identified. The gross changes seen in cortical porosis reflect changes in cellular remodeling activity, which are commonly assumed to result from a disturbance in the activation–resorption–formation sequence, with either a change in the rate of progression from one phase to another or in the number of active sites per unit volume.

Endosteal Envelope. To a large extent, the age-related changes in cortical bone, especially in adults, result from activity at the endosteal surface. In contrast to the periosteal or intracortical surfaces, the endosteum is highly labile, and bone comes and goes at different ages in shift-

ing phases of resorption and apposition, but rarely does the rate parallel activity at the periosteal surface. The progressive loss of cortical bone with age, therefore, can be traced to endosteal resorption with the severity of loss dependent on the degree that endosteal resorption outpaces periosteal apposition. The cause of bone loss at the endosteal surface could be related to the lack of adequate mechanical stimulation since the stresses generated by activity are least at the endosteum, or, as postulated by Frost, the adjacent marrow elements might have an adverse effect on bone, leading to slow resorption. Unless otherwise indicated, the following discussion refers to studies on the metacarpals.

During part of the first year of life, endosteal resorption exceeds periosteal apposition, leading to a decrease in the cross-sectional area of cortical bone; in effect, this might be considered a transient osteoporosis, probably associated with increased hematopoiesis. From 1 year of age to adolescence, periosteal apposition is greater than endosteal resorption, causing a net increase in cortical thickness and area; this entire period of life is one of endosteal resorption with progressive enlargement of the medullary canal. Even so, new bone formation may occur in selected areas to maintain the overall shape of a bone during modeling (such as the normal longitudinal curvature); in these areas, bone formation occurs on one side of the canal, but a greater amount of resorption occurs on other sides, resulting in an increased total canal diameter.

In adolescence, cellular activity at the endosteal surface shifts from resorption to apposition, a process mediated by increased steroid hormone production at this age. As a result, the medullary canal decreases in diameter to values seen earlier in childhood and often to values below those present at 1 year of age. The outer diameter of the bone continues to increase, causing a gain of cortical bone at both surfaces, so that net cortical thickness and area increase. Bone continues to be added at the endosteal surface until about 30 years of age, but differences in the age of onset and rate of apposition occur between males and females. As expected, the shift from endosteal resorption to apposition takes place earlier in girls than boys, similar to most developmental phenomena, but the difference is disproportionate compared to the usual 2-year delay of skeletal maturation between males (16 years) and females (14 years). The shift to endosteal apposition appears between the 10th and 16th year in girls (the age of onset varies in different racial and socioeconomic groups) and the 14th to the 20th year in boys. In the seven countries (the United States and six South American countries) studied by Garn et al. (1970), the age of onset differed by as much as 4 to 8 years between individual countries. In girls, this shift to endosteal apposition begins early in the steroid-mediated phase of sexual development, long before maximum bone size has been obtained, while in boys it is closer to skeletal maturation. Furthermore, during the steroid phase of development, the female appears to gain more bone than the male (at both the endosteal and the periosteal surfaces), resulting in a proportionately greater increase in cortical thickness and area. Garn found a similar pattern in all seven countries, suggesting that the endosteal surface is more responsive to estrogen than to testosterone. Steroid-mediated endosteal apposition may also be augmented by pregnancy. Serial measurements during pregnancy indicate that bone may be added rather than removed, and women of higher parity ultimately have narrower medullary canals, leading to a greater retention of bone in older age.

The adult phase of progressive bone loss begins at about 30 years of age with a reversal of endosteal activity from apposition to resorption. By 40 years of age, the medullary canal has enlarged in most, but not all, nationality and racial groups. When the adult stage begins, the initial rate of loss is small; however, it accelerates progressively with age, and by the sixth decade bone loss is rapid in both sexes. A similar pattern of bone loss has been found in all populations studied, differing only in rate. Thus, the amount of bone lost by blacks lags behind that for age-matched whites; nevertheless, the rate accelerates with age, paralleling that for whites. Sex-related differences in bone loss probably begin at the onset of the adult phase, but at 40 to 50 years of age, the rate markedly accelerates in females, and by 55 years the bone gained under steriod mediation from 12 to 30 years has been lost (Fig. 9–11). The long-term loss at the endosteal surface is two to three times greater in females, who, over a 50-year period beginning at 30 years of age, lose approximately one-third of the bone originally present; at that point, bone loss at the endosteal surface includes the periosteal bone laid down during the first few years of life.

Bone loss in the mid to distal radius of females has been reported to begin at 50 years of age, to accelerate, and to decrease after 65 years (Riggs et al., 1981). Trabecular bone in the distal radius may follow a similar curve. Bone

loss from the radius in males begins earlier, is slower, and is more uniform.

Trabecular Bone

General Features. In contrast to cortical bone, and possibly to trabecular bone loss in the appendicular skeleton, a progressive loss of trabecular bone begins in the axial skeleton soon after skeletal maturity. In the ilium, trabecular bone mass is greatest (40 percent of bone volume) during early childhood. It decreases rapidly during the first decade of life, leveling off to slightly more than 20 percent at maturity (Fig. 9–12).

In females, trabecular bone volume (the percentage of space occupied by trabeculae) in the ilium, though slightly higher than in males, decreases steadily in parallel with males until 5 to 10 years after menopause (whether natural or artificial), when a sharp decrease occurs. The increased rate of loss at this age appears transient, and 5 to 10 years later, it again parallels that for males. However, the amount of bone present remains significantly less in women than men, coinciding with the increased risk of fracture clinically. The acceleration of cortical bone loss in the female ilium appears to begin about 10 years earlier than the loss of trabecular bone or of cortical bone in the long bones.

In both sexes, the loss of trabecular bone in the ilium and in the vertebrae is due to a decrease in the number of trabeculae present, while the thickness of individual trabeculae remains unchanged (it may even increase).

A progressive loss of bone with age has also been found in dogs, but for some reason the trabeculae become thinner and do not decrease in number. In humans, over a 50- to 60-year period, males lose about 25 percent of the trabecular bone present at maturity, while females lose almost half. The amount of trabecular bone that is lost exceeds the loss of cortical bone, reflecting the increased metabolic activity of trabecular bone due to its greater surface area.

Vertebrae. In the vertebra, a progressive loss of mineral begins after skeletal maturity. This is accompanied by internal as well as external structural changes.

External Changes with Age. Vertebral height (the distance between end plates measured near their periphery) does not usually change with age, although it may decrease slightly in females. By contrast, the distance between the centers of the end plates decreases progressively in both sexes, but at a slightly higher rate in females, resulting in biconcavity of the vertebral bodies. The development of biconcavity can only occur if the internal trabeculae shorten, which probably results from repeated subclinical fractures of individual trabeculae followed by subsequent remodeling. As a result of this progressive biconcavity, the overall height of the individual decreases, a universal phenomenon of aging. Externally, the vertebral width as well as the height changes with age, but while the height decreases due to compressive forces, the width increases due to periosteal apposition. The increase in

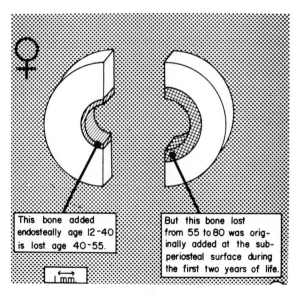

Figure 9-11. Two phases of adult bone loss in the female. The first phase of adult endosteal loss involves bone space laid down in adolescence and early adulthood. The second phase of endosteal loss erodes bone space added in infancy. *(From Garn, 1970, with permission.)*

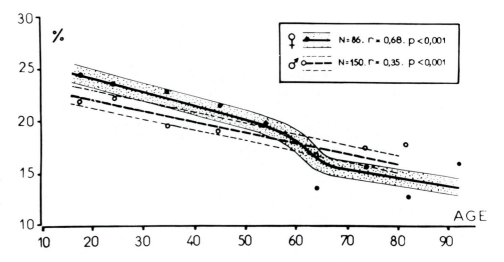

Figure 9-12. Changes in iliac trabecular bone volume with age and sex in 236 controls, illustrated by statistically smoothed curves. *(From Meunier and Courpron, 1976, with permission.)*

width is disproportionately greater at the ends than at the center, which produces flaring; this occurs at a slightly higher rate in males. The process of flaring is a manifestation of slowly developing osteoarthritic changes in the spine.

Internal Changes with Age. Bone loss with age follows a predictable pattern with little variation other than in the degree of severity found between individuals at any given age. Although changes occur simultaneously in both the vertical and horizontal trabeculae, each will be described separately.

The first detectable sign of aging is slight thinning of the horizontal trabeculae (transverse fenestrated plates) in the end zones; some of the innermost transverse fenestrated plates are resorbed, which shortens the end zones themselves (Fig. 9–13). Normally, the end zones shorten progressively until only one or two fenestrated plates remain, although they may be lost completely in advanced senile osteoporosis.

During the period when the first horizontal trabeculae disappear, the vertical plates in the central zone continue to expand (in length), and the enclosed cylinders reach a maximum. Pores and apertures then develop in the vertical cylindrical plates, beginning near their ends and progressing centrally. As the transverse and vertical trabeculae disappear, the pore size increases in the remaining transverse fenestrated plates. Resorption continues until mere fragments of plates remain, while at the same time, the absolute number of vertical trabeculae continues to decrease. As the trabecular bone mass decreases, enough vertical trabeculae are spared to retain adequate support against vertical compression forces. This function is aided by a redistribution of material leading to hypertrophy of the remaining vertical trabeculae, thereby partly compensating for the loss of other vertical, as well as horizontal, trabeculae. It has been estimated that the stabilization of each vertical trabecula against compression normally requires four times its mass in the form of horizontal trabeculae. Consequently, hypertrophy of the remaining

vertical trabeculae can restore a large part of the vertical strength with only small increases in their mass, even though total bone mass decreases markedly. Even so, the overall strength against other types of forces will be decreased.

The risk of compression fracture of the vertebra correlates with the density of the vertebral centrum. Yet, bone density is not uniform throughout the vertebral body (Edwards et al., 1986). Instead, it follows a selective pattern with less density anteriorly than posteriorly. In older individuals the density of bone in the anterior portion of the body is less than two-thirds that in the posterior portion, and the strength is less than half. Furthermore, the compressive strength of the vertebral body correlates best with the strength and apparent density of trabecular bone in the anterior half of the body. This suggests that the most sensitive indication of fracture risk is the density of trabecular bone in the anterior third of the vertebral body. Density measurements of the trabecular bone in this part of the body can be obtained using quantitative computed tomography.

OTHER AGE-RELATED CHANGES

Calcium Absorption

Techniques demonstrating radiocalcium absorption and calcium balance (Table 9–1) have demonstrated a decline in fractional calcium absorption with age (Gallagher et al., 1979). This decrease occurs in both sexes and is particu-

TABLE 9-1. AGE-RELATED CHANGES

Calcium absorption	↓
Lactase activity	±
$1,25\text{-}(OH)_2D_3$	↓
Parathyroid hormone	↓
Calcitonin	↓
Phosphate	↑
Estrogen in women	↓

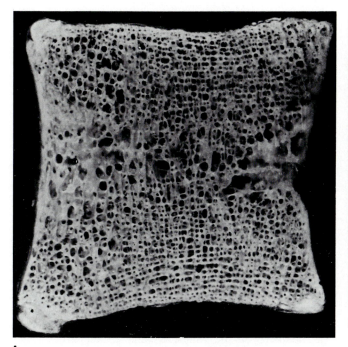

A

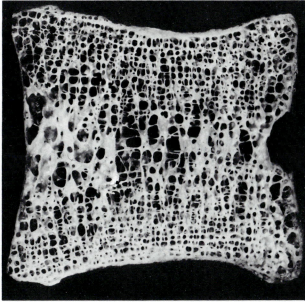

B

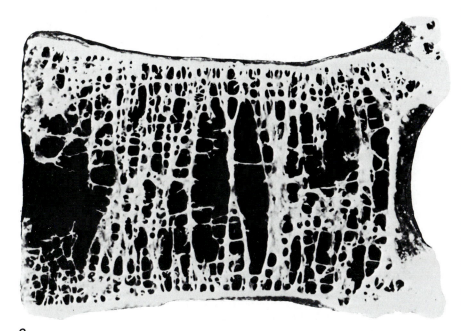

C

Figure 9-13. A. Photograph of a cleaned 2-mm-thick sagittal section of vertebra in the second decade of life revealing the platelike structures surrounding the basivertebral vein on the right and the platelike structures on the left, which form a fuzzy triangle on x-ray. The fenestrated plates of the end zones are seen as continuous, long transverse trabeculae in this view. **B.** A cleaned 2-mm-thick slab in the fifth decade of life. The spaces between the fenestrated plates and the longitudinal trabeculae appear larger, due chiefly to loss of trabecular structures. The plates of the anterior central zone remain prominent, showing more frequent perforations. **C.** A cleaned 2-mm-thick slab in the eighth decade of life from a patient with senile osteoporosis, revealing that "hypertrophied trabeculae" of osteoporosis are vertical plates. There is irregular atrophy of both transverse and longitudinal trabeculae. *(From Arnold, 1970, with permission.)*

larly prominent in the eighth decade. Not only is calcium absorption decreased, but also adaption to low calcium intake is impaired. In normal humans, 1,25-(OH)$_2$D is inversely correlated with calcium intake and is thus thought to be the mediator of intestinal calcium absorption. In most cases, the decrease in calcium absorption can be accounted for by a decrease in 1,25-(OH)$_2$D. An additional factor may be intestinal lactase activity, which may vary significantly from one individual to another (Pacifici et al., 1985).

Vitamin D and Metabolites

The importance of vitamin D in calcium absorption has been well documented. The active metabolite, 1,25-(OH)$_2$D$_3$, is significantly decreased in elderly subjects (Gallagher et al., 1979). Since serum 25-OH-D levels are normal in the elderly, an error in the metabolic pathway has been postulated as a cause for this decrease. More specifically, an age-related loss of activity of renal 25-OH-D$_3$-1-hydroxylase has been implicated by Zerwekh et al. (1983). This deficiency can be demonstrated by the failure of increased serum 25-OH-D$_3$ to cause significant increases in either serum 1,25-(OH)$_2$D$_3$ levels or intestinal calcium absorption in certain patients, who are thereby designated "nonresponders." Animal studies have also demonstrated this change in activity of the renal hydroxylase with aging (Armbrecht et al., 1980).

Alternatively, both decreased secretory reserve and possible end-organ unresponsiveness to endogenous parathyroid hormone have been suggested as factors in low 1,25-(OH)$_2$D$_3$ levels (Slovik et al., 1981). There is also the possibility that estrogen deficiency affects hydroxylase activity (Gallagher et al., 1980).

Parathyroid Hormone

The decrease in circulating levels of parathyroid hormone that occur with age have been attributed in the main to senescence of the gland. The mechanism of the decrease has not been elucidated. The possibility that the gland may lose its sensitivity to circulating calcium exists. On the other hand, a lack of secretory reserve or synthesizing ability may occur with age (Gallagher et al., 1980, Burtis and Lang, 1984).

Calcitonin

Women have lower circulating immunoreactive calcitonin (iCt) than men. They also exhibit a lower iCt response to calcium and pentagastrin than men (Gallagher et al., 1980; Avioli, 1982; Burtis and Lang, 1984). During treatment with estrogens, birth control pills, and during pregnancy and lactation, plasma iCt levels have been noted to rise.

The sex difference in calcitonin levels, and the fact that calcitonin levels decline with age has led to a postulated link between estrogen and calcitonin. In fact, calcitonin has been suggested as the mediator of the estrogen effect on bone. No definitive proof of this mediation has yet been published, and no definite acceleration in the decline of calcitonin levels has been demonstrated with menopause (Stevenson, 1981). Osteoporotic patients demonstrate a normal reserve of calcitonin (Tiegs et al., 1985). Because of our incomplete knowledge about the substance and its actions, calcitonin remains an intense area of interest.

Cellular Senescence

The skeleton is intimately involved in calcium and phosphorus homeostasis, which involves multiple organ systems. Alteration in the ability of the cells of any one of these systems to respond effectively could conceivably endanger the entire balance. At the cellular level in the skeleton, the osteoblast in particular has been singled out in discussions of senescence. If osteoblasts do not respond to whatever constitutes the recruitment stimulus, or if they fail to produce sufficient matrix to fill resorption cavities, skeletal incompetence may result. On the other hand, normal remodeling performs a crucial function in the adaptive ability of the skeleton. If osteoclasts do not initiate the remodeling sequence or if for some reason excessive resorption occurs, the biomechanical stability of the system may be at risk (Jaworski, 1984).

It is difficult to give credence to these effects on one organ system without expecting age to similarly affect all organs. Thus, consideration must be given to the hypotheses that the kidney cannot produce adequate 25-OH-D$_3$-1α hydroxylase, the parathyroid gland decreases its secretion of iPTH, the chief cells secrete less calcitonin, and lining cells of the intestine are imperfect in their response to 1,25-(OH)$_2$D$_3$. This paints a dismal picture indeed for the aging patient who wishes to avoid the sequelae of excessive bone loss.

Estrogen

Estrogens are steroid metabolites produced by the ovary. These compounds produce diverse effects on organs outside the reproductive system. At puberty, the vagina, uterus, and tubes enlarge, as do the external genitalia, due to estrogen stimulation. Fat deposition in the breasts, accompanied by stromal and ductal development also occur at puberty. The cervix begins secreting mucus, which is of low viscosity yet highly permeable to spermatozoa. The rounding of the female figure due to fat deposition in the buttocks and thighs is secondary to estrogen stimulation.

Puberty in the female is heralded not only by widening of the pelvic outlet and hastening of epiphyseal closure but by the onset of menses. Conversely, the menopause constitutes the cessation of menses, occurring near the mean age of 48 years. Premature menopause is that occurring before the age of 40. The human female of the twentieth century now survives many years beyond the function of her sex-steroid organs, a unique situation among mammals (Quigley, 1981). The cause of this disruption of the cyclic menses is unknown. There appears to be an extremely rapid depletion of oocytes and a corresponding loss of stimulation of the ovarian follicles. This in turn causes the release of FSH and LH to become uncoordinated, resulting in irregular menses. Hot flashes are a well known companion of the menopause and occur in 85 percent of menopausal women (McArthur, 1974).

The action of estrogen on bone causes a decrease in activation of remodeling units. Its effect on bone resorption and bone formation, therefore, is indirect. Normally, bone resorption is the first identifiable cellular change to occur in the remodeling cycle. Only later does bone formation occur, and this causes the resorption spaces to slowly fill-in with new bone. Therefore, the cellular pattern found in bone will vary, depending upon the time that has elapsed after treatment was started. Biopsy within the first 2 or 3 months will show a decrease in bone resorption because fewer remodeling units have been activated, but bone formation may still be unaffected. A decreasing amount of bone formation occurs as the duration of treatment increases. Yet an accurate evaluation can not be obtained until the duration of treatment exceeds the length of the remodeling cycle. At that point, all remodeling units present will have been activated after treatment began. Bone resorption and bone formation will then be found to be equally depressed.

The acceleration of bone loss that accompanies the menopause has been documented by many authors (Meema et al., 1975; Richelson et al., 1984). The rate of loss in postmenopausal women has not been significantly correlated with age (when artificial menopause in younger women is considered, as well as natural menopause in middle aged women), but it has been shown to correlate directly with estrogen deficiency. These findings support the model of age-related bone loss in the female, with accelerated bone-loss secondary to estrogen depletion superimposed upon it. The benefits and risks of therapy will be discussed in a later section.

OSTEOPOROSIS

Fuller Albright described the clinical features of osteoporosis in 1941 and postulated that an atrophy of bone matrix rather than disordered calcium metabolism was its basis. In his later dissertation (1947), he lay the blame for the matrix defect upon the osteoblast, and called attention to the association between postmenopausal estrogen deficiency and osteoporosis. His preliminary description and subsequent hypotheses have set in motion an era of intensive debate and investigation. Much progress has been made, but the multifactorial nature of the problem coupled with the time factor involved in longitudinal human studies has frustrated even the most ardent investigator.

Much new information is applicable to patient care, especially in situations where treatable disease entities are identified, but much is of theoretical interest only. The prevailing uncertainties surrounding both the etiology and treatment of osteoporosis illustrate the distance between different investigators studying a specific clinical problem, and emphasize the difficulty in clinical application of laboratory findings.

Definition

Osteoporosis literally means an increased porosity of bone, an inaccurate description of the types commonly seen; it can be more accurately defined as a clinical condition in which a progressive diminution of skeletal mass renders bone increasingly vulnerable to fracture. Not only do the diagnostic criteria generate controversy, but until secondary complications develop, such as vertebral collapse, hip fracture, loss of height, backache, or deformity, it may not even be possible to establish a definitive diagnosis. The term "secondary osteoporosis" has been used when a predisposing disease entity, such as malabsorption, can be identified, while the term *idiopathic* or *primary osteoporosis* applies to the larger group of individuals who have an accelerated rate of bone loss compared to an age-matched cross-section of the general population. Although numerous disease states can cause osteoporosis (Table 9–2), the following discussion concerns idiopathic osteoporosis.

Quantitative histologic, microradiographic, and radiographic measurements of age-related changes in "normal" bone demonstrate that a progressive loss of bone begins at 30 to 40 years of age, with the rate increasing at 40 to 50 years in females and 50 to 60 years in males (Fig. 9–14). These changes primarily affect trabecular bone and the endosteal surface of cortical bone, usually with a mild

TABLE 9-2. CLINICAL CONDITIONS ASSOCIATED WITH OSTEOPOROSIS

Menopause or aging
Disuse: immobilization, paralysis, weightlessness
Corticosteroid treatment
Cushing's syndrome
Osteogenesis imperfecta
Partial gastrectomy
Malabsorption syndromes
Chronic liver disease
Heparin treatment
Hyperparathyroidism
Hyperthyroidism
Rheumatoid arthritis
Acromegaly
Scurvy
Alcoholism
Diabetes
Lactase deficiency
Malignancy
Mastocytosis
Acid-rich diet
Decreased stress
Amenorrhea in runners
Smoking

disturbance in turnover balance that seems to favor resorption.

The rate of loss appears to differ between the axial skeleton (the vertebral column and pelvis) and the appendicular skeleton (the limbs). Bone loss in the axial skeleton begins earlier in life (20 to 30 years of age) than does bone loss in the limbs (about 40 years of age). Furthermore, it has been postulated that the loss of trabecular bone in the limbs (the distal radius) may resemble the pattern of cortical bone loss in the limbs rather than the pattern of trabecular bone loss in the spine, but more documentation is needed before this assumption can be accepted. Compare the pattern of bone loss in the vertebra (Fig. 9–4) to that seen in the ilium (Fig. 9–12), and both of these to cortical bone in the 2nd metacarpal (Fig. 9–10). Figure 9–10 illustrates the complex nature of cortical bone loss. The periosteal diameter increases progressively throughout life, whereas medullary canal diameter fluctuates until 20 to 30 years of age, after which it steadily enlarges. In effect, total cortical volume in older individuals depends on the rate of endosteal resorption. It is not known why this unremitting expansion of the medullary canal continues throughout most of adult life, nor whether periosteal expansion represents a protective response to decreasing bone mass.

Since the tendency toward increasing osteopenia appears to be a universal phenomenon, it is considered normal. This system of classification further widens the ill-defined border between normal and abnormal and magnifies the uncertainties of diagnosis. Presumably, the physiologic osteoporosis of aging becomes pathologic in individuals surviving to an age where the degree of bone loss becomes disabling in itself, whether due to fracture or to generalized frailty. In fact, if the leading causes of substrate levels are increased in all women who take estrogens, but there are no significant differences in these levels in normotensive compared to hypertensive women on estrogens (Judd et al., 1983). The association with hypertension has not led to an increased incidence of cerebrovascular accidents.

Other side effects of estrogen administration, such as thromboembolic disease and hyperlipidemia, have been linked to effects on the liver due to high estrogen concentrations in the portal circulation after oral administration of the drug (Laufer et al., 1983).

Recent studies of the transdermal route of administration of the drug have been encouraging, with adequate blood levels established to control hot flashes and vaginal atrophy, yet it produces no deleterious effect on the liver. Further study will be required to ascertain whether this dose form will give adequate protection from bone loss.

Given the encouraging advances in estrogen therapy, it would seem that the risk–benefit ratio for the patient is favorable. Even the group of so-called "rapid-losers" has been shown to respond to estrogen therapy (Christiansen and Ródbró, 1983). The optimum effect is achieved with early therapy in any group, but a response is seen even in patients five years after menopause (Christiansen et al., 1981). Some authors have demonstrated a beneficial effect from hormone therapy even after its cessation, while others have demonstrated loss of the protective effect (Horsman et al., 1979; Christiansen et al., 1981; Lindsay et al., 1981).

In summary, estrogen prevents the accelerated loss of bone that occurs at menopause, whether natural or artificially induced. The hormone achieves its effect by decreasing the activation of bone remodeling units. Therefore, early biopsy will erroneously show a decrease in bone resorption with no effect on bone formation, whereas biopsy after bone remodeling has reached a new equilibrium will show a decrease in both formation and resorption. Furthermore, it is now known that cyclical treatment with estrogen and progesterone does not cause an increase in uterine carcinoma as seen with continuous estrogen treatment. Even so, it must be kept in mind that treatment with estrogen does not replace bone that already has been lost, nor does it prevent the steady loss of bone universally seen in both males and females.

Parathyroid Hormone. One of the more fascinating theories concerns the role of parathyroid hormone (PTH). In the past, a low-calcium diet was found to produce osteoporosis by a parathyroid-dependent mechanism; conversely, the osteoporosis could be prevented by parathyroidectomy. A low-calcium intake causes a slight decrease in the plasma calcium concentration; the mild hypocalcemia stimulates PTH secretion, which restores the plasma calcium to normal, but at the expense of increased bone resorption, eventually leading to osteoporosis. The slight increase in resorption found histologically is compatible with this theory. In addition, the development of disuse osteoporosis in animals, whether from denervation or casting, can be markedly retarded by parathyroidec-

tomy. Since increased resorption is thought to occur in both disuse and idiopathic osteoporosis, parathyroidectomy might also be of benefit in idiopathic osteoporosis.

In contrast, the treatment of osteoporosis with low doses of PTH stands in direct opposition to parathyroidectomy. Reeve et al. (1976) reported a beneficial effect from PTH in four patients treated for up to 6 months. The rationale behind the use of PTH is twofold: PTH stimulates calcium absorption (by increasing l-hydroxylase activity in the kidney), and it stimulates DNA and RNA synthesis. It is felt that low doses of PTH will increase calcium absorption, which, together with the anabolic effect on bone, will increase bone mass. One additional rationale for the use of PTH in osteoporosis rests on Frost's concept that bone remodeling occurs in units or packets, with the cycle activated by a stimulus that initiates mitotic division in precursor cells. Osteoclasts are generated first with resorption preceding formation. Theoretically, bone formation cannot be stimulated without activating the entire system, and this can be done by giving an agent, such as PTH, that stimulates resorption. Once the bone turnover cycle has been activated, administration of proper medications allegedly can favor bone formation.

There are no available tissue techniques to study coupling of bone formation to bone resorption in vitro. In vivo studies in laboratory animals have demonstrated some interesting results. In parathyroidectomized rats, intermittent injection of PTH was noted to stimulate bone formation. When PTH was given as a continuous infusion, however, both resorption and formation were stimulated (Heersche, 1982). When osteoblast-like cells are exposed to parathyroid hormone in vitro, inhibition of bone formation results. In vivo exposure of these cells results in bone formation, thus bringing up the possibility of an indirect effect of PTH on bone.

Dietary Factors. Rates of bone loss leading to osteoporosis in the general population are in the neighborhood of 1 to 2 percent per year. Because negative calcium balance has been implicated as an etiologic factor in osteoporosis, the role of dietary calcium in relation to calcium balance has received much attention. Several authors have found no effect of calcium intake upon bone mineral content (Chalmers et al., 1967; Chalmers and Ho, 1970; Johnell and Nilsson, 1984). Conversely, the untreated osteoporotic patient was found to be in negative calcium balance by Thalassinos et al. (1982), compared to the positive balance which could be induced by high calcium intake. Heaney and Recker (1982a) reported a linear relationship between calcium intake and calcium balance. Matkovíc et al. in 1979 reported a much higher fracture rate associated with low calcium intake in a Yugoslavian community, compared to the fracture rate in residents with high calcium intake. The same study pointed out a significant difference in bone mass at age 30 between parallel communities that differed only in calcium intake. This points to the possible protective effect of increasing bone mass in childhood through high calcium intake, suggested by others (Parfitt, 1982).

Calcium has been accused of inducing a catabolic state and a possible negative energy balance (Lee et al., 1981). Other than this possible negative effect, and absorptive hypercalciuria, which occurs in less than 1 percent of postmenopausal women (Heaney and Recker, 1982b), there is little reason not to include supplemental dietary calcium in a treatment regime. As previously discussed, the efficiency of calcium absorption declines with age for a variety of reasons. Since most women are relatively calcium deficient throughout life, dietary supplementation is not only reasonable, but probably should start at a very early age.

The problem with attempting dietary change to increase calcium intake is that dairy products contain not only calcium, but also nitrogen and phosphorus. Meat products also contain both nitrogen and phosphorus. An increased nitrogen intake can cause an increased loss of calcium in the urine sufficient to produce a negative calcium balance. The etiology of the calciuria associated with high protein intake is thought to be mediated through an increase in acid load. Also, the catabolism of excess proteins causes an increase filtered load of calcium (Lutz and Linkswiler, 1981; Heaney and Recker, 1982). Other authors have confirmed this calciuretic effect with an increase in dietary protein (Margen et al., 1974), although wide variation was exhibited among individuals. With doubling of protein intake, the urinary calcium increased an average of 50 percent. It remains to be seen if elevated protein intake will be linked conclusively to osteoporosis.

When variations in nitrogen and calcium are factored out, phosphorous intake has been shown to have little effect on calcium balance. High phosphorous does not decrease the intestinal absorption of calcium when intake ranges from 200 mg to 2700 mg per day (Spencer et al., 1978). Regardless of the level of calcium intake, however, increased dietary phosphorous significantly decreases urinary calcium, probably from its renal effect. Phosphate is presumed to effect the osteoblast and stimulate collagen synthesis, bone formation, and mineralization. Because of the increased urinary calcium seen in immobilized patients, phosphate has been suggested as an agent to improve calcium balance in these patients. Conversely, low phosphorous intake may increase 1,25-(OH)$_2$D$_3$ synthesis with resultant increased calcium absorption and urinary calcium excretion. The effect of phosphate deprivation on 1,25-(OH)$_2$D$_3$ levels occurs by an unknown mechanism (Gray et al., 1983). It is possible that phosphorous may have some additional effect on calcium that is unknown, yet when combined with the calcium-saving effect of phorphorous on the kidney, causes a net change that is negligible.

Caffeine has been associated with a decline in calcium balance, and an increase in urinary calcium. Most study subjects exhibit an inverse relationship between the intake of caffeine-containing foods and dairy products. This makes interpretation of the significance of this factor difficult, especially since it has not been a consistent finding (Johnell and Nilsson, 1984).

The metabolites of vitamin D provide much interest both as causative factors and possible therapeutic modalities in osteoporosis. Previous mention was made of lower serum levels of 1,25-(OH)$_2$D$_3$ seen in the elderly. Osteoporotic patients as a group have significantly lower levels of 1,25-(OH)$_2$D$_3$ than age-matched controls (Gallagher et al., 1979). The serum levels of 25-(OH)D$_3$, however, remain normal or high (Loré et al., 1981). This illustrates a probable defect in the metabolic pathway from 25-(OH)D$_3$ to 1,25-(OH)$_2$D$_3$ for as yet unproven reasons. Loré et al., (1982) have postulated that an inadequate feedback inhibition of the liver 25-hydroxylase is responsible for high levels of 25-(OH)D$_3$ in osteoporotic women. This may be the reason that the elderly patient will lose the inverse correlation between calcium intake and serum 1,25-(OH)$_2$D$_3$, which is seen in young patients. The same loss of the inverse relationship between calcium intake and calcium absorption is seen in the elderly. Thus, vitamin D may be linked to PTH as a cause of osteoporosis in that a deficiency of 1,25-(OH)$_2$D$_3$ may lead to decreased calcium absorption, a slightly lower serum calcium, stimulation of parathyroid hormone excretion, and subsequent bone resorption.

Although treatment of osteoporosis with vitamin D would seem attractive based on the preceding discussion, there is little clinical evidence that it is efficacious. All metabolites of vitamin D have been used in clinical trials without any evidence that there is a positive effect on the skeleton (Hoikka et al., 1980; Jensen et al., 1982; Zerwekh et al., 1983). Both 1-(OH)D$_3$ and 1,25-(OH)$_2$D$_3$ were found to cause significant hypercalcemia in some patients, and 1,25-(OH)$_2$D$_3$ did not improve the response of bone to estrogen.

In rabbits, 1,25-(OH)$_2$D$_3$ had undesirable effects on fracture healing and osteoporosis caused by immobilization and prednisolone (Lindgren et al., 1984). These effects may not be applicable to human bone because of the differences between human and rabbit calcium metabolism.

Clinical trials with 24,25-(OH)$_2$D$_3$ resulted in double plasma levels of only that metabolite (Reeve et al., 1982). Calcium balance became more positive initially, then returned to baseline at 6 months. Plasma alkaline phosphatase and urinary calcium excretion were not changed.

Based upon the significant toxic effects of vitamin D and the lack of evidence supporting its use in treatment, most authors recommend only a dose of 400 to 500 IU per day.

Acid-Base Balance. Barzel (1970) proposed an entirely different etiologic mechanism for osteoporosis, with evidence to show progressive bone loss from the ingestion of acid. Bone contains large amounts of alkaline salts and probably participates in the maintenance of acid-base balance. The fact that urinary calcium excretion increases following acid loading, together with studies showing increased calcium loss in renal acidosis and starvation acidosis, suggests that bone is mobilized during acid loading and that its salts augment the buffering capacity of the ECF. It has been shown that chronic ingestion of ammonium chloride causes an increase in bone resorption (even tered to animals, probably because of rapid inactivation by pyrophosphatase. The diphosphonates, on the other hand, are resistant to pyrophosphatase, so they produce an equally effective response in vivo as in vitro.

Low dose diphosphonates have been found to have several effects on endosteal bone in rats (Evans et al., 1979). The level of activity of the osteoclast is reduced—this may occur by either an extracellular or cellular effect. Current evidence supports a toxic effect on the cellular level because of tissue culture studies, wherein fragmentation of osteoclast nuclei occurs with diphosphonate levels high enough to inhibit bone resorption (Rowe and Housemann, 1976). The result of this cellular effect is an increase in production of osteoclasts as a form of compensation for the reduced activity. The summed effect is reduced formation of bone at the endosteal surface.

For this reason, diphosphonates have been administered experimentally to prevent mineral deposition in patients with myositis ossificans and calcinosis universalis, and they have been given to enhance mineral deposition in patients with osteoporosis. Each of the many diphosphonates that have been studied has a slightly different action; some of them, such as disodium etidronate (EHDP), might be useful in osteoporosis except for undesirable side effects (particularly osteomalacia) produced by an optimum dose. Unless future studies can identify a place for these compounds in the treatment of osteoporosis, they must be viewed as a fascinating group having a limited clinical role in spite of their profound effects on the musculoskeletal system.

Fluoride. Skeletal fluorosis was initially recognized and described in 1937 in cryolite miners (Roholm). Later reports of osteosclerosis in patients living in areas with high concentrations of fluoride in the water supply, especially India (Singh et al., 1963), stimulated interest in fluoride as a beneficial agent for the treatment of osteoporosis. Subsequent metabolic studies demonstrated a variable effect of fluoride on calcium balance. Fluoride stimulates osteoblastic function in bone and stabilizes the hydroxyapatite crystal (Lane et al., 1984). The resulting histologic picture of increased osteoid border width, failed mineralization of cement lines, enlarged osteocyte lacunae, and increased cellularity of the new bone has been described by many investigators (Jowsey et al., 1968; Vigorita et al., 1983; Lane et al., 1984). The administration of fluoride alone induces histologic osteomalacia, in direct contrast to a more normal pattern of mineralized bone when calcium with or without vitamin D is included in the treatment regime. Even so, normal structure is never achieved, although abnormalities of bone morphology remodel to some extent with the cessation of fluoride intake.

An increase in bone resorption has been reported by many authors, but this effect is not as great as that seen in hyperparathyroidism, and there is also absence of paratrabecular fibrosis. It may be that calcium supplementation serves as a parathyroid gland suppressant during fluoride therapy. Concomitant administration of calcium and fluoride lowers serum fluoride levels, probably due to chelation (Jowsey and Riggs, 1978). This effect of calcium on fluoride absorption is quantitatively similar regardless of the dosage level.

The histologic picture of fluorosis has generated justifiable concern that the structural integrity of the bone may be undermined. Because increased crystallinity and possibly decreased elasticity have been observed in fluoridic bone (Wolinsky et al., 1972), new bone formation cannot automatically be equated with greater strength. High levels of fluoride in bone (5000 ppm or more) decrease its ultimate strength and modulus of elasticity compared to normal bones of equal density (see Fig. 7-4). A similar relationship probably exists for bones containing moderate levels of fluoride (1500 to 2000 ppm).

Numerous recent studies of osteoporotic patients treated with fluoride have demonstrated beneficial effects. Although the new bone thus produced is not normal, it represents nonetheless an increase in bone mass and as such provides some protection against fracture and pain (Grove and Halver, 1981; Harrison et al., 1981; Riggs et al., 1982; Williams, 1982; Lane et al., 1984). The crucial factor seems to be actual fluoride retention—evidenced by a serum fluoride level of 5.0 μmol/1 or greater. The protective effect of fluoride is delayed clinically by 12 to 18 months, probably reflecting the time necessary for mineralization of new osteoid. Later mineralization has been shown to occur in patients after cessation of fluoride therapy. Despite encouraging results, optimism must be tempered by reports of side effects in up to 42 percent of patients (Riggs et al., 1980, 1982). Side effects range from edema and arthralgias to recurrent vomiting, blood loss anemia, painful plantar fascial syndrome, and rheumatic synovitis. These side effects occur when dosage levels are in the 40 to 70 mg range. The gastrointestinal symptoms can be lessened with ingestion of fluoride with food. Rheumatic problems generally resolve with lowering of the dose, which can be slowly increased later.

Fluoride continues to be a promising agent for the treatment of osteoporosis. Its use requires supplemental calcium and vitamin D as well as careful monitoring of the clinical course. Patients who are nonresponders to treatment need to be identified. Further study may elucidate the reason for this nonresponse, and whether it represents a correctable deficit in the osteoblast or elsewhere.

Coherence Treatment: ADFR (activate-depress-free-repeat). The current accepted theory of bone remodeling emphasizes the importance of the basic multicellular unit (bone remodeling unit) that couples bone formation to bone resorption (Frost, 1966b, 1979, 1981). More than 95 percent of an adult's annual bone turnover is supplied by these units, and approximately 10^6 units are active in an adult skeleton at any one time (Frost, 1985). Quantum theory has been used to describe this system because all remodeling activity is carried out by discrete remodeling units that have a life of their own. Once a unit is activated, it remodels a known volume of bone (0.05 to 0.1 cu mm) within a discrete period of time (3 to 4 months), and once it has completed its task it is no longer active in bone remodeling. Each remodeling unit, therefore, represents a quantum (packet) of remodeling activity that in effect is the indivisible quantity of bone remodeling and it functions as an all or none phenomenon.

This raises questions about the efficacy of continuous treatment protocols for osteopenia. Normally, bone remodeling units are said to be "incoherent" because each is in a different stage of development, so cellular activity differs in each packet of cells with some remodeling units resorbing bone, some forming bone, and some in a latent phase. Most agents appear to act on more than one type of cell, but surprisingly little is currently known about this subject. Therefore, if an agent were given continuously, the net gain should be close to zero.

The concept of coherence treatment is to manipulate the cell "packets" so they are marching in step, with all cells in the same phase (Frost, 1981, 1984). A pulse of drug is given for a few days to activate new remodeling units, followed by a short course of treatment with a second drug to depress the resorption phase. No treatment is given during the bone formation phase. The cycle can be repeated every few months (the time lapse should be greater than the length of the remodeling cycle). Theoretically, the cells should form a normal amount of bone, but the resorption cavities will be shallower, and the net effect will be a gain in bone mass.

Early work with coherence treatment has shown encouraging results. In one study phosphate served as the activator and diphosphonate as the depressor. Phosphorus activates bone remodeling units by causing a slight decrease in ionized plasma calcium concentration, which leads to an increase in PTH secretion. Diphosphonate depresses bone resorption. In patients treated for 1½ years or more, trabecular thickness increased between 50 percent and 162 percent (Anderson et al., 1984).

The possibility of manipulating bone cell populations for therapeutic purposes heralds a new era in the treatment of bone disease. As a result, an unprecedented surge of interest in and knowledge of bone disease is likely to occur within the foreseeable future. The only information capable of dampening such a trend would be documented evidence that the concept of the "bone remodeling unit" is erroneous, a theory that has gained wide acceptance based on the types of studies performed in the past 25 years. Yet, a serious dearth of information exists regarding the specific effects of most drugs on the bone remodeling system. Much work will be needed to identify the most suitable drugs and to delineate the correct time intervals for treatment, which may vary from individual to individual, and from decade to decade of life.

The possibility exists that the etiology of osteoporosis will prove to be relatively unimportant once effective agents capable of influencing the various populations of bone cells have been identified. Finally, this theory offers numerous possibilities for treating afflictions of bone other than osteoporosis. Once enough is known about the specific action of various agents on bone it may be possible to manipulate coherent bone cell populations in order to remove excess bone (myelofibrosis, osteopetrosis, Engel-

mann's disease), to increase the turnover rate (elimination of toxic materials), and even to treat regional problems using special techniques (spinal or intracranial stenosis, dental problems, and other regional abnormalities).

Miscellaneous. Countless other forms of treatment have been attempted, including various types of diets and numerous medications, but none have proven efficacious. Calcitonin, due to its inhibitory effect on bone resorption, continues to hold interest, but further documentation is needed before its value can be determined. Recent results of a study by Rasmussen et al. (1980) demonstrated a 37 percent increase in absolute bone volume (85 percent increase in active bone formation surface and 64 percent increase in osteoid surface) in patients treated with oral phosphate and calcitonin. This study reported results after only 6 months of treatment, and obviously longer studies must be performed.

In conclusion, the recent flurry of activity in the investigation of osteoporosis has resulted in a bewildering mass of knowledge that serves to underscore the multi-factorial nature of the problem. Understandable frustration is thus engendered in the physician attempting to treat or prevent osteoporosis. The basic approach to the problem is still predicated upon the exclusion of unsuspected but treatable disease such as hyperparathyroidism, an "adequate" intake of calcium and vitamin D, and the encouragement of maximum physical activity. Certainly, the regime of calcium, vitamin D and fluoride with or without estrogen and progesterone can significantly decrease the incidence of new fractures (Lane et al., 1984). With more longterm studies, and further investigation of the ADFR concept, a more hopeful scenario may yet develop for the patient with osteoporosis.

REFERENCES

Albright F. Osteoporosis. Ann Intern Med 27:861, 1947.

Albright F, Smith PH, Richardson AM: Post menopausal osteoporosis: Its clinical features. JAMA 116:2465, 1941.

Anderson C, Cape RDT, Crilly RG, et al.: Preliminary observations of a form of coherence treatment for osteoporosis. Calc Tiss Res 36:341, 1984.

Anderson JJB, Milin L, Crackel WC: Effect of exercise on mineral and organic bone turnover in swine. J Appl Physiol 30(6):810, 1971.

Armbrecht HJ, Zenser TV, Davis BB: Effect of age on the conversion of 25-hydroxyvitamin D_3 to 1,25-dihydroxyvitamin D_3 by kidney of rat. J Clin Invest 66:1118, 1980.

Arnold JA: External and trabecular morphologic changes in lumbar vertebrae with aging. In Whedon GD, Cameron JR (eds): Progress in Methods of Bone Mineral Measurement. Washington, D.C., Gov Printing Office, 1970, p 352.

Avioli LV: Calcitonin therapy for bone disease and hypercalcemia. Arch Intern Med 142(12):2076, 1982.

Barzel US: The role of bone in acid base metabolism. In Barzel US (ed): Osteoporosis. New York, Grune, 1970, p 199.

Bassett CAL: Biophysical principles affecting bone structure. In skeleton or in most extracellular calcium deposits. The concentration differences are maintained by membrane function, especially the plasma membrane and the mitochondrial membrane. A microsomal fraction (these intracellular inclusions probably contain remnants of the endoplasmic reticulum) also accumulates calcium, but its role is less certain. A 5000- to 10,000-fold difference in calcium ion concentration can be maintained across the cell wall. Cellular calcium homeostasis, however, is probably controlled and regulated at the mitochondrial level, rather than at the plasma membrane (Borle and Anderson, 1976), since changes in this compartment often precede other cellular effects and the magnitude is greater. In addition, the calcium transport velocity and capacity of mitochondria is much larger than that of the plasma membrane, and the surface area of the mitochondrial inner membrane is 30 to 100 times greater than the plasma membrane surface. The mitochondrial calcium pool appears to serve the same general function in the cell as the bone mineral pool does in the body. Both serve as reservoirs with important buffer functions.

CALCIUM AND PHOSPHORUS INTAKE

Sources

Milk and milk products are the major sources of calcium. To exceed a dietary calcium intake of 1 g/day requires a large consumption of these food products, but there are many individuals whose intake is negligible. Green leafy vegetables, although not a good source, are probably second in importance to milk products, followed by calcium-enriched bread (Table 10–10). Most other items of the diet do not supply much calcium but are often rich in phosphorus.

There are, however, unappreciated sources of calcium, which, in many adults, can supply a high percentage of the daily intake. Water contains calcium and may supply up to 100 mg/liter; a six-pack of beer contributes 72 mg of calcium; most brands of toothpaste are rich in calcium; and many medications contain significant amounts (for instance, an antacid tablet may contain 200 mg).

Calcium supplements, given to augment intake, provide varying amounts of calcium depending on the compound (Table 10–11). On a per weight basis, calcium

TABLE 10-11. CALCIUM SUPPLEMENTS

Calcium Compound	Molecular Weight	Calcium Content (mg Ca/g compound)	Grams Needed to Provide 1 g Ca
Carbonate	100	400	2.5
Chloride	111	360	2.8
Phosphate	172	230	4.4
Citrate	570	211	4.7
Lactate	308	130	7.7
Gluconate	448	89	11

carbonate, a basic component of antacids, is the most efficient. It is also effectively absorbed by most people, so well, in fact, that an excessive intake may lead to hypercalcemia, soft-tissue calcification, and renal damage. The type of calcium compound given influences the amount absorbed. For example, a greater amount of calcium citrate is absorbed than calcium compound, as measured by urinary excretion after equal doses of calcium (Nicar and Pak, 1985). Particle size also influences absorption. Compounds of calcium carbonate with particles larger than 147μ are not as well absorbed as smaller particles, and those under $74\ \mu$ are even better absorbed (Anderson et al., 1984). Nevertheless, the differences in absorption between various compounds probably have little clinical importance.

Phosphorus is so widely distributed in foodstuffs that, in normal subjects, phosphate deficiency can only be produced artificially. Phosphorus is provided by milk, poultry, fish, and meat, as well as grains. Cold beverages are also high in phosphorus (20 mg/100 ml), but contain almost no calcium. There is a surprising discrepancy in the reported values of calcium and phosphorus contained in the average American diet, basic data that one might assume would be accurate. For instance, Lutwak (1975) stated that the level of phosphorus in the average American diet has progressively increased, as calcium intake has decreased. He reported that the Ca:P ratio in the American diet was 1:2.8 in 1955, and that milk consumption has decreased and meat consumption has increased since then, leading to a Ca:P ratio approaching 1:4.

In contrast, Page and Friend (1978) found that the intake of calcium increased between 1909 and 1957 with no significant change over the next 20 year period, whereas the intake of phosphorus was remarkably steady during the entire period. Therefore, little change occurred in the Ca:P ratio which was 1:1.9 in 1909, 1:1.55 in 1947, and 1:1.67 in 1976. These discrepancies underscore the difficulty of collecting data on dietary intake. Information for large population studies has usually been taken from economic data on commodities and food, or from surveys on food consumption of individuals. More recently, the Health and Nutrition Examination Survey (HANES) recorded food intake for the preceeding day only, a technique that would be expected to increase accuracy. The data shows a Ca:P ratio of 1:2 or greater with a lower intake of both calcium and phosphorus in older individuals (Table 10–12).

TABLE 10-10. SOURCES OF CALCIUM

Source	Calcium (mg/100 g)	Phosphorus (mg/100 g)
Cow's milk	120	100
Cheese	700–800	500–800
Cottage cheese	95	180
Lean meat	13	200
Eggs	54	205
Leafy vegetables	30–200+	30–80
Seeds	20–200	100–475
Fruits	6–20	10–50
Water	0.5–10	

TABLE 10-12. CALCIUM AND PHOSPHORUS INTAKE IN THE UNITED STATES

	N	Calcium (mg)		Phosphorus (mg)		Ca:P Based on	
		Mean	*50th Percentile*	*Mean*	*50th Percentile*	*Mean*	*50th Percentile*
Females							
25–44 years	2014	622	524	1008	925	1:1.6	1:1.8
45–74 years	3508	557	475	890	830	1:1.6	1:1.7
Males							
25–44 years	1812	923	768	1623	1500	1:1.8	1:2
45–74 years	3116	771	662	1307	1222	1:1.7	1:1.8

(From U.S. Dept. HHS (HANES-2), 1983.)

Numerous dietary constituents can alter the bioavailability of calcium or can influence the process of absorption. This topic will be discussed in part in this section and supplemented in the section on absorption.

More than 40 years ago it was discovered that whole wheat products contained an "anticalcifying factor" that caused a negative calcium balance (McCance and Widdowson, 1942). For several decades, this factor was thought to be phytic acid (inositol hexaphosphoric acid) or phytin (the calcium magnesium salt) which is present in cereals and seeds (Fourman and Royer, 1968). Phytic acid combines with calcium to form an insoluble salt, leading to the recommendation that it be used as a therapeutic agent to reduce calcium absorption in such conditions as sarcoidosis, vitamin D poisoning, and idiopathic hypercalcemia.

The subject is complicated by the fact that bacterial action in the large intestine digests some of the phytate, freeing calcium that is then available for absorption. It has been found that the ingestion of an equivalent amount of phytic acid as that present in whole grain bread has a neglible effect on calcium balance, indicating that some component other than phytin may play a major role.

It is now known that fiber itself impairs calcium absorption (Allen, 1982), and that the ingestion of foods that contain fiber, such as whole grain products, fruits, vegetables, soy beans, and unpolished rice decreases the amount of calcium absorbed. Fruits and vegetables supply about 12 percent of the calcium ingested in the American diet. Because of their fiber content, these foods cause a greater loss of calcium than they contribute to the diet. This adversely affects calcium balance.

Fiber contains structural components of the plant cell wall (cellulose, noncellulosic polysaccharides, and lignin), and nonstructural polysaccharides (pectins, gums, mucilages, and algal polysaccharides) (Southgate, 1978). Many of these components can bind calcium, but current evidence suggests that the common denominator may be uronic acids, which are associated with various components of fiber in concentrations that vary with the source of the fiber.

It has been calculated that the typical Western diet contains 17 g of fiber and 12 mM of uronic acids, capable of binding 152 mg of calcium. A high fiber diet contains 50 to 150 g of fiber and 30 to 110 mM of uronic acid, enough to bind all of the calcium in the diet, and a vegetarian diet contains enough uronic acid to bind 360 mg of calcium. Even so, 80 percent or more of the uronic acid ingested is fermented in the intestine and the calcium that is released also becomes available for absorption.

The influence of fiber components on calcium absorption has commonly been dismissed as an issue of little practical importance, yet numerous studies have shown that the addition of reasonable amounts of whole wheat, cellulose, fruits, or vegetables to normal diets consistently causes a negative calcium balance despite an adequate calcium intake. This suggests that the current trend to increase fiber intake in order to decrease the incidence of colon cancer may reflect adversely on the skeleton, especially on the development of osteoporosis. Further insight must await clearer elucidation of the interrelationships between varying dietary components and absorption. In any case, it seems wise to avoid the intake of calcium-rich foods, in particular calcium supplements, at the same time of day as foods high in fiber are consumed, to decrease the likelihood of interference. For practical purposes, calcium supplements should be the easiest to schedule in this manner.

Other dietary factors can influence the availability of calcium. Oxalate occurs in tea, as well as in green, leafy vegetables such as spinach, kale, and rhubarb, where it binds all of the calcium found in the leaves. Oxalate, however, does not interfere with the absorption of other sources of calcium ingested at the same time. Therefore, the calcium present in foods containing oxalate should be considered unavailable physiologically, and in this light oxalate would not contribute to a negative calcium balance. In effect, it simply removes a potential source of calcium from consideration.

Lactose improves calcium absorption in normal individuals (Fig. 10–12). The effect is greatest in the ileum where it enhances transport by diffusion, rather than active, vitamin D-dependent transport. As a result, long-term feeding of lactose to calcium-replete rats causes a decrease in mucosal calcium binding protein (CaBP) due to the enhanced calcium absorption.

A more complex mechanism exists in patients with lactase insufficiency and lactose intolerance. These patients develop gastrointestinal symptoms, such as flatulence, bloating, and diarrhea from milk. They also have an increased incidence of osteoporosis. Absorption studies using [47]Ca show a decrease in calcium absorption from milk (which contains lactose) with normal calcium absorption from lactose-free milk (Fig. 10–13). Yet the total there is some evidence it may be similar (Lutwak and Coulston, 1975). The mechanism of action might not be related to calcium absorption directly, but to increased phosphate absorption with a secondary depression of the serum calcium, thereby stimulating PTH secretion. A large body of information exists documenting various mechanical and physiologic effects caused by changes in the Ca:P ratio of animals, especially rats; the ratio is of greater importance in insuring normal bone mineralization than are the absolute amounts of the salts themselves (Bethke et al., 1932; Brown et al., 1932; Carttar et al., 1950; Schlicke, 1969).

For any given calcium intake, whether high or low, the percent ash content of bone decreases as the Ca:P ratio increases, due to inadequate mineralization and increased osteoid (rickets). The level of calcium intake also has an effect, but it is less important; for a given Ca:P ratio, the percent ash of bone increases as the calcium and phosphorus intake increases (except at higher levels of intake, if the ratio approximates 1:1). The changes seen in bone are most apparent in younger animals and decrease with time, even if the deprivation diet is continued (probably because the demand for calcium and phosphorus is greatest during periods of rapid growth). The most favorable Ca:P ratio ranges between 1.00 and 2.00; for an ideal ratio, such as 1.5, there is an optimum level of intake for calcium and phosphorus. A diet containing an optimum Ca:P ratio and an optimum intake produces maximum growth and a longer life span (in animals); in addition, the requirement for vitamin D is at a minimum, and histologic studies of bone show the least amount of osteoblast and osteoclast activity. Calcium and phosphorus intake levels lower than optimum can still support "normal" growth and reproduction, but the bones are shorter though of good quality. Severe restriction of calcium and phosphorus intake markedly impairs growth, and rickets develops. It is well known that rickets can be produced in animals by restricting the intake of phosphorus; however, a decrease in phosphorus increases the Ca:P ratio unless calcium is restricted as well. It is difficult to produce rickets if the intake of calcium is decreased proportionally to phosphorus (so an ideal Ca:P ratio is maintained). Rickets also develops if the intake of phosphorus is adequate but calcium intake increases enough to raise the Ca:P ratio above 5 to 6:1; the associated changes which occur include decreased growth, increased serum calcium (1 to 2 mg percent or more), decreased serum phosphate (1 mg percent), increased serum alkaline phosphatase, and decreased total body calcium and phosphorus. This condition has been termed "high-calcium rickets." As might be expected, corresponding changes occur in the physical properties of bone. In fact, measurable differences in the structural integrity of bone may precede unequivocal changes in mineral content. Many authors feel that the Ca:P ratio is not very important in humans, compared to animals. Unfortunately, today's fragmented knowledge of this subject often generates unjustified assumptions and erroneous conclusions that mislead, rather than enlighten. It is known that an increased load of phosphorus lowers the Ca:P ratio that at some ill-defined level stimulates para-

thyroid hormone secretion, probably due to an increase in plasma phosphorus and a decrease in calcium. This in turn increases the number of active bone remodeling units. The point of contention seems to be the level at which such an effect occurs and whether this mechanism ever becomes clinically important. If the Ca:P ratio does prove to be important in humans, as well as in animals, the phosphorus content of the American diet could have significant implications for the future, particularly in regard to osteoporosis.

Garn (1970) has approached the question of what constitutes an adequate calcium intake from an entirely different and possibly more meaningful direction. He performed extensive x-ray studies on normal individuals in eight different countries, including the United States, and calculated the amount of bone gained or lost at different ages throughout the life span. After comparing the changes in skeletal mass with the level of calcium intake, he has concluded that "it is no longer reasonable to assume that a high calcium diet promotes the integrity of compact bone or that a low calcium diet speeds bone loss either on a population basis or on an individual basis."

The extra skeletal benefits of calcium must not be overlooked as an additional bonus to calcium supplementation. A variety of medical problems improve with an increased intake of calcium. These include high blood pressure (McCarron et al., 1984), severe atherosclerosis, mortality from coronary heart disease, and the blood lipid profile (Renaud et al., 1983).

Infant. In the premature and possibly in the full-term infant calcium absorption occurs mainly by diffusion, because the mechanism needed for active absorption of calcium is not fully developed. The capacity for active absorption appears to be present in the premature, but it fails to respond normally to vitamin D stimulation.

The human body, like that of any other species, is calcium poor at birth. The fetal requirements for calcium and phosphorus accelerate after the 28th week, when the fetal skeleton contains approximately 5.5 g of calcium, since at term it contains about 30 g. During the first 2 years of life, the demands for both calcium and phosphorus are particularly high, since large amounts of these minerals are needed to insure postnatal growth and mineralization of the skeleton. If an infant is receiving milk in quantities sufficient to supply adequate calcium (125 to 150 mg per kilogram body weight per day), the requirements for phosphorus (95 mg per kilogram body weight per day) will be met. Such an infant will store about 40 mg of calcium per kilogram body weight per day.

There are subtle as well as obvious differences between cow's milk and human milk, which undoubtedly are related to species differences between the two animals (Table 10–14). Cow's milk contains about four times as much calcium, and six times as much phosphorus, as human milk; therefore, an infant receiving cow's milk has a much higher intake of calcium but an even higher intake of phosphorus. Since an infant absorbs an average of 30 percent (range 10 to 55 percent) of the calcium in cow's milk, and 60 percent (range 50 to 70 percent) in human

TABLE 10-14. COMPOSITION OF HUMAN AND COW'S MILK

	Human	Cow
Calories (per 100 g)	70	66
Carbohydrate (g/100 g)	7	5
Protein (g/100 g)	1.5	3.5
Fat (g/100 g)	4.0	3.5
Calcium (mg/100 g)	25–40	120
Phosphorus (mg/100 g)	16	95–100

milk, the lower calcium content of human milk is partially compensated. Likewise, an infant absorbs about 20 percent of the phosphorus in cow's milk and 50 percent of that in human milk. These differences in absorption could be due to the lower casein, the higher lactose, or the relatively higher albumin content of human milk compared to cow's milk. Babies receiving cow's milk lose less calcium in the urine, and it is possible that the low phosphorus content of human milk might be the limiting factor in calcium (and also magnesium) retention (Irving, 1973). Although much remains to be learned, there are indications that the calcium retention of babies fed human milk may not be adequate, and that the skeletal growth of babies on cow's milk may exceed that of breast-fed babies (Garry and Wood, 1946). This limitation of skeletal growth in breast-fed babies could be due to the lower phosphorus content of human milk, since studies of babies from the fifth to the eighth day of life have shown that phosphorus supplements to breast milk can increase calcium absorption and decrease urinary excretion. It is of interest that the rate of growth for various animals correlates with the calcium content of milk (Table 10–15).

Child and Adolescent. The calcium and phosphorus requirements of children can not be determined by balance procedures, since children normally maintain a positive balance due to growth, but the degree desirable is unknown. The daily calcium and phosphorus requirements per kilogram of body weight progressively decrease with age, while the total requirements increase because of increasing size. The maximum total requirement is reached during the adolescent growth spurt, in both males and females.

Adult. Several studies of adults have shown that calcium balance is in equilibrium on an intake of 10 mg calcium per kilogram body weight per day. However, the progres-

sive loss of bone (and of calcium) which begins in the fourth or fifth decade of life suggests that this assumption may be fallacius (unless some of the calcium is deposited extraskeletally, which would invalidate the balance studies). The universal occurrence of progressive bone loss in adults, regardless of the level of calcium intake, indicates that unknown factors are of equal or greater importance. Therefore, any specific recommendation of dietary calcium requirement is probably meaningless. For instance, the calcium intake of Bantu women is approximately half that of English women, but femoral neck fractures are less than one-tenth as frequent. In the United States the calcium intake of blacks is considerably less than that of whites (Table 10–16), but the bones of whites are more osteoporotic (Fig. 10–14) (Garn et al., 1976; Cohn et al., 1977; Mangaroo et al., 1985). If the level of calcium intake were the determining factor in osteoporosis, this information suggests that the calcium intake of whites may be excessive. Based on these results, it would be more logical to recommend a lower, not a higher, calcium intake for osteoporotic bones. The point is there are other factors besides calcium intake, for instance genetic predisposition, that determine bone strength.

CALCIUM AND PHOSPHORUS BALANCE

Classically, metabolic balance studies have been used for an overall assessment of calcium and phosphorus metabolism, but they do not provide information about intervening events within the organism. The addition of kinetic methods using labeled isotopes has contributed greatly to the understanding of calcium and phosphorus balance.

Balance studies are very different to perform accurately, making confinement in a metabolic unit essential in order to accurately measure intake and output. The studies must extend over a sufficient period of time to balance out inevitable errors in collection and measurement;

TABLE 10-15. WEIGHT INCREASE RATE OF INFANTS COMPARED TO CALCIUM CONTENT OF MOTHER'S MILK

Species	Days to Double Birth Weight	Calcium in Mother's Milk (%)
Man	180	0.02–0.03
Cow	47	0.12
Dog	7	0.32
Rabbit	6	0.517

TABLE 10-16. CALCIUM INTAKE OF BLACKS AND WHITES IN THE UNITED STATES

	N	Calcium (mg)	
		Mean	*50th Percentile*
Females			
White			
25–44 years	2840	659	544
45–65+ years	2753	591	506
Black			
25–44 years	669	421	356
45–65+ years	559	435	360
Males			
White			
25–44 years	1242	1021	844
45–65+ years	2476	779	661
Black			
25–44 years	206	727	607
45–65+ years	509	563	483

(From: U.S. Dept. HEW (HANES-1), 1979.)

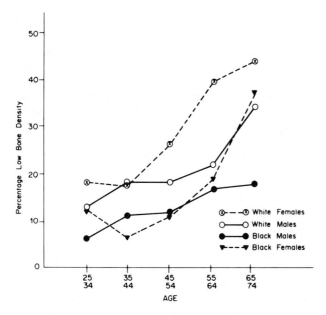

Figure 10–14. Percent of population with low bone density by age, sex, and race. U.S. adults, ages 24 to 75, Hanes/Survey, 1971–1975. Middle phalanx, little finger. Low bone density: less than 0.2 mm Al equivalence. *(From Mangaroo et al., Bone 6(3):135–138, 1985, Pergamon Press, Ltd, with permission.)*

the patients must be in a state of metabolic equilibrium, which negates studies following illness, fracture, or any change in the patient's normal routine. Arithmetically, the weakness of the method is greater when small differences are present, as in patients with idiopathic osteoporosis, where a daily deficit of 20 or 30 mg of calcium can be significant over a 30- or 40-year period. Even small errors can mask small deficits when the total calcium intake is 1000 g or more per day. All intake and output must be rigidly monitored, including vitamins, mouthwash, and toothpaste. Because of the lag period between ingestion and excretion in the stool, colored markers can be given for better differentiation between the beginning and end of study periods. Serious errors can occur from calcium lost in perspiration. This cannot be measured accurately but can be accommodated for by performing studies in an environment where the temperature and humidity are carefully monitored and controlled. With forced sweating, 0.64 mg calcium/10 ml of sweat has been measured by Vellar (1968) with a loss of 8 mg/hour. Consolazio et al. (1962) have reported that as much as 20 mg/hour could be lost under hot conditions, and with heavy sweating the loss might be 30 percent of the total excretion. The loss of phosphorus in sweat is negligible, as are other dermal losses of calcium and phosphorus (hair and nails). Much of the literature pertaining to balance studies at different ages has been summarized by Irving (1973).

In general, obligatory endogenous losses of calcium total 250 to 280 mg/day, which includes 100 to 130 mg/day in the stool, 150 mg/day in the urine, and 15 mg/day in sweat. These endogenous losses are relatively unaffected by the level of dietary calcium, so in the absence of other factors that alter the endogenous loss, calcium balance is largely regulated by the amount of calcium absorbed.

Morgan (1972, 1973) has conceptualized the metabolism of calcium and phosphorus into three components—*fluxes*, in intestine, kidney, and bone; *controllers*, which influence the fluxes; and *homeostatic systems*, which buffer the ECF concentrations against changes in the fluxes. The major net movements (fluxes) of calcium and phosphorus include:

1. The net absorption of calcium and phosphate from the intestine (the difference between intake and fecal excretion)
2. The rate of renal tubular reabsorption of calcium and phosphate
3. The rates of bone formation and bone destruction
4. The difference between the rates of bone formation and bone destruction (net bone formation and net bone destruction)

The magnitude of these fluxes has been tabulated for normal individuals (Table 10–17). The relation between the body and its external environment depends upon net movements of calcium and phosphate in the intestine, kidney, and bone and is measured by balance studies. Exchanges between the various compartments within the body can be estimated using kinetic analytic methods (Bauer et al., 1955; Heaney, 1964; Bronner, 1973), but major assumptions must be made regarding the compartments measured and interpretation of results. The theoretical problems inherent in kinetic studies can be minimized by coordinating other methods of investigation, such as morphologic studies of bone. However, each additional step greatly increases the complexity of investigation and must be measured against the expected return.

TABLE 10–17. RELATIVE MAGNITUDE OF THE MAJOR VARIABLES OF CALCIUM AND PHOSPHATE METABOLISM IN MIDDLE-AGED PERSONS

	Calcium		Phosphate	
	mg/day	%	mg/day	%
Intake	1000	—	1200	—
Intestine				
Net absorption	220	—	750	—
Bone				
Formation	200	—	100	—
Destruction	230	—	115	—
Net destruction	30	—	15	—
Kidney				
Filtered load	8000	100	4300	100
Tubular reabsorption	7750	97	3550	82
Urinary excretion	250	3	765	18

(From Morgan, 1972, with permission.)

ADAPTATION

It has been known for more than thirty years that animals, including man, can adapt to wide variations in dietary calcium, and that the proportion of calcium absorbed increases on a low-calcium diet (Nicolaysen et al., 1953). The net absorption of oral calcium rises considerably during growth, fracture healing, the treatment of rickets with vitamin D, or after removal of a parathyroid adenoma, and at such times almost all ingested calcium can be retained. Humans have been reported to be in equilibrium on calcium intakes as low as 100 to 200 mg per day. It has been noted that calcium retention depends upon the previous calcium intake, and when subjects are put on a low-calcium diet after subsisting at a high-calcium level, the bowel is unable to adapt immediately, leading to a negative calcium balance, which becomes less negative with time. The influence of dietary calcium on calcium absorption is probably mediated by PTH, causing an increase in the renal synthesis of 1,25-dihydroxycholecalciferol (1,25-[OH]$_2$D$_3$) (assuming there is an adequate vitamin D intake). The mechanisms by which calcium deprivation stimulates absorption could involve a marginal reduction of plasma ionized calcium concentration, leading to a stimulation of PTH secretion, which in turn activates 1-hydroxylase activity in the kidney, resulting in an increase in circulating 1,25-(OH)$_2$D$_3$ and thus to increased calcium transport in the intestinal cell.

ABSORPTION

The ultimate source of calcium and phosphorus is food, and specific mechanisms have evolved for extracting these nutrients in the intestine. The epithelial cells that control the entrance of various substances into the body contain a number of subcellular structures and organelles in common with other cells, but they also have their own unique features. The cells are polarized with microvilli on one surface, the nucleus in the basal portion, and relatively smooth lateral and basement membranes. The microvilli are covered with a mucopolysaccharide coat (glycocalyx) that contains anionic groups that might complex calcium or other ions.

Although little if any calcium is absorbed in the stomach, it is in the stomach that much of the calcium is brought into solution, presumably to facilitate absorption. Due to hydrochloric acid, the gastric contents are acidic, with a pH of about 2.0. The acidic medium favors the liberation of calcium ions, preparatory to absorption in the small bowel. The rate of absorption is probably greatest in a mildly acid or moderately alkaline pH (below 8.5).

It has long been assumed that gastric acid enhances calcium absorption and that achlorhydria has an adverse effect. Recent evidence indicates that the presence of gastric acid may not be as critical to calcium absorption in humans as was formerly thought (Bo-Linn et al., 1984). Yet it is known that skeletal problems often occur in post gas-

trectomy patients, and this suggests that calcium absorption may be deficient, as well. It appears that a relative decrease in calcium absorption occurs. In the absence of gastric acid, soluble forms of calcium, such as calcium chloride or calcium gluconate can be absorbed normally, but less soluble forms such as calcium carbonate or tricalcium phosphate are not absorbed as well (Mahoney et al., 1975). Furthermore, gastrectomy patients absorb calcium in calcium gluconate better than in food, and the calcium in calcium lactate better than in milk.

In the presence of food, the pH is approximately 6.0 in the proximal jejunum, and 7.6 (never below 6.5) in the mid and lower ileum.

A number of mechanisms have been proposed to describe the transport of calcium across the intestinal mucosa, and the overall process has been extensively investigated. Yet studies of absorption are difficult to perform, and progress has been hampered by the practical difficulties encountered in experimental studies, whether in vivo or in vitro. The most widely used in vitro technique has been the inverted intestinal sac preparation, but it rapidly loses its structural integrity (at 30 minutes, 50 to 75 percent of the mucosal epithelium disappears), and this may account for some of the discrepancies in the literature. Nevertheless, it has been repeatedly demonstrated that calcium is absorbed by at least two processes: (1) a saturable, carrier-mediated, energy dependent (and vitamin D dependent) process, and (2) a nonsaturable process of diffusion. Total calcium absorption is the sum of saturable and nonsaturable functions, and it is an exponential function of intake (Pansu et al., 1980). From a practical standpoint: (1) At a given intraluminal calcium concentration, absorption is regulated by factors that effect the saturable component (calcium, vitamin D status, age, pregnancy, and lactation); (2) absorption by diffusion is a linear function of the luminal calcium concentration with about 25 percent absorbed regardless of the activity of the saturable component; and (3) diffusion is relatively unimportant at lower luminal calcium concentrations, but it becomes increasingly important as calcium concentration increases.

All segments of the bowel appear capable of active calcium transport, as well as of diffusion. The efficiency of absorption (the amount of calcium absorbed per unit length of bowel) in the small intestine is greatest in the proximal duodenum and decreases progressively distally. Efficiency correlates with the amount of CABP in the bowel wall. The highest concentrations are found in the first part of the duodenum with lower levels distally, but measurable levels are still present in the ileum (Sommerville et al., 1985).

It is now known that active calcium absorption occurs in the colon, at least in the ascending and descending colon of the rat, but not in the transverse colon (Favus et al., 1980). Active calcium absorption in the colon also occurs in humans and normal absorption may be present in patients with extensive small bowel resections, as long as the colon is intact and the patient does not have an ileostomy (Hylander et al., 1980). In most species, absorption

Present evidence indicates that calcitonin if given in large enough doses will increase urinary phosphate excretion, probably through a direct action on the kidney. In addition, it increases the renal content and urinary excretion of cyclic AMP, it activates renal adenylate cyclase, it inhibits the conversion of 25-(OH)D_3 to 1,25-(OH)$_2D_3$, and it can produce hypercalcuria. These effects, however, are of questionable significance physiologically, as suggested by the failure of thyroidectomy to produce any unique alterations in urinary electrolyte excretion that can be specifically corrected by the administration of calcitonin.

In the gastrointestinal tract calcitonin inhibits the secretion of gastric acid, pepsin, pancreatic enzymes, and insulin. This provides a mechanism for protecting against excessively rapid absorption of calcium in order to avoid hypercalcemia. In addition, certain gastrointestinal hormones, such as gastrin and cholecystokinin, are powerful stimulants of calcitonin secretion, but the responsible mechanisms and ultimate implications remain uncertain.

The interaction of calcitonin with other glands and hormones is complex and incompletely defined. Calcitonin and PTH are antagonistic in their effects on the concentration of serum calcium, on the rate of transfer of calcium and phosphate from bone to blood, and on the rate of bone resorption. Both hormones show a similar phosphaturic effect on the renal handling of inorganic phosphate, although the effect of PTH is within the physiologic range, whereas a larger dose of CT is required. PTH conserves calcium by promoting reabsorption by the renal tubule, while CT increases urinary excretion. Interactions with adrenal cortical hormones, estrogens, androgens, and thyroid have received considerable interest but need to be better defined.

The final explanation for the action of calcitonin probably lies in a clearer understanding of the cellular and subcellular response. Only then will it be possible to integrate isolated observations of CT action, such as the stimulation of phosphate uptake in bone cells, the enhancement of CT effect by simultaneous infusion of phosphate, the stimulation of urinary cyclic AMP (similar but less pronounced than with PTH), and the production of hypophosphatemia (by calcitonin) without a significant hypocalcemia. It is possible that a simultaneous increase of phosphate uptake into the cell or the mitochondria, with a stimulation of calcium ion efflux and adenylate cyclase activation, could cause a decrease in cytosol or mitochondrial Ca^{2+} concentration and an increase in HPO_4^{2-} concentration, which would explain the observed responses (Borle, 1975; Rasmussen et al., 1976).

Consider the action of calcitonin in its day-to-day role in the conservation of calcium. A calcium-rich food is consumed, and this stimulates the secretion of calcitonin, whether due to the release of gastrointestinal hormones in the blood, to calcium absorption that causes a mild increase in serum calcium, or to some other factor. Calcitonin then inhibits secretory functions in the bowel that delays further calcium absorption, and it blocks osteolysis, which also decreases the release of calcium into the blood. These actions serve to prevent hypercalcemia. During periods of high calcium intake, the conservation ac-

tion of calcitonin becomes superfluous, as other mechanisms are active. Therefore, the end organs escape, but the ability of the system to respond is restored once the calcium-rich period is over.

One additional characteristic of calcitonin is a gradual loss of effect, or an adaptation to the hormone that occurs on repeated administration. The duration of exposure, therefore, seems to be important for end organ reactivity, as the osteoclasts escape from the inhibition imposed by calcitonin. In vitro studies show that PTH-stimulated resorption can only be prevented for about one day by adding calcitonin, and in vivo rat studies show that calcitonin prevents the rise in serum calcium only for one day. The escape phenomenon of osteoclasts appears to characterize normal, but not abnormal, cells. For instance, the osteoclasts in Paget's disease do not escape. Adaptation has also been demonstrated in the bowel (Ziegler et al., 1984).

In summary, calcitonin is more active physiologically after acute than chronic administration, and it probably plays a more important role in calcium homeostasis during periods of low calcium intake.

CALCIUM AND PHOSPHORUS HOMEOSTASIS

The term "homeostasis" refers to the biologic regulatory mechanisms that maintain the internal environment of the body in a relatively steady state. The internal environment is represented by the blood and the various interstitial (intercellular) tissue fluids, including that which permeates the ground substance of bone. Since the calcium and phosphate content of the diet may vary considerably, and since bone resorption, accretion, and mineral exchange may show wide fluctuations under normal conditions, as well as in disease, an elaborate system is required to control intestinal absorption, membrane transfer, and renal excretion. These mechanisms carefully guard the concentration of calcium and phosphate in plasma and extracellular fluid and are critical to the health of the individual and the integrity of the skeletal system. Wide fluctuations in plasma calcium concentration can adversely effect any of its multiple functions; the most critical problems occur at the neuromuscular junction, which becomes hyperexcitable when calcium is insufficient in amount, and this can result in tetany and convulsions. In fact, the plasma calcium concentration is preserved at the expense of the skeleton.

A useful distinction that can help clarify the increasing and often confusing information available on this subject is the distinction between skeletal and mineral metabolism. Although the skeleton represents the major mineral pool, and as such is common to both systems, it is possible to conceptualize skeletal function separately from mineral metabolism, even though a change in one inevitably is reflected by a change in the other. Skeletal metabolism maintains the supporting framework for normal musculoskeletal function, whereas mineral metabolism maintains ion concentrations within the limits necessary for normal physiologic and cell function.

Because the extracellular fluid compartment contains

concentrations of ionized calcium and phosphate that are supersaturated with respect to bone, a constant calcium gradient exists from blood to bone. Since the rate of calcium uptake by bone is usually greater than the rate of absorption by the gut, a continuous return of calcium from bone to extracellular fluid must be maintained, a process controlled by PTH. In the absence of this hormone, extracellular fluid calcium levels fall, but the reverse does not occur in the absence of calcitonin. Without calcitonin, the fine control of plasma calcium may be decreased, but the overall loss of control is negligible.

The level of serum calcium is controlled by a series of feedback mechanisms involving three endogenous hormones—PTH, calcitonin, and 1,25-(OH)$_2$D$_3$, a highly potent sterol derivative, which, by its control of calcium-binding protein synthesis, mediates the transport of calcium into and out of the extracellular space, including plasma. Plasma phosphate is partly controlled by the action of PTH and vitamin D on bone, in addition to the exquisite sensitivity of renal phosphate reabsorption to PTH. Therefore, the interactions of the three hormones maintain calcium and phosphate levels within the narrow range necessary for normal function of the neuromuscular system. In addition, three exogenous factors (calcium, phosphorus, and vitamin D) also affect homeostasis, yet the specific requirements of these are unknown.

There is evidence that the response of the individual cell is the common denominator regulating calcium-dependent processes, whether skeletal, extracellular, or cellular. Therefore, extracellular calcium homeostasis depends on a complex relationship between cellular activity and ionic concentrations, particularly of Ca^{2+}, H$^+$, and HPO$_4^{2-}$. These ions are part of an interrelated ionic network, within and without the cell, such that a change in the concentration of one results in systematic, though incompletely understood, changes in the others. The hormones controlling calcium and phosphate metabolism, namely PTH, calcitonin, and 1,25-(OH)$_2$D$_3$, do so through their effects on cellular activity and on ion concentration.

Regulation of calcium in the extracellular fluids is achieved by controlling its flux across the renal tubule, the intestinal mucosa, and bone. For theoretical purposes, the calcium control mechanisms are often considered similar at the three sites, though significant differences exist. PTH acts at all three sites (its action in the intestine may be indirect through the control of 1,25-[OH]$_2$D$_3$ synthesis in the kidney), causing a movement of calcium into the ECF and thereby increasing the plasma calcium concentration. The action of PTH on bone and on intestine is accompanied by a movement of phosphate into the plasma, while PTH action on the proximal renal tubule moves phosphate out of the plasma and increases urinary phosphate excretion; overall, this not only prevents hyperphosphatemia, but may cause hypophosphatemia. The decrease in plasma phosphate concentration facilitates the effect of PTH on plasma calcium by inhibiting bone mineral deposition and enhancing resorption.

The sequence of events set in motion by a change in the plasma calcium is illustrated by hypocalcemia (see Fig. 10–8). When the blood becomes slightly hypocalcemic, the parathyroids respond by secreting PTH into the peripheral circulation. A transient fall in plasma calcium concentration occurs initially (clinically, this is masked by an increase in plasma and urine calcium) due to the uptake of calcium by renal and bone cells. The increased cytosol calcium concentration activates the calcium pump, resulting in the release of calcium into the general ECF and plasma. The ECF calcium concentration then rises progressively after a 1- to 2-hour lag period. The resulting increase in plasma calcium inhibits PTH secretion, thus restoring balance.

In contrast to hypocalcemia, an increase in the plasma calcium concentration inhibits PTH secretion, but it stimulates calcitonin secretion by the C cells in the thyroid (see Fig. 10–9). These two hormones work in an opposing manner to control the calcium concentration, and the action of both is interrelated to that of vitamin D. In the absence of vitamin D, PTH cannot mobilize bone mineral in order to elevate the plasma calcium concentration, nor can vitamin D mobilize bone mineral in the absence of PTH. Calcitonin, however, is able to lower the plasma calcium in the absence of vitamin D; in fact, the presence of calcitonin decreases the activity of vitamin D by inhibiting the conversion of 25-(OH)D$_3$ to 1,25-(OH)$_2$D$_3$.

A number of theories have been proposed to explain the mechanisms that regulate bone mineral mobilization. The more prevalent concepts include the following: (1), 1,25-(OH)$_2$D$_3$ induces the formation of one or more proteins that transfer calcium from bone fluid to bone cells; (2) PTH increases the rate of calcium uptake by the cells, while calcitonin has the opposite effect; (3) in vitamin D deficiency, the entrance of calcium into the cells is limited and PTH has little influence. Basically, these theoretical actions could shift the balance between bone mineral deposition and dissolution by fine adjustments of calcium levels in the interstitial fluid of bone. The action of vitamin D on bone mineral mobilization is blocked completely by actinomycin D, providing evidence that RNA protein synthesis has a crucial role in this process.

Until relatively recently, there was no satisfactory explanation for two basic problems of mineral metabolism: (1) the role of bone mineral in calcium homeostasis and (2) the interaction of bone with a plasma calcium × phosphate product that is supersaturated with respect to the mineral phase (the solubility product of apatite crystals is much lower than the calcium and P$_i$ concentrations in plasma).

Indirect evidence now suggests that two separate fluid compartments exist in bone, separated by a continuous layer of cells, variously called the bone membrane, the resting or surface osteoblast layer, or the surface layer (see Fig. 10–3). Except in areas of increased cellular activity, this lining or envelope may be only one cell thick, although it is possible that areas of low reactivity exist where the surface is devoid of cells and coated with pyrophosphate or other material. The percentage of such "bare" areas on the total bone surface appears to increase with age.

One compartment contains bone fluid (bone ECF) in direct contact with the bone mineral; it possesses different be used to describe the change in the vasculature in response to fracture, rather than "hyperemia." While they suggested that there was a "coordinated effort" between the vessels and osteogenic cell proliferation, they carefully avoided conclusions regarding cellular origin.

Rhinelander (1968, 1974; Rhinelander and Baragry, 1962; Rhinelander et al., 1968) extensively studied the blood supply of healing fractures using a microangiographic technique similar to that used by Trueta. He noted differences in the vascular pattern in response to nondisplaced and displaced fractures. In the former, the medullary vessels always seem to play the major role in providing blood supply to the callus and necrotic bone ends. In displaced fractures, the periosteal network derived from torn muscles about the fracture was paramount in the first week, although endosteal callus provided the earliest osseous union. During later stages of healing, the medullary network became more important than the periosteal network, as with the nondisplaced fractures.

Soft tissue vasculature also plays a major role in fracture healing, particularly in surgically treated fractures. Whiteside and Lesker have demonstrated that extraperiosteal dissection compromised the collateral circulation to crushed (but not uncrushed) muscle (1978a), and that the radiographic union rate in their rabbit tibial model was much lower (7 percent versus 71 percent) with extraperiosteal versus subperiosteal dissection (1978b). The surgeon who chooses to treat fractures by open methods should be aware of the importance of the extraperiosteal circulation.

Most of the emphasis on the role of blood supply has been in the early stages of fracture healing. Sim and Kelly (1970) pointed out, however, that the vasculature continues to be regulated throughout the healing process and in their experimental model was related to bone remodeling. They further suggested that there might be some metabolic factor linking flow to the tissue's need for nutrients.

While the gross morphologic changes of limb vasculature with fracture have been reasonably well described, the concomitant physiologic effects are less well identified and understood. Among the altered metabolic conditions are a low oxygen tension and normal oxygen consumption with increased blood flow as measured by platinum microelectrodes implanted in healing bone defects (Heppenstall et al., 1975). This finding is consistent with a recent report by Paradis and Kelly (1975), who found that increased bone blood flow and increased mineral deposition after fracture are closely related. In the dog, they demonstrated a peak blood flow approximately five times the control value at 10 days. The timing of this peak correlates with the peak vascular volume found by Wray and Lynch in the rat, although one might anticipate some differences in fracture healing in the rat and dog from a temporal standpoint. The findings of Heppenstall and his colleagues led them to suggest that new formation occurs under anaerobic conditions that persist until the vascularity matches the cellularity. These conclusions are consistent with Goldhaber's (1958) report of bone formation in cell culture under low oxygen tension.

Brookes (1971) suggested that the pH is decreased and the P_{CO_2} is increased initially after fracture. As new vessels grow into the fracture area and blood flow increases, the pH becomes elevated and the P_{CO_2} diminished. With decreasing vascularity, the pH and P_{CO_2} tend toward normal. Furthermore, Brookes believed that a low pH and reduced blood flow favored the formation of compact bone, while a high pH and blood flow favored the formation of trabecular bone. Heppenstall et al. (1975) demonstrated only minimal changes in the P_{CO_2}, and the changes did not parallel those suggested by Brookes. These metabolic changes have an impact on the early milieu that results in cellular proliferation and differentiation. It seems likely, given available information, that the gross vascularity has less to do with whether or not a fracture will heal, than on the metabolic conditions the vascularity creates. Since manipulations and surgery, as well as soft tissue swelling, all have the capacity to adversely affect the vascularity, and indirectly the metabolic milieu, the physician must insure that the advantages of any interventions outweigh their potential harmful effects.

Cell Origin

Marchand, in 1902, suggested that osteoblasts arise from mesenchymal cells, and Baschkirzew and Petrow, in 1912, further suggested that mesenchymal cells were pluripotent (Bassett, 1962). There is no reason to doubt that fibroblasts, chondroblasts, and osteoblasts (and indeed their mature forms) are derived from pluripotent mesenchymal cells (Hall, 1971; Bassett, 1972). The source of the mesenchymal cells remains unclear, however, and there are conflicting opinions. It seems likely that primitive cells from muscle and fascia (Brookes, 1971), periosteum (Tonna and Cronkite, 1961b; Chalmers et al., 1975), endothelial or perivascular cells (Trueta, 1961, 1963), marrow cells, and circulating cells (Ostrowski and Wlodarski, 1971) may all be responsible for the formation of bone-forming cells. Bone-forming cells, however, may also arise directly from fibrous tissue (Ruedi and Bassett, 1967) and cartilage cells (Bohatirchuk, 1969; Mindell et al., 1971), as well as from the more primitive cells. Evidence suggesting multiple origins requires a potential of cellular differentiation that allows cells of mesenchymal origin to be readily interconvertible into various primitive and mature forms, or at least to take on different morphologic and structural characteristics under different stimuli (Urist et al., 1965; Becker and Murray, 1967; Hall and Shorey, 1968; Hall, 1971). Furthermore, the placement of dead bone graft within a millipore chamber with resulting bone formation surrounding, but not within the chamber suggests that new living bone cells are of host origin, and that the bone graft contains some diffusible bone inducing agent (Algire et al., 1954; Goldhaber, 1961).

Perhaps more complex than the question of cell origin is the identification of those factors that stimulate osteoprogenitor cells (the cells from which osteoblasts arise) to differentiate into the more specialized forms. Many specific as well as nonspecific agents (e.g., drugs) have been demonstrated to affect fracture repair and it is increasingly apparent that the regulation of bone formation is extremely complex (Raisz and Kream, 1983). Systemic factors (e.g., calcium parathormone) and local factors (Levander, 1938; Urist, 1972) both affect osteogenesis at its many stages. Chalmers and his associates (1975) suggested three requirements for osteogenesis: (1) an inducing agent, (2) an osteogenic precursor cell, and (3) a permissive environment.

The in vitro technique of bone-cell culture introduced by Dame Honor Fell in 1928 (Fell, 1969) greatly enhanced the study of osteogenesis owing to the exquisite control of environmental variables. For example, Bassett and Herrmann, in 1961, using cell cultures, demonstrated that compaction and high oxygen content lead to bone formation from primitive mesenchymal cells, confirming Glucksman's earlier observations (1939). Compaction and low oxygen content, on the other hand, resulted in cartilage formation, while mechanical tension and high oxygen content formed fibrous tissue. The studies of Johnson and Southwick (1960) have also suggested that tension leads to fibroplasia. Recently, Yeh and Rodan (1984) demonstrated that osteoblasts submitted to tensile forces produced markedly increased quantities of Protaglandin E. Prostaglandins are known to be intercellular mediators and can stimulate osteoblastic activity as well as in vitro bone resorption (Raisz and Kream, 1983) and they may therefore be an important link between mechanical stimulation and cellular responses. Cell cultures have also been utilized to study the effects of other variables such as pH, parathormone, and vitamins on osteogenesis (Bassett, 1971). Although one must exercise some caution in drawing conclusions about in vivo bone formation based purely on cell culture observations, it is clear that bone formation and repair are dependent on both the mechanical and chemical environment.

Evidence to date suggests that a variety of local factors regulate or stimulate osteoprogenitor cells. Urist and his colleagues have identified a 17,000 Dalton, diffusible protein ("bone morphogenetic protein" or BMP) in bone that stimulates the formation of osteoprogenitor cells (Urist et al., 1982, 1983). This inducing agent has been shown to stimulate bone formation under a wide variety of experimental conditions and to result in the healing of large defects in rat fibulas that did not usually heal with grafts (Oikarinen and Korhonen, 1979). Bone also contains a neutral protease which can degrade BMP (Urist et al., 1972). A larger 83,000 Dalton protein ("human skeletal growth factor" or HSGF) has been reported to be a potent stimulus to the proliferation of osteoprogenitor cells (Farley and Baylink, 1982; Farley et al., 1982). In addition, Puzas et al. (1981a, 1981b) have identified a small (6,000 to 14,000 Dalton) polypeptide in bone that inhibits the proliferation of cells without affecting their ability to synthesize proteins, and Drivdahl et al. (1981) (in the same group of researchers) have identified a 12,000 Dalton substance in bone that stimulates the proliferation of cells. This latter substance may or may not be related to BMP. Thus, it appears that there are a number of substances in bone that allow local regulation.

In addition to local factors in bone, Hulth (1980) has recently postulated, based on empiric evidence, that damaged soft tissues can stimulate the formation of either bone or fibrous tissue by some as yet unidentified mechanism. Rubin (1985) and others (e.g., Sheldrake, 1981) have suggested that the differentiation of cells is controlled in part by "morphogenetic fields." The nature of such fields has not been explored or identified, but they may be thought of as analogous to an electrical field. While the experimental evidence to support this hypothesis is limited, available evidence is clearly consistent with such a notion as are the clinical facts reviewed by Hulth (1980).

Production of Extracellular Matrix

As the appropriate cellular milieu is being formed for fracture repair, the new cells begin producing their characteristic extracellular matrix (Duthie and Barker, 1955a, 1955b; Carneiro and Leblond, 1959; Nusgens et al., 1972). Some of the factors responsible for cellular differentiation or proliferation may act to stimulate cells to form a matrix, but there are undoubtedly factors that affect only the synthetic activity of cells. Only recently have any of these factors been identified. For example, variation in electrostatic fields seems to strongly affect collagen synthesis by fibroblasts (Hall, 1968; Bassett and Herrmann, 1968), while Actinomycin D is known to diminish protein synthesis in osteogenic cells (Brazell and Owen, 1971).

Regardless of what stimulates matrix production in healing fractures, it is clear that along with cellular proliferation (and DNA production), there is an increase in the synthesis of proteins as reflected by an increase in RNA (Deutsch and Gudmundson, 1971). This rise in RNA precedes the production of the collagenous and noncollagenous proteins in the callus. In the rat, there is a peak production of mucopolysaccharides at 1 to 2 weeks postfracture, followed by a fall to normal levels at 4 to 7 weeks (Udupa and Prasad, 1963; Lane et al., 1979a). It is presumed that this early rise is related to matrix production, primarily by the cartilage cells participating in the repair process, although fibroblasts and bone cells are also known to produce mucopolysaccharides (Godman and Porter, 1960; Moore and Schoenberg, 1960).

Collagen production (as determined by [C-14]-L-proline incorporation and hydroxyproline levels), while also peaking at one to two weeks, does not diminish as rapidly and is probably related to the cellular activity of both fibroblasts and osteoblasts in the fracture callus (Udupa and Prasad, 1963; Stacher and Firschein, 1967; Kuhlman and Bakowski, 1975). The prolonged elevated production levels of collagen are undoubtedly related to osteoblastic activity during the repair and remodeling phases of healing. The studies, however, of Lane et al. (1979b) suggest temporal differences in the amount of collagen (and hexosamines) produced in immobilized versus nonimmobilized rats. Thus, the matrix production appears to be dependent on a specific situation (e.g., species, type of immobilization, and perhaps even the particular bone). There is also evidence to suggest that the early collagen production by the osteoblasts is high in hydroxylysine content and, therefore, more like embryonic than adult bone collagen (Ellis et al., 1976). Furthermore, the type of collagen (i.e., type I or type II) may be dependent on the degree of immobilization since principally Type I collagen was seen in while in other bones ultimate torsional strength or toughness might be more pertinent. The appropriate determination of strength should therefore include an array of selected tests that would reflect relevant properties.

Owing to the difficulties of comparing fracture healing in animal models, Lindsay and Howes (1931), reported the use of a standardized model for mechanically testing healed tibial fractures in rats. Their study had the obvious limitations previously noted, but it represented a new direction. Later studies by McKeown et al. (1932) and Eskelund and MunkPlum (1950) clearly showed the poor correlation between the radiographic findings and histology and breaking strength.

Recent investigators have made use of many mechanical properties to study fracture healing (Falkenberg, 1961; Laurin et al., 1963; Bourgois and Burny, 1972; Jorgensen, 1972a, 1972b; Lightowler and Swanson, 1972; Hernandez-Richter et al., 1973). The general correlation of "elasticity" with "ultimate strength" has resulted in the common use of stiffness as a nondestructive criterion for healing (Mather, 1967), although it is not entirely satisfactory from all aspects. At least one observer (Jernberger, 1970) has used an invasive technique to study the changes in the stiffness of fracture callus in humans.

Floriani et al., in 1967, noted that the physical properties of bone were related to the velocity of sound across it. Specifically, the ultrasonic properties of bone are directly related to its elastic properties, which are in turn determined by the organic as well as inorganic constituents of the material. Several groups have subsequently used ultrasound techniques to study fracture healing (Abendschein and Hyatt, 1972; Gerlanc et al., 1975). Markey and Jurist (1974) reported that the resonant frequencies of vibrated bone might be a useful means of assessing fracture strength. Lewis and Tarr (1975) assessed healing by determining the acceleration of healing bone after impact and, using similar principles, Saha and Pelker (1976) determined the state of healing by measuring stress–wave response of a healing bone to impact loading. The development of similar nondestructive, noninvasive techniques that correlate with mechanical and chemical properties of fracture callus could potentially be of great help in more objectively studying the healing fracture, both for experimental studies and for clinical assessments. However, the practical problems associated with them (e.g., the errors created by overlying soft tissues and the variability of data from differing sorts of callus) have not been solved.

Delayed Union and Nonunion

In any group of patients with similar fractures, the healing times for the majority will be reasonably uniform (i.e., within a matter of weeks of each other). A minority of the group will have healing times much longer than "usual" or "normal," or indeed, may fail to heal. When fractures require longer than the usual time to heal but are still showing definite signs of progression in healing, a delayed union exists. A nonunion is present when the fracture is unhealed beyond the "ordinary" time that would be anticipated, and shows no tendency toward further healing.

There are certainly as many reasons for delayed union or nonunion as there are factors affecting fracture healing. In most clinical cases, those factors likely to influence nonunions can be identified (Table 11–1). For example, inadequate immobilization (either in terms of type or length of time) may be responsible in human fractures if the fracture then heals after subsequent satisfactory immobilization. Soft-tissue interposition has been clinically and experimentally shown to retard fracture healing (Altner et al., 1975). While impaired blood supply is often thought to be a cause of slow healing, Laurnen and Kelly (1969) and Rhinelander et al. (1968) have shown increased blood flow to limbs with delayed unions. Less often, some pathologic condition such as malignancy or infection, may interfere with normal union. In spite of the fact that slow healing rates may be explained in many fractures, however, there remain some that have no discernible explanation for their failure to heal.

It is of interest to note that there are relatively few experimental studies of nonunions in animal models (Pearse and Morton, 1931, 1937; Kindred and Adams, 1965). This is because nonunions are so rare in small animals and, in fact, difficult to produce. Lindholm et al. (1969) produced nonunions in rats by daily manipulation of femur fractures, but found they all healed if manipulation was stopped. They stated nonunion "has not been observed" in immobilized rats. Altner and his associates (1975) were able to produce nonunions in 9 out of 10 of their experimental dogs in whom they had interposed muscle tissue in a 3 to 5 millimeter defect in the ulna. Cavadias and Trueta (1965) produced nonunions of osteotomies in the radius of dogs when the periosteal vessels and either nutrient vessels or metaphyseal vessels were disrupted. Whiteside and Lesker (1978b) were able to produce nonunions in rabbit tibias with extensive extraperiosteal dissection. More recently, Fuentes et al. (1984) produced delayed union (i.e., 12 weeks postoperatively) in the radius of 25 of 40 dogs with simple osteotomy and in 39 of 50 dogs with bone resection followed by weight bearing without immobilization. Thus, significant sur-

TABLE 11–1. FACTORS RELATED TO DELAYED UNION OR NONUNION

Factors associated with fracture
   Location
   Soft tissue damage
   Soft tissue interposition
   Bone loss
   Contamination, infection
   Tumor

Factors associated with treatment
   Inadequate reduction
   Inadequate fixation (external, internal)
      Inadequate extent of fixation
      Inadequate time of fixation
   Distraction
   Damage to blood supply with open reduction
   Postoperative infection

Unexplained

gical efforts are required to produce nonunions in small animals. The lack of good animal models of closed nonunions has hampered our knowledge about the cellular and chemical characteristics of nonunions.

Nonetheless, there are a few studies that provide some clues to the chemical processes occurring in nonunions in man. The early studies of Wendeberg (1961) suggest that mineral uptake is not markedly different from that in normally healing fractures. His findings have been substantiated by Puranen et al. (1975). Shaffer et al. (1971) demonstrated increased strontium uptake in the nonunion of a child, again documenting that failure to mineralize tissues is probably not a cause of nonunion.

Bohr (1971) showed that tetracycline uptake is increased in nonunions, suggesting increased bone formation. Since he could not demonstrate increased resorption, he thought mechanisms other than mineralization were responsible for the nonunions. This study supports those reporting normal or even increased mineral uptake in nonunions.

Brighton (1972) reported consistently higher oxygen tensions in delayed unions compared to normally healing fractures. This finding is consistent with the finding of increased blood flow in some established nonunions (Laurnen and Kelly, 1969; Paradis and Kelly, 1975). Poor blood supply per se may not be as important in producing nonunions as once believed, although the loss of blood supply in the critical early stages of fracture repair may lead to nonunions.

Several investigators have suggested that the rate of nonunion in certain fractures is decreased by delayed internal fixation as compared to immediate internal fixation (Charnley and Guindy, 1961; Lam, 1964; Emery and Murakami, 1967). Whether or not this hypothesis is correct, the practice of delayed internal fixation has not become widespread. The factors responsible for this phenomenon have not been identified, although it is presumed that the motion at the fracture site between the time of fracture and fixation results in more callus, or "better" callus, than would be present if the fracture were fixed initially.

Two recent studies have resulted in interesting hypotheses regarding the development of delayed unions. The first study demonstrated positive cutaneous electrical potentials on the thighs of 40 percent of normal subjects, negative potentials in 36 percent, and mixed potentials in 24 percent (Wilber and Russell, 1979). After femur fractures in 89 patients, all cutaneous potentials became negative, but 1 to 5 days were required for this electronegativity to occur in some cases. While all patients were treated operatively, the delayed and nonunion rate was 36 percent in patients treated 0 to 5 days after injury, while only one instance of delayed union occurred in the group treated after 5 days. The authors hypothesized that the trauma initiates an afferent, direct-current autonomic signal. When the signal exceeds a threshold, it excites an efferent cerebral signal. The efferent direct current signal then acts to augment the local forces of bone healing and is perhaps responsible for the changes in biopotentials after fractures. These investigators imply that surgery prior to reversal of the cutaneous potentials somehow affected the triggering of the efferent signal, perhaps by anesthesia, and thus prevented the normal conditions needed for healing. This theory is particularly fascinating in view of the possibility of changing adverse biopotentials (i.e., those associated with high rates of delayed union) with biofeedback.

The second report centers around the relative degrees of soft tissue and bony injury (Hulth, 1980). Hulth postulates that injured tissues (soft tissues or bone) stimulate (possibly by molecular determinants) the structural genes of undifferentiated cells to produce messenger RNA and proteins for either fibrous repair or bony repair in a specific way. In injuries with extensive soft tissue damage, there may exist a greater stimulus for fibrous repair and a lesser stimulus for bony repair, leading to delayed union or even nonunion. Some experimental support for Hulth's theory comes from the results of the recent studies of Whiteside and Lesker (1978a, 1978b). They demonstrated significantly higher (93 percent versus 29 percent) delayed union rates at 3 weeks in rabbit tibial osteotomies with extraperiosteal dissection compared to subperiosteal dissection (as might be expected based on clinical observations). In groups of animals where muscle transection had also been carried out (as a model of muscle damage), however, the delayed union rate was high with both extraperiosteal and subperiosteal dissection. Furthermore, calcium levels in the callus of the muscle trauma groups were lower than those with only subperiosteal dissection, and hydroxyproline levels were lower in the group with only subperiosteal dissection. These findings clearly suggest that injured soft tissues play a role in delayed unions.

Delayed unions or nonunions may be treated by prolonged external immobilization (cast or brace), internal fixation, bone grafting, electrical stimulation, or some combination. Internal fixation alone is likely to be successful when there is substantial callus formation but inadequate immobilization. Bone grafting is generally used when there has been (or is likely to be) an inadequate amount of callus. The precise mechanisms of bone grafting are not well understood, but the implanted bone may transplant osteogenic cells (if fresh autograft), or may serve as a lattice work for new bone, or may provide some inducing agent.

Electrical stimulation of delayed unions or nonunions is an exciting, relatively new treatment (Lavine et al., 1972; Bassett et al., 1981, 1982; Brighton, 1981; Brighton et al., 1981) with most reports suggesting a positive effect. There are three general methods by which these delayed unions or nonunions may be electrically stimulated: direct current through implanted electrodes; alternating currents induced by time-varying electromagnetic fields (pulsed electromagnetic fields or PEMFs); and constant or pulsed capacitively coupled fields (Brighton, 1981). (The results in fresh fracture are mixed, with some positive reports [Friedenberg et al., 1971a, 1971b; Wahlstrom, 1984] and some negative reports [Hinsenkamp et al., 1978].) The clinical reports seem rather uniformly positive about the efficacy of electrical stimulation for the treatment of nonunions. It must be noted, however, that only one of the clinical reports is a prospective, random, double-blind (active and dummy pulsed magnetic field stimulators) clinical trial, and that report is a preliminary one with only 16 patients (Barker et al., 1984). In that study, five of nine patients with an active unit and five of seven patients with a dummy unit healed their fractures during the study time of 24 weeks. These results suggest that the immobilization or nonweightbearing are the important aspects of the treatment of the nonunions rather than the magnetic fields. Furthermore, it seems that the responsiveness is dependent on the particular bone, with the humerus having lower success rates than the tibia (Marcer et al., 1984). Since large, well-designed randomized and blinded studies have not been performed, the question of efficacy is as yet unanswered.

While delayed unions are quite common, their counterparts, accelerated unions, are not often identified. Many investigators, however, have attempted to produce accelerated union by venous tourniquets (Pearse and Morton, 1931, 1937; Hutchinson and Burdeaux, 1954; Colt and Iger, 1963; Kruse and Kelly, 1974), drugs (DeGubareff and Platt, 1969; Gudmundson and Lidgren, 1973; Schneider et al., 1973), sympathectomy (McMaster and Roome, 1934; Lowenstein et al., 1958; Herzig and Root, 1959), hormones (Ewald and Tachdjian, 1967; Wray, 1967; Herold et al., 1971; Harris et al., 1975), exercise (Heikkenen, 1974), and electrical stimulation (Minken et al., 1968; Friedenberg et al., 1971a, 1971b; Lavine et al., 1971, 1972; Jorgensen, 1972b; Hinsenkamp et al., 1978). Most of these attempts have not produced consistent enough results to be clinically useful.

STRESS FRACTURES

The skeleton's ability to withstand the extremes of functional activity in the absence of damage is primarily the result of the bone's capacity to adapt to changes in the mechanical environment. The primary benefit of the extremely sensitive adaptive response is that the skeleton is "tuned" to each individual's current functional demands. Under normal circumstances, this relationship between structure and function results in "appropriate" levels of bone mass, promising pain-free use.

The onset of a stress fracture indicates a failure of this structure:function relationship; the functional demands of the individual have somehow surpassed the structural capacity of the bone. While stress fractures have been a military concern for well over 100 years, a civilian stress fracture epidemic has paralleled the recent emphasis on health and fitness. Stress fractures often occur in well-trained athletes "peaking" towards the limits of their potential, as well as in poorly trained people, particularly women, following an abrupt increase in the level of their physical activity. Recently, this distinction has become more evident as the military has experienced an enlistment shift in the sexual population; there are more female recruits now than ever before.

Even among the highly motivated female recruits included in the cadet training program for the U.S. Military Academy, up to a 10 percent incidence of stress fractures was observed in 102 female trainees (Protzman and Griffis, 1977). Indeed, stress fractures are the leading cause of time lost in the military, incapacitating 1 to 5 percent of the male and 7 to 20 percent of the female recruits (Scully and Besterman, 1982). But even with the large number of people suffering from this condition, no one is certain of its origin or true incidence.

The conventional view of the etiology of the "training up" type of stress fracture is that the increased activity engenders microdamage within critical areas of the cortex, and accumulates until the structural integrity of the bone is compromised. This scenario is not unlike the bending of a paper clip until sufficient "microdamage" builds up that the wire breaks. This analogy has indeed lead to the names we give this phenomenon: "stress fractures" or "fatigue fractures." In the skeleton, such a sequence would be aggravated by the relatively slow remodeling process, incapable of rapidly repairing areas of the damaged cortex before continued loading caused structural fatigue failure. Once sufficient structural failure occurred, according to this view, evidence of a defect or an area of bone rarefaction appears radiographically or by bone scan. Reduction of activity or immobilization then allows the reparative remodeling to run its course, following which higher levels of activity could be gradually resumed.

This conventional view implies that the fatigue life of bone is very poor, and that cyclic loading would quickly accumulate sufficient damage within the bone tissue to cause failure (Carter et al., 1981). By linear extrapolation of their in vitro data, it would appear that relatively vigorous physiologic levels of activity (i.e., running) would lead to fatigue failure in bone (30 percent loss of stiffness) in approximately 100,000 cycles, or 100 miles. These rather pessimistic conclusions, however, are based on in vitro fatigue observations made on machined bone specimens at levels of strain well beyond those measured during vigorous activity. More importantly, they deny the bone the one major benefit of being a tissue—that it is alive and has the intrinsic capacity to adapt. Indeed, a study of the in vivo fatigue behavior of bone has demonstrated that live bone enjoys an "endurance limit," a level of strain in which the cycles to failure curve increases dramatically towards infinity (Seireg and Kempke, 1969). This suggests that alternative explanations of the "fatigue fracture" phenomenon must be considered.

In monitoring the remodeling response of bone to excessive repetitive loading, a new etiology could be hypothesized. Rubin et al. (1984) observed large structural defects generated by this sort of regime that were not cracks or microdamage, but rather resorption spaces and expansion of vascular channels. These spaces, combined with exuberant periosteal new bone formation, presented a similar histological picture to that observed in human cases (Harris et al., 1986). Surprisingly, however, the region of the most consistent and extensive intracortical remodeling was not that subjected to the greatest strain (the area of the cortex most likely to "accumulate microdamage"), but rather was located about the bone's neutral axis (the area of cortex subjected to the smallest normal strains).

These data would suggest that the most extensive and demonstrable bone defects associated with "training up" are not distinct cracks resulting from material failure. Rather, the resorption of the cortex and the eventual structural failure of the bone, which may result from the decrease in effective load bearing area, appears to be a consequence of the bone tissue's remodeling response to the prevailing strain situation, rather than a failure of the bone material due to fatigue. Thus, this in vivo evidence suggests that the conventional view of stress fractures is inappropriate, and that the terms "stress" or "fatigue" fractures are misnomers.

This new theory of stress fractures could explain an array of poorly defined musculoskeletal complaints associated with normal radiographic appearances. While purely speculative at this time, it is possible that some cases of "shin splints," heel pain, and "groin pulls" represent early stages of bone resorption as described above, with remodeling and "repair" occurring before radiographic findings are evident. It is well known that bone scans are more sensitive in detecting "stress fractures" than plain radiographs and that not all cases detected by scan develop radiographic changes if treated early. It is also likely that some cases might not cause sufficient tissue changes to result in increased uptake on scans, but cause mild, vague symptoms and then resolve (i.e., remodel) spontaneously.

SUMMARY

Nature has provided remarkable mechanisms for healing fractures. In most smaller animal species, nonunions are rare, and, in fact, difficult to produce experimentally unless radical steps are taken. Animals seemingly have the instinct to protect the injured part until it can be used more or less normally. (Of course, it can be expected that many of these fractures heal in a position that would be interpreted as a cosmetically unacceptable deformity in humans even though the limbs probably have reasonable function.) In contrast to most animals, humans seemingly have a higher chance of developing delayed unions. Given the generally universal mechanisms in biologic species, it is not likely that the differences in union rates are owing to different repair mechanisms in humans. Rather, it is more likely that humans use the injured parts too soon, or in inappropriate ways, or that our "therapeutic" interventions interfere with nature's processes.

It is critical to realize that any intervention, including something as seemingly innocuous as a "gentle" closed reduction, has the potential to interfere with the repair process by whatever mechanisms. This fact has received very little emphasis in the surgical literature since, by their very training, doctors tend to intervene in most situations. Surgical intervention most certainly affects the repair process by destroying critical blood supply, altering the electrical environment, possibly interfering with the appropriate differentiation of pluripotential cells, and by preventing small amounts of motion that may act as a stimulus for the repair process. This is not to say that there are not specific indications for surgery (e.g., to restore dis-placed joint surfaces, to reduce the rate of nonunions of femoral neck fractures), but rather to say that we must realize that each intervention is possibly deleterious to the repair process. The decision to intervene (with its liabilities) must therefore be carefully weighed against its potential gains.

How might interventions interfere with the repair process? One possible mechanism might be in altering the soft tissue milieu suggested by Hulth (1980), or the morphogenetic fields suggested by Sheldrake (1981). Another possibility is that we have not found the correct balance between rest, immobilization, and function. Animals seemingly have the instinct to begin using the injured part at a time when function is critical in the repair process. Humans, on the other hand, probably do not use function early enough owing to pain, immobilization, or advice from the doctor. There is increasing evidence that function is a critical factor in the repair process (Dehne, 1980; Sarmiento et al., 1984), and our interventions may not be taking enough advantage of this natural healing factor.

Ideally, fracture treatment should seem to demand a quantitative understanding of the many factors affecting fracture healing, as well as an appreciation of the complex manner in which they interact. These factors should include the effects of any anticipated interventions. Many of these factors have been discussed in greater or lesser detail in the preceding portions of this chapter (Table 11–2). The composite response ("healing time") of bone to a fracture could theoretically be expressed by a complex mathematical function, assuming each variable was understood quantitatively:

$$\text{Healing time} = f(L,\ 1/C,\ M,\ A,\ S,\ E.\ .\ .\ .)$$

where L, equals loads (compression, tension, bending, torsion, shear); C, capillary blood supply (volume, surface area, flow, etc.); M, motion; A, age (a factor at least relevant before skeletal maturity); S, surface area (or number of exposed pluripotential cells); E, electrical environment, etc. Of course, many other variables could be important in such a function. While it might seem overwhelming to attempt a quantitative understanding of the interaction of so many factors, some are undoubtedly of much greater importance than others. By attempting to isolate the effects of specific variables, recent research has afforded us a more complete insight into fracture healing. While we are beginning to understand the effects of some of those variables, however, we have not yet reached a state of sophistication that would afford us an understanding of their interactions.

On the other hand, our understanding of the fracture repair processes is rapidly growing, and when placed in a historic perspective, that understanding has added significantly to the modes of therapy and to the avoidance of some natural sequelae of the fractures. Much of our knowledge has been necessarily accumulated by trial and error in treating patients. This is owing to the complexity of the problem and the difficulties in formulating research questions, techniques, and experiments that can provide sufficiently clear answers. It is perhaps also in part owing to our failure, both experimentally and clinically, to view icles that also contain collagen. Then the vesicle contents are extruded from the cell and the completed proteoglycan molecules form attachments through charge interactions to collagen fibers in the cartilage matrix (Shepard and Mitchell, 1976). Little is known about the mechanisms that control proteoglycan synthesis although proteoglycan synthesis appears to be controlled by a feedback mechanism in the microenvironment of the chondrocyte. The cells may respond both to the biomechanical requirements of the tissue or to the concentration of the proteoglycans surrounding it. Proteoglycan synthesis in suspended cells can be stimulated by high concentrations of chondroitin sulfate and proteoglycans (Dorfman, 1981). Yet proteoglycan synthesis in chondrocytes is inhibited by hyaluronic acid (Muir, 1979). Other researchers have found that high levels of extracellular proteoglycans inhibited proteoglycan synthesis and that low levels increased synthesis (Lash and Vasan, 1983). The conditions under which the studies were done are very important. In vivo and in vitro studies have been reported that give contradictory results. Factors contributing to these results may be methods used and age of tissue (Lash and Vasan, 1983).

A biomechanical feedback is inferred from older reports of increased thickness following exercise and decreased thickness following immobilization. Moreover, the chondrocytes (Edwards and Michael, 1977) respond to a depletion of their matrix proteoglycan by production of increased quantities of proteoglycan. The presence of E prostaglandins, however, will prevent this normal synthesis response to proteoglycan depletion and may be, therefore, a contributing factor in the pathogenesis of cartilage fibrillation and osteoarthritis (Fulkerson and Damiano, 1983).

Distribution

There is moderate variation in the concentrations of the various glycosaminoglycans within articular cartilage. The concentrations of chondroitin sulfate and keratosulfate rapidly rise as one progresses from the surface to one third of the depth of the cartilage and then it gradually diminishes (Lipshitz et al., 1976a). The absence of proteoglycans at the surface of the articular cartilage might be due in part to suppression of proteoglycan synthesis by synovial hyaluronate. This suppression has been described in tissue-culture (Wiebkin and Muir, 1975). The content and ratios of chondroitin sulfate and keratosulfate vary topographically over the articular cartilage of a joint (Bjelle, 1974) and also between different joints in the same animal (Wright et al., 1973). The greatest differences in chemical composition of cartilage, however, are found between different individuals (Maroudas, 1975). The physiologic significance of these variations in glycosaminoglycan content remains elusive.

Permeability

The proteoglycan constituent of the cartilage matrix is primarily responsible for its fine porous structure. Whereas small nutrient and water molecules readily diffuse through the cartilage matrix, larger molecules such as some immunoglobulins may be excluded under normal circum-

stances. The loss of proteoglycan in the cartilage matrix that follows an insult to articular cartilage might permit greater access into the cartilage matrix of potentially destructive immunoglobulins and enzymes in the synovial fluid; these enzymes include neutral proteases, cathepsin D, collagenase, and hyaluronidase (Howell, 1976).

Histochemistry

Proteoglycans can be identified in cartilage histochemically. Each ester sulfate and each carboxylate group on the glycosaminoglycan molecule has a negative charge. Various dyes combine with the negative groups on the glycosaminoglycans. Safranin-O, for instance, can be used to determine the relative concentration of proteoglycan in different histologic sections of uniform thickness (Rosenberg, 1971). One molecule of the dye binds to each negatively charged group on the glycosaminoglycan if dye-dye interaction is blocked with an ethanol wash (Rosenberg, 1971). Other dyes will form dye–dye interactions after binding to the negative charges on polysaccharides and, in so doing, change from their original (orthochromatic) to another (metachromatic) color (Mathews, 1965). These include toluidine blue, alcian blue, azure A, and crystal violet.

Immunology

Cartilage proteoglycans have antigenic properties, and free glycosaminoglycans seem to play a role in inflammatory joint diseases. Three antigenic components of human proteoglycans that can evoke a cell-mediated response have been identified (Herman and Carpenter, 1975). The nature of this response in various arthritides will be considered later in this chapter.

Degradation

Degradation of proteoglycans can occur as part of normal development, accompany various arthritides, and result from immobilization, exercise or load bearing (Lash and Vasan, 1983). The catabolism of proteoglycan within normal articular cartilage is probably accomplished by both lysosomal and nonlysosomal enzyme systems contained within the cartilage (Chrisman and Fessel, 1962; Ali, 1964; Chrisman et al., 1967; Chrisman et al., 1981).

Neutral enzymes, particular metalloproteases, are primarily responsible for articular cartilage breakdown. Enzymes secreted from synovium are important in this process, but prostaglandins (Fulkerson et al., 1979) and catabolin (Dingle, 1981) may cause cartilage depletion through enzyme release directly from chondrocytes (Steinberg and Sledge, 1979). Prostaglandin mediated effects may be modulated by cyclic nucleotide activity in chondrocytes (Houston et al., 1982; Malemud et al., 1982).

Since trauma to articular cartilage causes release of arachidonic acid, a precurser of prostaglandins, it is likely that proteoglycan depletion of articular cartilage by prostaglandins will follow significant trauma (Chrisman et al., 1981; Donohue et al., 1983).

Although a majority of the proteoglycan population in articular cartilage has a lifespan of approximately 600 days (Hall et al., 1977), a small portion of cartilage proteoglycans are rapidly degraded and resynthesized. Experiments using labeled glycine and sulfate show that 9.5 percent of the proteoglycan in mature rabbits have a half-life of only 6.8 days (Hall et al., 1977), implying an active remodeling system by chondrocytes.

PHYSICAL AND MECHANICAL PROPERTIES

In 1944, Hirsch studied the compressive properties of cartilage and discovered that there was an instantaneous deformation upon load application, followed by further time-dependent deformation. Removal of the load again produced a time-dependent recovery phase. Hence, cartilage behaves as a viscoelastic material. The elasticity implies instantaneous deformation proportional to the load applied with a reversibility of this deformation on removal of the load. With a prolonged load, further deformation, or creep, occurs. As a viscoelastic tissue, the response of cartilage to a load is thus time-dependent. When rapidly loaded, the cartilage modulus of elasticity is quite high, demonstrating that the rate of load application will change the mechanical response of cartilage. This is one reason that a cushioned heel is important in running shoes; the potentially damaging impact of running on pavement will be delivered more gradually to articular cartilage, at a lower strain rate, thereby permitting better adaptation to the applied stress.

THE ROLE OF PROTEOGLYCANS

The compressive modulus of articular cartilage is directly proportional to proteoglycan content (Roth et al., 1981). Kempson et al. (1971) found that the stiffest cartilage had the highest concentration of glycosaminoglycans (chondroitin sulfate and keratosulfate). Both the electrostatic and osmotic properties of the proteoglycans contribute to cartilage elasticity. The negative charges on the glycosaminoglycan arms of the branching proteoglycan molecules repel each other. In order to obtain maximum separation of these negatively charged branches, proteoglycan aggregates attempt to occupy the largest possible domain (McDevitt, 1973) (Fig. 12–10).

Proteoglycans hold water in the cartilage matrix osmotically and impede the loss of water from loaded cartilage both osmotically and by controlling matrix permeability. The high "fixed charge density" due to the negatively charged groups on the proteoglycans leads to considerable "swelling pressure" within cartilage (Maroudas, 1976). As a result, 65 to 80 percent (by weight) of cartilage is relatively incompressible fluid. Proteoglycans also provide some resistance to the flow of water through the matrix of loaded cartilage.

THE ROLE OF THE FLUID PHASE

The relatively incompressible fluid bound in cartilage matrix bears much of the axial load crossing the joint and contributes to the high initial stiffness of cartilage on im-

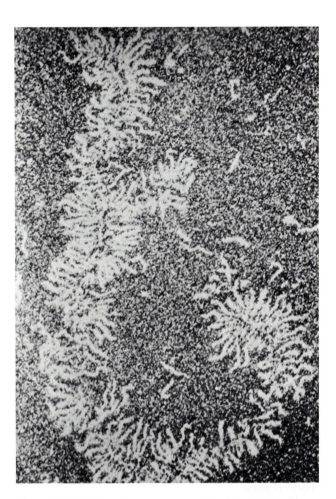

Figure 12–10. Proteoglycan aggregate. See Figure 12–8 for explanation. (*Courtesy of Lawrence Rosenberg, M.D.*)

pact loading (Maroudas, 1973; McDevitt, 1973). In response to a prolonged mechanical load (and pressure gradient), fluid may rapidly flow laterally or be exuded through the cartilage surface (Mulholland, 1974). This flow of fluid away from the loaded area is partially responsible for the viscoelastic response to compressive loads (Linn and Sokoloff, 1965). The relatively large gaps between collagen fibers are filled with proteoglycans, which are the most important factor in determining permeability (Fig. 12–11). Resistance to fluid flow is therefore proportional to proteoglycan concentration (Muir, 1970). Hence, a reduction in proteoglycan concentration will reduce the compressive stiffness of cartilage, reduce the modulus of elasticity excessively, increase the rate of creep (Kempson, 1976) and allow greater deformation under load. Lateral permeability to fluid flow is also dependent on the state of strain and pressure within the tissue. Lateral permeability decreases as cartilage is compressed (Mansour and Mow, 1976).

THE ROLE OF COLLAGEN

The contribution of collagen architecture to the mechanical properties of articular cartilage has been debated at

Bonne W, Johnson H, Malanov C, Bryant M: Changes in the lipids of human articular cartilage with age. Arthritis Rheum 18:401, 1975.

Brighton CT, Irwin JT, Lipton MA, Lane JM: Application of tissue culture techniques to the storage of viable articular cartilage. Trans Orthop Res Soc 2:93, 1977.

Brighton CT, Lane JM, Koh JK: In vitro rabbit articular cartilage organ model: Sulphate-35 incorporated in various oxygen tensions. Arthritis Rheum 17:245, 1974.

Brower T: Normal articular cartilage. Clin Orthop 64:9, 1969.

Bullough P, Goodfellow J: The significance of the fine structure of articular cartilage. J Bone Joint Surg 50B:852, 1968.

Bullough PG, Jagannath AL: The morphology of the calcification front in articular cartilage. J Bone Joint Surg 65B:72, 1983.

Burgeson R: Articular cartilage, intervertebral disc, synovia. In JB Weiss, MIV Jayson (eds): Collagen in Health and Disease. New York, Churchill Livingstone, 1982, p 335.

Candolin T, Videman T: Surface changes in the articular cartilage of rabbit knee during immobilization. Acta Pathol Microbiol Scand 88(5):291, 1980.

Cheung HS, Cottrell WH, Stephenson K, Nimni ME: In vitro collagen biosynthesis in healing and normal rabbit articular cartilage. J Bone Joint Surg 60:1976, 1978.

Chrisman OD: Biochemical aspects of degenerative joint disease. Clin Orthop 64:77, 1969.

Chrisman OD: The effect of growth hormone on established cartilage lesions. Clin Orthop 107:232, 1975.

Chrisman OD, Fessel JM: Enzymatic degradation of chondromucoprotein by cell-free extracts of human cartilage. Surg Forum 13:444, 1962.

Chrisman OD, Ladenbauer-Bellis I-M, Fulkerson JP: The osteoarthritic cascade and associated drug actions. Sem Arth Rheum XI(1)Suppl 1:145, 1981a.

Chrisman OD, Ladenbauer-Bellis I-M, Panjabi M: The relationship of mechanical trauma and the early biochemical reactions of osteoarthritic cartilage. Clin Orthop 161:275, 1981b.

Chrisman OD, Semonsky C, Bensch KG: Cathepsins in articular cartilage. In Robinson RA (ed): The Healing of Osseous Tissue. Washington, D.C., Natl Acad Sci, 1967, p 169.

Chrisman OD, Snook GA, Wilson TC: The protective effect of aspirin against degeneration of human articular cartilage. Clin Orthop 84:193, 1972.

Clarke IC: The microevaluation of articular surface contours. Ann Biochem Eng 1:31, 1972.

Clarke IC: Articular cartilage: A review and scanning electron microscope study. II. The territorial fibrillar architecture. J Anat 118(2):261, 1974.

Clarke IC: Planes of weakness in articular cartilage. Trans Orthop Res Soc 3:71, 1977.

Coelho R, Chrisman OD: Sulfate metabolism in cartilage II. J Bone Joint Surg 42A:165, 1960.

Coletti JM, Akeson WH, Woo SLY: A comparison of the physical behavior of normal articular cartilage and the arthroplasty surface. J Bone Joint Surg 54A:147, 1972.

Collins DH: The Pathology of Spinal and Articular Disease. London, Arnold, 1949, p 74.

Collins DH, McElligott TF: Sulfate $^{35}SO_4$ uptake by chondrocytes in relation to histologic changes in osteoarthritic human articular cartilage. Ann Rheum Dis 19:318, 1960.

Crelin ES, Southwick WO: Mitosis of chondrocytes induced in the knee joint articular cartilage of rabbits. Yale J Biol Med 33:242, 1960.

Curtiss PH, Klein L: Destruction of articular cartilage in septic arthritis: in vivo studies. J Bone Joint Surg 45A:797, 1963.

Daniel D, Akeson W, Amiel D, et al.: Lavage of septic joints in rabbits: effect of chondrolysis. J Bone Joint Surg 58A:393, 1976.

Dingle JT: Catabolin—A cartilage catabolic factor from synovium. Clin Orthop 156:219, 1981.

Donohue JM, Buss D, Oegema TR, Thompson RC: The effects of indirect blunt trauma on adult articular cartilage. J Bone Joint Surg 65A:948, 1983.

Dorfman A: Proteoglycan Biosynthesis. In Hay ED (ed): Cell Biology of Extracellular Matrix. New York, Plenum Press, 1981, p 115.

Edwards J: Physical characteristics of articular cartilage. Proc Inst Mech Eng 181:16, 1967.

Edwards CC, Hill TA: The natural history of treated and untreated fungal arthritis—a chemical and ultrastructural study. Surg Forum 28:497, 1977.

Edwards CC, Michael R: The effect of intra-articular amphotericin-B on articular cartilage. Trans Orthop Res Soc 2:29, 1977.

Ehrlich MG, Mankin HJ, Treadwell BV: Uridine diphosphate (UDP) stimulation of protein-polysaccharide production: A preliminary report. J Bone Joint Surg 56A:1239, 1974.

Enneking WF, Horowitz M: The intra-articular effects of immobilization on the human knee. J Bone Joint Surg 54:973, 1972.

Evanson JM, Jeffrey JJ, Krane SM: Human collagenase: Identification and characterization of an enzyme from rheumatoid synovium in culture. Science 148:499, 1967.

Fell HB, Dingle JT: Studies on the mode of action of vitamin A. Lysosomal protease and the degradation of cartilage matrix. Biochem J 87:403, 1963.

Freeman MAR: Adult Articular Cartilage. New York, Grune & Stratton, 1974.

Freeman MAR: Adult Articular Cartilage, London, Pitman Publishing Co., 1979.

Friedlander GE, Ladenbauer-Bellis I-M, Chrisman OD: Cartilage matrix components as antigenic agents in an osteoarthritic model. Trans Orthop Res Soc 5:170, 1980.

Fuji K, Kuboki Y, Sasaki S: Aging of human bones and articular cartilage collagen. Gerontology 22:263, 1976.

Fulkerson JP, Damiano P: Effect of Prostaglandin E_2 on adult pig articular cartilage slices in culture. Clin Orthop 179:308, 1983.

Fulkerson JP, Ladenbauer-Bellis I-M, Chrisman OD: In vitro hexosamine depletion of intact articular cartilage by E-prostaglandins: Prevention by chloroquine. Arthritis Rheum 22(10):1117, 1979.

Furukawa T, Eyre DR, Koide S, Glimcher MJ: Biochemical studies on repair cartilage resurfacing experimental defects in the rabbit knee. J Bone Joint Surg 62A:79, 1980.

George RC, Chrisman OD: The role of cartilage polysaccharides in osteoarthritis. Clin Orthop 57:259, 1968.

Ghadially FN, Lalonde JM: Long term effects of myochrysine in articular cartilage. Arch Cell Pathol 28(1):31, 1978.

Hall D, Mankin HJ, Lippiello L: Turnover of proteoglycan of adult rabbit articular cartilage. Trans Orthop Res Soc 2:10, 1977.

Harris ED Jr, Faulkner CS III, Brown FE: Collagenolytic systems in rheumatoid arthritis. Clin Orthop 110:303, 1975.

Harrison MHM, Schajowicz F, Trueta J: Osteoarthritis of the hip: A study of the nature and evolution of the disease. J Bone Joint Surg 35B:598, 1953.

Hascall VC, Kimura JH: Proteoglycans: Isolation and Characterization. In Cunningham LW, Frederiksen DW (eds): Methods of Enzymology, vol. 82. New York, Academic Press, 1982, p 760.

Havdrup T, Telhag H: Mitosis of chondrocytes in normal adult joint cartilage. Clin Orthop 153:248–252, 1980.

Herman JH, Carpenter BA: Immunobiology of cartilage. Semin Arthritis Rheum 51:1, 1975.

Herman JH, Nutman TB, Nozoe M, et al.: Lymphokine-mediated suppression of chondrocyte glycosaminoglycan and protein synthesis. Arthritis Rheum 24:824, 1981.

Higuchi M, Masuda T, Susuda K, et al.: Ultrastructure of articular cartilage after systemic administration of hydrocortisone in the rabbit. Clin Orthop 152:296, 1980.

Hirsch C: The pathogenesis of chondromalacia of the patella. A physical, histologic and chemical study. Acta Chir Scand 90:1, 1944.

Hoaglund FJ: Experimental hemarthrosis effect on articular cartilage. J Bone Joint Surg 49A:285, 1967.

Hollander JL, McCarty DJ Jr (eds): Arthritis and Allied Conditions, 8th ed. Philadelphia, Lea and Febiger, 1972, p 1140.

Homer R, Thompson RC: The nutritional pathways of articular cartilage. J Bone Joint Surg 54A:742, 1972.

Hopwood J, Robinson II: The structure and composition of cartilage keratan sulfate. Biochem J 141:517, 1974.

Horwitz AL, Dorfman A: Subcellular sites for synthesis of chondromucoprotein of cartilage. J Cell Biol 38:258, 1976.

Houston JP, McGuire M, Meats J, et al.: Adenylate cyclase of human articular chondrocytes. Biochem J 208:35, 1982.

Howell DS: Osteoarthritis—etiology and pathogenesis. AAOS Symposium on Osteoarthritis. St. Louis, C.V. Mosby, 1976.

Hultkrantz JW: Über die spalthrichturger der gelenkknorpel. Verh Anat Ges 1898.

Hunter JA, Finley B: Scanning electron microscopy of connective tissues: Articular cartilage. Int Rev Connect Tissue Res 6:242, 1973.

Janoff A, Feinsten G, Malemud CJ, Elias JM: Degradation of cartilage proteoglycan by human leukocyte granule neutral protease—A model of joint injury. J Clin Invest 57:615, 1976.

Jones IL, Klamfeldt A, Sandstrom T: The effect of continuous mechnical pressure upon the turnover of articular cartilage proteoglycans in vitro. Clin Othop 165:283, 1982.

Jubb RW: breakdown of articular cartilage by vascular tissue. J Pathol 136:333, 1982.

Jubb RW, Fell HB: The breakdown of cartilage by chondrocytes. J Pathol 130:159, 1980.

Kempson GE, Freeman MAR, Swanson SAV: Tensile properties of articular cartilage. Nature 20:1127, 1968.

Kempson GE, Spivery CJ, Swanson SAV, Freeman MAR: Patterns of cartilage stiffness on normal and degenerate human femoral heads. J Biomech 4:597, 1971.

Kempson GE, Tuke MA, Dingle JT, et al.: The effect of proteoglycolytic enzymes on the mechanical properties of adult human articular cartilage. Biochem Biophys Acta 428:741, 1976.

Krystal G, Morris GM, Sokoloff L: Stimulation of DNA synthesis by ascorbate in cultures of articular chondrocytes. Arthritis Rheum 25:318, 1982.

Kuettner KE, Eisentein R, Sorgeinte N: Lysozyme in calcifying tissues. Clin Orthop 112:316, 1975.

Lapiere CM, Lenaers A, Kohn LD: Procollagen peptidase: An enzyme exercizing the co-ordination of peptide of procollagen. Proc Natl Acad Sci USA 68:3054, 1971.

Lash JW, Vasan NS: Glycosaminoglycans of cartilage. In Hall BK (ed): Cartilag vol I, Structure, Function and Biochemistry. New York, Academic Press, 1983, p 215.

Layman DL, McGoodwin EB, Martin GR: Transport form of collagen. Proc Natl Acad Sci USA 68:4541, 1971.

Linn FC, Sokoloff L: Movement and composition of interstitial fluid of cartilage. Arthritis Rheum 8:481, 1965.

Lippiello L, Hall D, Mankin HJ: Collagen synthesis in normal and OA human cartilage. J Clin Invest 59:593, 1977.

Lippiello L, Yamamota K, Robinson D, Mankin H: Involvement of prostaglandins from rheumatoid synovium in inhibition of articular cartilage metabolism. Arthritis Rheum 21:909–917, 1978.

Lipshitz H, Etheredge R, Glimcher MJ: Changes in the hexosamine content and swelling of articular cartilage as a function of depth from the surface. J Bone Joint Surg 58A:1149, 1976a.

Lipshitz H, Glimcher MJ, Mow VC, Torzilli PA: On the stress relaxation of articular cartilage. Trans, Orthop Res Soc 1:208, 1976b.

Lothe K, Spycher MA, Ruttner JR: Human articular cartilage in relation to age, a morphometric study. Exp Cell Biol 47:22, 1979.

Lutfi AM, Kosel K: Effects of intra-articularly administered corticosteriods and salicylates on the surface structure of articular cartilage. J Anat 127:393, 1978.

Malemud CJ, Moskowitz RW, Papay RS: Correlation of the biosynthesis of prostaglandin and cyclic AMP in monolayer cultures of rabbit articular chondrocytes. Biochim Biophys Acta 715:70, 1982.

Malemud CJ, Sokoloff L: The effect of prostaglandins on cultured lapine articular chondrocytes. Prostaglandins 13(5):845, 1977.

Mankin HJ: Localization of tritiated thymidine in articular cartilage of rabbits. III. Mature articular cartilage. J Bone Joint Surg 45A:529, 1963.

Mankin HJ: Effect of systemic corticosteroids on rabbit articular cartilage. Arthritis Rheum 15:593, 1972.

Mankin HJ: Biochemical abnormalities in osteoarthritic human cartilage. Fed Proc 32:1478, 1974a.

Mankin HJ: Water binding in articular cartilage. J Bone Joint Surg 56A:1031, 1974b.

Mankin HJ: The response of articular cartilage to mechanical injury. J Bone Joint Surg 64A:460, 1982.

Mankin HJ, Baron PA: The effect of aging on protein synthesis in articular cartilage of rabbits. Lab Invest 14:658, 1965.

Mankin HJ, Dortman J, Lippiello L, et al: Biochemical and metabolic abnormalities in articular cartilage from osteoarthritic hips. J Bone Joint Surg 53A:523, 1971.

Mankin HJ, Lippiello L: Biochemical and metabolic abnormalities in articular cartilage from osteoarthritic hips. J Bone Joint Surg 52A:424, 1970.

Mankin HJ, Lippiello L: The glycosaminoglycans of normal and arthritic cartilage. J Clin Invest 50:1712, 1971.

Mankin HJ, Thrasher AZ: Water content and binding in normal and osteoarthritic human cartilage. J Bone Joint Surg 57A:76, 1975.

Mansour JM, Mow VC: The dependence of articular cartilage permeability on strain and pressure. Trans Orthop Res Soc 1:71, 1976.

Mansour JM, Mow VC, Redler I: In Pope MH, McLay RW, Asher RC (eds): Proc N Engl Bioeng Conf. Burlington, Vt, University of Vermont, 1973, p 183.

Maroudas A: Cartilage of the hip joint. Ann Rheum Dis 32:1, 1973.

Maroudas A: Glycosaminoglycan turn-over in articular cartilage. Phil Trans R Soc Lond B271:293, 1975.

Maroudas A: Balance between swelling processes and collagen tension in normal and degenerate cartilage. Nature 260:803, 1976.

Maroudas A, Bullough P, Swanson SAV, et al: The permeability of articular cartilage. J Bone Joint Surg 50B:166, 1968.

Martinex A, Arguelles F, Cervera J, Bomar F: Sites of sulfation in the chondrocytes of the articular cartilage of the rabbit. Virchow's Arch (Cell Pathol) 23:53, 1977.

Mathews MB: The interaction of collagen and acid mucopolysaccharides: a model for connective tissue. Biochem J 96:710, 1965.

McCarty DJ Jr: Pseudogout. In Hollander JL, McCarty DJ Jr (eds): Arthritis and Allied Conditions, 8th ed. Philadelphia, Lea and Febiger, 1972, p 1140.

McDevitt CA: Biochemistry of articular cartilage. Ann Rheum Dis 32:364, 1973.

McKenzie LS, Horsburg BA, Ghorh P, Taylor TF: Effect of anti-inflammatory drugs on sulfated glycosaminoglycan synthesis in aged human articular cartilage. Ann Rheum Dis 35:487, 1976.

McKibbin B, Maroudas A: The Matrix. In Freeman MAR (ed): Adult Articular Cartilage, 2nd Edition. London, Pitman Publishing Co. Ltd., 1979, p 1.

Meachim G: The effect of scarification on articular cartilage in the rabbit. J Bone Joint Surg 45B:150, 1963.

Meachim G, Denham D, Emery IH, Wilkinson PH: Collagen alignments and artificial splits at the surface of human articular cartilage. J Anat 118:101, 1974.

Meachim G, Ghadially FN, Collins, DH: Regressive changes in the superficial layer of human articular cartilage. Ann Rheum Dis 24:23, 1965.

Mitchell N, Shepard N: The resurfacing of adult rabbit articular cartilage following multiple drill holes through the subchondral bone. J Bone Joint Surg 58A:230, 1976.

Mitchell N, Shepard N: Healing of articular cartilage in intra-articular fractures in rabbits. J Bone Joint Surg 62A:628, 1980.

Mitrovic D, Lippiello L, Gruson F, et al.: Effects of various prostanoids on metabolism of bovine articular chondrocytes. Prostaglandins 22(3):503, 1981.

Mow VC, Mansour JM: The nonlinear interaction between cartilage deformation and interstitial fluid flow. J Biomech 10:31, 1976.

Muir H: Chemistry and metabolism of connective tissue glycosaminoglycans (mucopolysaccharides). Int Reve Connect Tissue Res 2:101, 1964.

Muir IHM: Biochemistry. In Freeman MAR (ed): Adult Articular Cartilage, 2nd ed. London, Pitman Publishing Co. Ltd. 1979, p 145.

Muir H, Bullough P, Maroudas A: The distribution of collagen in human articular cartilage with some of its physiological implications. J Bone Joint Surg 52B:554, 1970.

Mulholland R: Lateral hydraulic permeability and morphology of articular cartilage in normal and osteoarthrosic cartilage. Proc Sym Inst Orthop Lond, 1974.

Myers ER, Mow VC: Biomechanics of cartilage and response to biomechanical stimuli. In Hall BK (ed): Cartilage vol. I Structure, Function, and Biochemistry. New York, Academic Press, 1983, p 313.

Nimni M, Desmukh K: Differences in collagen metabolism between normal and osteoarthritic human articular cartilage. Science 181:751, 1973.

Nole R, Munson N, Fulkerson J: Bupivacaine and saline effects on articular cartilage. Arthroscopy 1(2):123–127, 1985.

Oronsky AL, Sherry H, Gold V, et al.: Destruction of cartilage matrix by enzymatic constituents derived from human polymorphoneuclear leukocytes. Trans Orthop Res Soc 2:4, 1977.

Palmoski MJ, Brandt KD: Effects of some nonsteroidal anti-inflammatory drugs on proteogylcan metabolism and organization in canine articular cartilage. Arthritis Rheum 23:1010, 1980.

Palmoski MJ, Brandt KD: Benoxaprofen stimulates proteoglycan synthesis in normal canine knee cartilage in vitro. Arthritis Rheum 26:771, 1983.

Person DA, Sharp JT: The etiology of rheumatoid arthritis. Bull Rheum Dis 27:888, 1976.

Pugh JW, Radin EL, Rose RM: Quantitative studies of human subchondral cancellous bone. J Bone Joint Surg 56A:313, 1974.

Radin EL, Ehrlich MG, Chernack RS, et al.: Effect of repetitive impulse loading on the metabolism of rabbit articular cartilage and its relationship to bone stiffness. Trans Orthop Res Soc 2:74, 1977.

Radin EL, Paul IL, Rose RM, Simon SR: The mechanics of joints as it relates to their degeneration. AAOS Symposium on Osteoarthritis. St. Louis, C.V. Mosby, 1976.

Radin EL, Swann DA, Weisser PA: Separation of a hyaluronate-free lubricating fraction from synovial fluid. Nature 228:327, 1970.

Reagan B, McIneray V, Mankin, H., et al.: Irrigating solutions for arthroscopy. J Bone Joint Surg 65A:629–631, 1983.

Redler I: A scanning electron microscopic study of human normal and ostoarthritic articular cartilage. Clin Orthop 103:262, 1974.

Redler I, Mow VC, Zimny ML, Mansell J: The ultra-structure and biochemical significance of the tidemark of articular cartilage. Clin Orthop 112:357, 1975.

Repo RV, Mitchell N: Collagen synthesis in mature articular cartilage of the rabbit. J Bone Joint Surg 53B:541, 1971.

Robinson HC, Telser A, Dorfman A: Studies on biosynthesis of the linkage region of chondroitin sulphate-protein complex. Proc Natl Acad Sci USA 56:1859, 1966.

Rosenberg L: Chemical basis for the histological use of Safranin-O in the study of articular cartilage. J Bone Joint Surg 53A:69, 1971.

Rosenberg L, Hellmann W, Kleinschmidt AK: Macromolecular models of protein polysaccharides from bovine nasal cartilage based on electron microscopic studies. J Biol Chem 245:4123, 1970.

Roth V, Mow VC, Lai DR, Eyre DR: Correlation of intrinsic compressive properties of bovine articular cartilage with its uronic acid and water content. Proc Orth Res Soc 6:49, 1981.

Rubacky GE: Inheritable chondromalacia of the patella. J Bone Joint Surg 45A:1685, 1963.

Salter RB, Simmonds DF, Malcolm BW, et al.: The effects of continued passive motion on the healing of articular cartilage defects. J Bone Joint Surg 57:570, 1975.

Salter RB, Simmonds DF, Malcolm BW, et al.: The biological effect of continuous passive motion on the healing of full thickness defects in articular cartilage. J Bone Joint Surg 62A:1,232, 1980.

Santer V, White RJ, Roughley PJ: Proteoglycan from normal and degenerate cartilage of the human tibial plateau. Arthritis Rheum 24:691, 1981.

Scheinberg RD, Ehrlich MG, Lippiello L, Mankin HJ: Degradative enzyme activity in isolated chondrocyte populations. Clin Orthop 164:279, 1982.

Schwarz ER, Ogele RC, Thompson RC: Aryl sulfatase activities in normal and pathologic human articular cartilage. Arthritis Rheum 17:455, 1974.

Shepard N, Mitchell N: The localization of articular cartilage proteoglycan by electron microscopy. Anat Rec 187:463, 1976.

Simmons DP, Chrisman OD: Salicylate inhibition of cartilage degeneration. Arthritis Rheum 8:960, 1965.

Simon WH: The Human Joint in Health and Disease. University of Pennsylvania Press, 1978.

Simon WH, Friedenberg S, Richardson S: Joint congruence. J Bone Joint Surg 55A:81, 1614, 1973.

Sledge CB: Growth hormone and articular cartilage. Fed Proc 32:1503, 1973.

Sokoloff L: Elasticity of articular cartilage: Effect of ions and viscous solutions. Science 141:1055, 1963.

Sokoloff L: Cell biology and the repair of articular cartilage. J Rheum 11:9, 1974.

Starkey PM, Barrett AJ, Burleigh ML: The degradation of articular collagen by neutrophil proteinase. Biochem Biophys Acta 483:386, 1977.

Stastny P, Rosenthal M, Andreis M, Ziff M: Lymphokines in the rheumatoid joint. Arthritis Rheum 18:237, 1975.

Stecker RM: Heberden's nodes. N Engl J Med 222:300, 1940.

Steinberg J, Sledge CB, Noble J, Stirrat CR: A tissue culture model of cartilage breakdown in rheumatoid arthritis. Biochem J 180:403, 1979.

Stockwell RA: The cell density of human articular and costal cartilage. J Anat 101:753, 1967.

Stockwell RA: Structural and histochemical aspects of the pericellular environment in cartilage. Phil Trans R Soc Lond B 271:293, 1975.

Stockwell RA, Meachim G: The Chondrocytes. In Freeman MAR (ed): Adult Articular Cartilage, 2nd Edition. London, Pitman Publishing Co. Ltd., 1979, p 69.

Stockwell RA, Scott JE: Observation on the acid glycosaminoglycan content of the matrix of aging cartilage. Ann Rheum Dis 24:341, 1965.

Swann DA, Slayter HS, Silver FH: The molecular structure of lubricating glycoprotein I, the boundary lubricant for articular cartilage. J Biol Chem 256(11):5921, June, 1981.

Tanzer ML: Crosslinking of collagen. Science 180:561, 1973.

Teitz CC, Chrisman OD: The effect of salicylate and chloroquine on prostaglandin-induced articular damage in the rabbit knee. Clin Orthop 108:264, 1975.

Thompson RC, Robinson HJ: Articular cartilage matrix metabolism. J Bone Joint Surg 63A:327, 1981.

Trippel SB, Ehrlich MG, Lippiello L, Mankin HJ: Characterization of chondrocytes from bovine articular cartilage. J Bone Joint Surg 62A:816, 1980.

Vane JR: Inhibition of prostaglandin synthesis as a mechanism of action for aspirin-like drugs. Nature (New Biol) 231:232, 1971.

Videnian T, Michelsson JE, Raukamaki R, Langenskiold A: Changes in 35 Sulphate uptake in different tissues in the knee and hip regions of rabbits during immobilization. Acta Orthop Scand 47:290, 1976.

Volastro P, Malawista S, Chrisman OD: Chloroquine protective and destructive effects on injured rabbit cartilage in vivo. Clin Orthop 91:243, 1973.

VonKuhn R, Leppelmann JJ: Galaktosamin und gluocosamin im knorpel in abhangigkeit vom lebensalter. Liebig's Ann Chem 611:254, 1958.

Walker DG, Lapiere CM, Gross J: A collagenolytic factor in rat bone promoted by parathyroid extract. Biochem Biophys Res Commun 15:397, 1964.

Watson M: The suppression effect of indomethacin on articular cartilage. Rheumatol Rehabil 15:25, 1976.

Weightman BO, Freeman MAR, Swanson SAV: Fatigue of articular cartilage. Nature 244:303, 1973.

Weiss C: Light and Electron Microscopic Studies of Normal Articular Cartilage. In Simon, WH (ed): The Human Joint in Health and Disease. University of Pennsylvania Press, 1978.

Weiss C, Rosenberg L, Helfet AJ: An ultrastructural study of normal young adult human articular cartilage. J Bone Joint Surg 50A:663, 1968.

Weissmann G: Lysosomal mechanisms of tissue injury in arthritis. N Engl J Med 286:141, 1972.

Wiebkin OW, Muir H: Influence of the cells on the pericellular environment. Phil Trans R Soc Lond B 271:283, 1975.

Woessner JF Jr: Acid cathepsins of cartilage. In Bassett CAL (ed): Cartilage, Degradation and Repair. Washington DC., Natl Acad Sci, 1967, p 99.

Woo SLY, Akeson WH, Jemmott GF: Measurements of nonhomogenous, directional mechanical properties of articular cartilage in tension. J Biomech 9:785, 1976.

Woo JT, Ladenbauer-Bellis I-M, Fulkerson JP, Chrisman OD: Hexosamine depletion of articular cartilage slices by arachidonic acid. Trans Orthop Res Soc 5:5, 1980.

Wright V, Dowson D, Kerr: The structure of joints. IV. Articular cartilage. Int Rev Connect Tissue Res 6:109, 1973.

Young PC, Stack MT: Estrogen and glucocorticoid receptors in adult canine articular cartilage. Arthritis Rheum 25(5):568, 1982.

SUGGESTED READINGS

Freeman MAR: Adult Articular Cartilage. London, Pitman Publishing, 1979.

Hall BK: Cartilage vol. I, Structure, Function and Biochemistry. New York, Academic Press, 1983.

Simon WH: The Human Joint in Health and Disease. University of Pennsylvania Press, Philadelphia, 1978.

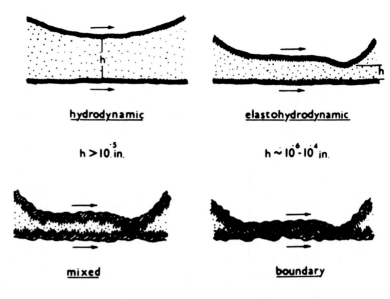

hydrodynamic

$h > 10^{-5}$ in.

elastohydrodynamic

$h \sim 10^{-6} \text{-} 10^{-4}$ in.

mixed

boundary

Typical dimensions of surface films

30 Å boundary lubricant molecule $(10^{-7}$ in.$)$

10-50 Å oxide layer $(0.2 \text{-} 2 \times 10^{-7}$ in.$)$

Figure 13-9. Dimensions of surface films for various kinds of lubrication. (*Reprinted courtesy American Society of Mechanical Engineers.*)

to the Royal Society, he stated "The synovial fluid is a proper fluid for the lubrication of joints." From the standpoint of understanding the precise mechanisms of joint lubrication, however, no significant advances were made until well into the twentieth century. In 1925, Benninghoff (who had earlier described the arcades of collagen fibers in cartilage) suggested that the elasticity of cartilage was perhaps due to the exudation and reabsorption of synovial fluid. This work apparently went unnoticed for many years.

In 1932, MacConaill noted the importance of engineering concepts in the understanding of joint lubrication. In considering the known principles of lubrication to joints such as the knee, he surmised that the geometry of the surfaces and viscosity of the lubricant lent themselves to a hydrodynamic type of lubrication.

Several years later, Jones (1934, 1936) experimentally measured the coefficient of friction of joints and found that it was quite low, of the order of 0.02 to 0.1. (More recent measurements have been in the range of 0.005 to 0.01.) The hydrodynamic theory was of some concern to Jones, owing to the fact that joints were not always in motion and did not reach the high velocities required for a hydrodynamic system. He recognized that joints at the start of motion were in contact, yet even in slow motion had a low coefficient of friction. Based on his studies of decay curves of joints that had been placed in swinging motion, he felt that joints were lubricated by mixed lubrication, i.e., a fluid film (hydrodynamic), during movement and solid friction or boundary lubrication at the starting and stopping points. However, he was not able to show that synovial fluid possessed the necessary "oiliness" required to satisfy the usual boundary conditions.

The next important observations were made on the lubricant rather than the mechanisms of lubrication. Karl Meyer and his associates reported in 1934 the isolation and chemical characterization of mucin from the vitreous humor of the anterior eye chamber and called the substance "hyaluronic acid" (Meyer, 1947). Ropes et al., in 1939, demonstrated that synovial fluid was essentially a dialysate of plasma with the addition of mucin (which had long been recognized as a constituent of synovial fluid). They, as others, felt that the mucin was responsible for the viscous nature and presumably lubricant qualities of synovial fluid. While they did not know its chemical composition, they suggested that the origin of mucin was either the connective tissue about the synovial membrane or the hyaline cartilage of the joint but favored the former explanation. Meyer, in the same year, isolated hyaluronic acid (mucin) from synovial fluid and suggested that it came from synovial cells (Meyer, 1947). While a controversy raged in the 1940s and early 1950s about the origin of hyaluronic acid, the chemical and physical nature of synovial fluid was well characterized during that time (Bauer et al., 1940; Ropes et al., 1940; Meyer, 1947; Gardner, 1952; Ogston and Stanier, 1953a, 1953b).

Since at least the time of Hunter, it seemed apparent that the lubricating properties of synovial fluid were related to its viscous nature. Ogston and Stanier (1953a, 1953b), in their studies on synovial fluid, concluded that a major function of the hyaluronic acid might be its contribution to joint lubrication. The thixotropic nature of the fluid seemed to substantiate that claim.

In the 1950s attention turned away from synovial fluid and back to the lubricating mechanisms. MacConaill (1950), who had first suggested the possibility of the hydrodynamic theory, began to doubt its validity as the sole mechanism responsible for the incredibly efficient joint lubrication system. Initially, he had not addressed the question of the relatively low velocities of moving joints. Nonetheless, he still felt that with the addition of such intra-articular structures as menisci and fat pads, converging wedges of lubricant could be developed at lower speeds and with the gliding and rotating movements of the joints. Gardner (1953) agreed with MacConaill on the importance of the hydrodynamic principles, but like Jones, importantly recognized that in certain situations conditions of boundary lubrication could exist.

John Charnley (1959), while looking for solutions to the failure of arthroplasties in the 1950s, began to study lubrication mechanisms. He proposed that boundary lubrication, rather than hydrodynamic lubrication, was the primary mechanism of the joint's efficiency, but he recognized (as did others) that the deformability of articular cartilage probably played an important role in the lubrication mechanism and that the mechanism was most likely complex (Charnley, 1960; Frost, 1960; White, 1963a, 1963b). The likelihood of boundary lubrication has been more recently suggested by Davis and his colleagues (1978), based on the fact that lubricating efficacy was independent of the synovial fluid viscosity, a feature consistent with most boundary lubrication theories.

The fact that basic engineering lubrication theories were controversial even among engineers had been almost ignored by those studying joints. By 1960, however, a number of workers recognized that the physical and chemical characteristics of the joint surfaces and lubricant were as important as the geometry and mechanical characteristics. This led to significant departures from previous approaches to explain the efficiency of joints.

RECENT OBSERVATIONS RELATIVE TO JOINT LUBRICATION

A recognition of the roles of cartilage and synovial fluid in joint lubrication as well as the availability of current technology has stimulated new interest and ideas. The transmission and scanning electron microscopes have provided insight into the ultrastructural characteristics of articular cartilage, and the general morphologic concepts are well accepted (Anderson, 1962; Weiss et al., 1968, 1975; McCall, 1969; Meachim and Roy, 1969; Muir et al., 1970; Clarke, 1971; Mow et al., 1974a, 1974b; Redler, 1974; Redler et al., 1975). Most investigators have subdivided the four zones (superficial, middle, deep, calcified) of articular cartilage in various ways (Fig. 13–10). The surface layer appears to be distinct from the remainder of the superficial zone, and this layer has perhaps received the greatest attention owing to its role in joint lubrication. Parallel ridges have been identified in many specimens (McCall, 1969; Clarke, 1971; Mow et al., 1974a; Redler, 1974) (Fig. 13–11). Whether these ridges represent parallel fibers is open to question. They may represent artifacts of fixation or preparation or may be a functionally important feature of the lubricating mechanism. Most authors agree that the superficial layer consists of tightly packed tangential colla-

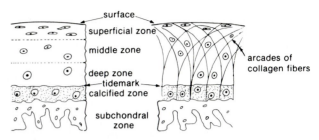

Figure 13–10. Articular cartilage—four zones on left, Benninghoff's model of collagen arcades on right.

gen fiber bundles. The fibers of the middle zone are more random in orientation, less closely packed, and larger than those in the superficial zone. The deep layer has fibers that have a more or less radial orientation (Fig. 13–12). This general morphology fits Benninghoff's description, although recent evidence suggests more random orientation of fibers than Benninghoff postulated (Torzilli, 1976).

The physical properties of cartilage are intimately related to its chemical composition. The superficial layer of articular cartilage contains little water or glycosaminoglycans (Muir et al., 1970; Lipshitz et al., 1975). There are increasing amounts of both in the middle and deep layers. The distribution of water is determined by the amount of polyanionic glycosaminoglycans and is probably not closely related to the distribution of collagen (Maroudas and Muir, 1970; Muir et al., 1970; Snowden and Maroudas, 1974). The flow of interstitial fluid, important in cartilage nutrition, is probably related to the distribution and character of the proteoglycan-water gel (Linn and Sokoloff, 1965; Jaffe et al., 1974; Maroudas, 1974; Mullholland, 1974). The movement of interstitial fluid with cartilage (i.e., permeability) is normally quite low (on the order of 10^{-13} cm^4/dyne-sec) and the permeability decreases with

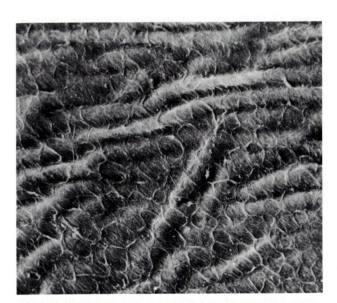

Figure 13–11. Surface of articular cartilage. Scanning electron microscopic view of cartilage showing parallel ridges. (*Courtesy of Dr. Redler.*)

continuation of the collagen fibrils of the epimysium, per-imysium, and endomysium into the tendon (see Fig. 14–1) and through interdigitation of muscle cell membranes with collagen fibrils at the boundary between the muscle cell and the tendon. The interdigitation of muscle cell and tendon looks much like interlocking fingers (Fig. 14–3) and transmits tension directly from the muscle cells to the tendon (Elliot, 1965). Collagen fibrils never enter the muscle cells, but lie adjacent to the basement membrane of the muscle cell (Mair and Tomé, 1972). The plasma membrane of muscle cells thickens at the muscle tendon junction and myofilaments extend directly into it. This thickened region of cell membrane corresponds to the terminal Z-line of the myofibril (Mair and Tomé, 1972).

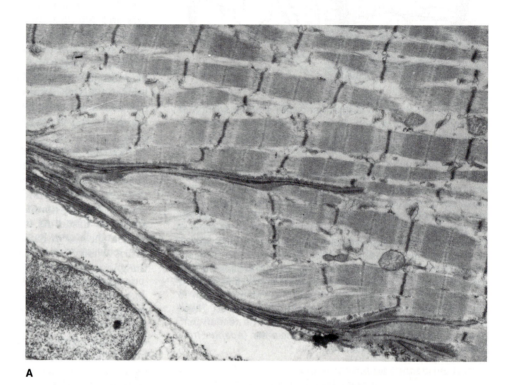

A

B

Figure 14–3. Electron micrographs of tendon attachment to muscle. **A.** A muscle cell approaching its tendon. The collagen fibrils lying on the surface of the cell and interdigitating with the cell continue into the tendon. (Original magnification × 10,000). **B.** Complex interdigitations between a muscle cell and the collagen fibrils at the attachment site of muscle and tendon. (Original magnification × 17,000).

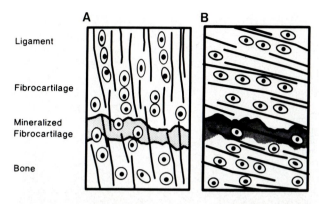

Ligament

Fibrocartilage

Mineralized
Fibrocartilage

Bone

Figure 14–4. Schematic diagrams illustrating the tendon, ligament, or capsular insertion into bone. Four zones can be identified: tendon or ligament, fibrocartilage, mineralized fibrocartilage, and bone. Although almost all insertions of tendon, ligament, and capsule pass through these zones, the angle of insertion varies. For example, in the medial collateral ligament of the knee the collagen fibrils of the femoral insertion make almost a 90-degree angle with the bone surface (**A**), while the collagen fibrils of the tibial insertion pass obliquely along the bone for a long distance and superficially may be continuous with the periosteum. **A.** A perpendicular insertion into bone. **B.** An oblique insertion into bone.

Tendon Insertions

At its other end, tendon inserts into bone (Fig. 14–4). This insertion presents a problem not found in the attachment of muscle to tendon: it must allow the transition from the flexible, pliable tendon to the rigid bone. This is accomplished by the tendon collagen fibrils passing through zones of increasing stiffness: tendon, fibrocartilage, mineralized fibrocartilage, and bone (Cooper and Misol, 1970). Ligament and capsular insertions follow a similar pattern.

As Clopton Havers reported in 1691 (Cooper and Misol, 1970), insertions vary in the obliquity of the angle between the collagen fibrils of the tendon, ligament or capsule, and the bone such that some of the dense fibrous tissues insert primarily into periosteum while others insert directly into bone (Figs. 14–4 and 14–5). The medial collateral ligament of the knee provides an example of this variability. The collagen fibrils of the proximal insertion penetrate the bone at an angle almost perpendicular to the bone surface while at the tibial insertion they pass obliquely along the bone, many of them continuing distally as part of the periosteum. Studies of ligament insertions suggest that these differences may affect the response of the insertion to loading and immobilization (Laros et al., 1971; Noyes et al., 1974a, 1974b).

CAPSULE AND LIGAMENT

Capsule and ligament have similar structures and functions. Like tendon, both of them consist primarily of highly oriented densely packed collagen fibrils but unlike tendon they more often assume the form of layered sheets or lamellae. The orientation of collagen fibrils that form adjacent lamellae may differ slightly but usually fibrils from one layer intertwine with those in adjacent layers binding one lamella to the next. Ligament and capsule both serve to attach adjacent bones across synovial joints and yet allow motion between the bones. They consist of a proximal bone insertion, the substance of the ligament or capsule, and the distal bone insertion (Fig. 14–6). In most instances they prevent excessive or abnormal joint motion yet allow a normal range of movement.

Muscles also stabilize joints but muscles cannot contract fast enough, either voluntarily or by tendon or ligament reflex, to stabilize a joint subjected to the sudden unexpected loads that might occur in sports or in accidents (Pope et al., 1979). However, muscles apparently can stabilize joints and protect the ligaments and capsule if the load is expected. Lewis and Shybut (1981) measured the forces in the knee collateral ligaments of dogs dropped from a height of 30 cm. They found that the ligament forces were less than when the dogs were walking, suggesting that the dogs anticipated the drop and absorbed the resulting force with the muscles crossing the joint. When the dogs walked or trotted, ligament forces were minimal. The greatest ligament forces occurred during tests of ligamentous laxity. Thus, during normal activity, muscle contractions and joint shape provide most of the joint stability. When the muscles are relaxed, ligaments, capsule, and joint shape are the primary restraints of excessive joint motion or joint displacement.

Joint Capsule

The joint capsule forms a dense fibrous cuff around a synovial joint. Synovial membrane lines the interior and loose areolar tissue covers the exterior. This loose tissue contains small vessels that supply the capsule similar to the arrangement between nonsheathed tendon and paratendon. Capsules may be reinforced by both tendons and articular ligaments. For example, the expansion of the semimembranosis tendon helps form the posterior oblique ligament of the knee and part of the knee joint capsule, and the medial collateral ligament of the knee lies closely applied to the knee joint capsule. Capsules may be penetrated by vessels and nerves and occasionally allow synovial protrusions.

Ligaments

Ligaments may be intracapsular, capsular or extracapsular. Intra-capsular ligaments like the cruciates of the knee or ligamentum teres of the hip can be easily identified as separate structures. Capsular ligaments represent thickening of capsular tissue and may be so closely applied to the capsule that they cannot be easily identified as discrete structures. Areolar connective tissue covers their exterior along with the joint capsule. Extracapsular ligaments such as the coracoacromial ligament, the coracoclavicular ligaments, or costoclavicular ligaments lie at some distance from a synovial joint. Yet, their function remains that of stabilizing the relationship between adjacent bones or reinforcing the stability of a joint.

tissue but the direction and that they modify their matrix in response to alterations in their mechanical environment.

INJURY AND REPAIR

Lacerations, tears, ruptures, and inflammatory swelling and weakening of the dense fibrous tissues cause especially difficult treatment problems. The disability caused by flexor tendon lacerations or ligamentous and capsular injuries to the ankle, knee, and shoulder frequently attracts attention. Injuries to the spinal ligaments, facet joint capsules, and annuli fibrosi can be as unstable as fractures and more difficult to diagnose and treat. In any site, injury of the specialized dense fibrous tissues initiates a response that can, under favorable circumstances, restore them to a functional state. Without this response even relatively minor injuries would produce severe disability and surgical procedures involving these tissues could not succeed. The repair response determines how soon a patient can resume normal activity after injury and whether injuries are best treated with immobilization, protected motion, surgical intervention, or a combination of these treatments.

Fractures heal by restoration of bone that remodels and eventually cannot be distinguished from normal bone. Currently available evidence indicates that no matter what treatment the physician elects, the skeletal fibrous tissues heal by scar formation rather than by restoration of normal tissue. The eventual result of scar tissue healing cannot be predicted. It can restore normal function but it also may restrict motion. Under some circumstances the scar tissue contracts and under others it may stretch. Optimal treatment of diseases and injuries of the dense fibrous tissue must not only restore their structure, but make the repair tissue assume the properties of normal tissue.

A variety of factors influence the ultimate result of an injury to dense fibrous tissue including the type, duration, and extent of injury; specific tissue type; type of surrounding tissue; type of treatment; medications such as steroids; and the age, general health, and nutritional status of the patient. Despite these variations, the injury response of dense fibrous tissue follows a sequence very similar to that found in other vascularized connective tissues (Mason and Shearon, 1932; Mason and Allen, 1941; Flynn and Graham, 1962; Potenza, 1962, 1964, 1975; Postacchini et al., 1978, 1980; Ross and Benditt, 1965; Clayton et al., 1968; Ketchum, 1977; Frank et al., 1985). This sequence consists of four overlapping phases: injury, inflammation, repair, and remodeling.

By damaging cells and matrix the injury initiates inflammation: the cellular and vascular response to injury that helps defend against infection and remove necrotic tissue. Repair begins during the inflammatory response and eventually fills the wound space with a collagenous matrix. Maturation or remodeling of this matrix occurs as the cells and matrix increasingly align themselves so that they resemble the uninjured tissue, the density of collagen increases, the collagen cross-linking increases, and the cel-

lularity, vascularity, and tissue edema decrease. Repair may be apparently complete within six weeks, but the remodeling process requires years and may never duplicate the original tissue.

The frequently investigated example of a lacerated or torn capsular ligament illustrates the injury and repair response in dense fibrous tissue (Miltner and Hu, 1933; Miltner et al., 1937; Jack, 1950; Clayton and Weir, 1959; O'Donoghue et al., 1961; Clayton et al., 1968; Frank et al., 1983; Frank et al., 1985).

The laceration or rupture kills cells, disrupts the collagenous matrix, and damages blood vessels. Cell death results in the release of a complex mixture of inflammatory mediators including histamine, kinins, and prostaglandins. The inflammatory mediators induce vascular dilation and increased vascular permeability that increases the exudation of fibrinogen and other macromolecules. Mediators also stimulate migration of inflammatory cells within vessels, migration of these cells from the vessels to the site of injury, and neovascularization. Vessel injury and disruption of the matrix exposes the clotting factors and platelets to collagen, activating the clotting mechanism, the complement and kinin systems, plasmin generation, and stimulating platelet degranulation. A hemorrhagic exudate fills the wound and within minutes forms a firm clot that seals the defect. The clot consists of fibrin, platelets, red cells, and cell and matrix debris. Fibrin not only provides a framework for fibroblast attachment and stretching but it may attract fibroblasts to the injury site and stimulate fibroblast proliferation (Graham et al., 1984). The presence of lymphocytes, platelets, and plasma also may increase fibroblast migration (Graham et al., 1984).

Within hours polymorphonuclear neutrophils and lymphocytes invade and populate the injury site. Monocytes follow them and become tissue macrophages. At the same time fibroblasts around the margins of the wound swell, assume irregular shapes with multiple cytoplasmic processes, and increase their volume of endoplasmic reticulum. These cells proliferate and begin to migrate into the defect spreading along the fibrin mesh of the clot.

Within 2 to 3 days following injury the cells at the site of the defect begin proliferating rapidly and synthesizing new collagen (Ross and Benditt, 1965). The uninjured tissue surrounding the defect becomes edematous as the vessels dilate and inflammatory cells appear. Simultaneously, endothelial cells of surrounding vessels enlarge and proliferate forming vascular buds that follow the course of the migratory fibroblasts. At this point, 2 to 3 days after injury, the ligament ends have retracted slightly and phagocytes release enzymes that begin to digest the exudate, the fibrin clot, and cell debris and allow resorption of this material. The clot attaches the ligament ends but slight tension will disrupt it. The vascular buds soon canalize to allow blood flow and may restore vascular connections across the laceration site within 3 to 4 days of injury.

By 7 to 10 days the normal ligament tissue surrounding the injury becomes more swollen, cellular, and vascular (Fig. 14–15). Within the defect, vascular granulation

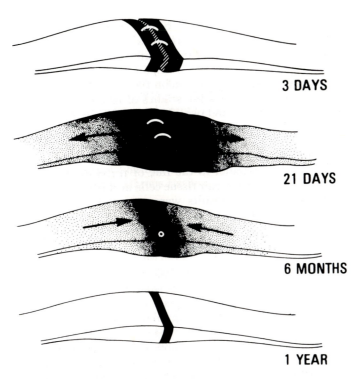

3 DAYS

21 DAYS

6 MONTHS

1 YEAR

Figure 14-15. Schematic drawing of ligament healing. Dark areas indicate regions of ligament damage, inflammation or scaring. At 3 days after injury and repair, sutures connect the damaged ligament ends. The area of inflammation and injury is sharply limited. By 21 days the ligament has swollen and the area of inflammation and edema has extended into the previously normal ligament and may involve the entire ligament from insertion to insertion. At 6 months the swelling and the scar mass have decreased. By 1 year the scar has contracted to a thin but distinct band with normal ligament on either side.

tissue fills the gap and now may be strong enough to unite the ligament ends. Many vessels now cross the defect. The population of active fibroblasts within the granulation tissue continues to increase as the density of inflammatory cells decreases. The granulation tissue will hold the ends of the ligament together but the edema and inflammation of the uninjured ligament ends weaken the ligament substance. These alterations may explain the clinically observed "softening," weakening, and retraction of the fibrous tissues that decrease the ability of the tissue to hold sutures under tension.

By 3 weeks following injury, the edema and increased cellularity extends throughout the uninjured portions of the ligament to its insertions as does the vascular dilation and increased vascularity. The wound remains extremely vascular and has considerably increased the mass of granulation tissue. Fibroblast proliferation achieves the maximum density of these cells. The new matrix and the cells appear poorly oriented relative to the collagen fibrils and cells on either side of the defect. At this point, the tensile strength of the repair tissue has increased considerably despite its appearance.

By 6 weeks following injury, the edema, cellularity,

and vascularity of the uninjured tissue decreases and within the injury site new collagen fibrils blend with the older fibrils. The new fibrils still lack a high degree of orientation but the strength of the repair tissue continues to increase.

Six months following injury the cellularity and vascularity of the repair tissue have decreased further. The fibroblasts demonstrate a greater degree of orientation relative to the cells on either side of the defect and they still synthesize new collagen.

At 1 year following injury, the cells still actively remodel the repair tissue although the cell density has declined. The cells and matrix show a higher degree of orientation and many of the small blood vessels have disappeared. The edema, vascularity, and cellularity of the uninjured ligament have returned to normal but the remodeling process at the injury site continues for at least another year.

Although the mature repair tissue looks much like the normal tissue it usually can be identified as scar tissue rather than normal ligament and it probably differs from normal tissue in composition, mechanical properties, and innervation. At present we have very little understanding of the significance of these differences but we appreciate that their clinical importance depends on the specific tissue injured and the functional demands placed on the repair tissue.

In the preceding example, the vascular response to injury and invasion of the laceration site by granulation tissue contributed significantly to the inflammation and repair following injury. Because of the limited vascularity and cellularity of the dense fibrous tissues some authors have assumed that these tissues, particularly tendons within sheaths, have limited intrinsic capacity for repair. Potenza (1975) stressed that sheathed digital flexor tendons heal " . . . by the reparative cellular response of the sheath and surrounding tissues and not by any intrinsic response of their own." Peacock (1976) indicated that "fibrocytes found in uninjured mature tendon apparently are end cells which have little capacity to divide or synthesize protein in amounts necessary to develop strong union between tendon ends" and therefore isolation of injured tendons from the surrounding tissues will result in failure of healing and may cause tendon necrosis. He stressed that wounds of skin, subcutaneous tissue, tendon, and other structures form a single wound container that fills with the products of the healing process.

The combination of the "one wound–one scar" concept and the apparent limitations of intrinsic tendon healing implied that injured tendons will necessarily adhere to surrounding structures as they heal and that these adhesions are an essential part of the healing process. Indeed, as described in the example of a ligament laceration, it appears that dense fibrous tissues under many circumstances depend primarily on the invasion of granulation tissue for their repair rather than on their own cells and vessels. This creates problems in tendon healing since the invading granulation tissue may bind the tendon to surrounding tissues, particularly if it is immobilized for a prolonged period of time (Duran and Houser, 1975). After the

The following general scheme of transmission at the NMJ is accepted by most neurobiologists. Depolarization of a presynaptic nerve terminal causes calcium to enter the terminal from the extracellular fluid, and somehow this leads to release of large numbers of transmitter molecules into the synaptic cleft, across which they diffuse to receptors on the postsynaptic membrane. Despite a great deal of effort in the last two decades, the precise reasons why release is calcium-dependent remain unknown. Calcium must be present in the extracellular fluid for release to occur. Any kind of depolarization will cause it to enter the cell; under normal circumstances the source of the depolarization is an action potential, but transmitter can be released equally well by depolarization induced experimentally by current passage or elevation of potassium concentration after the action potential mechanisms have been abolished. Calcium probably traverses the membrane through specific calcium conductances, which are denser on the terminal than on the axon leading to it. A plausible reason for the greater calcium conductance of this part of the cell is the need for calcium in the release process. At this point, however, uncertainties about the intimate nature of the process begin to proliferate. Calcium may not enter the cell exclusively through specific conductances of the kind involved in action potential generation; part of its entry may be carrier mediated. Only a fraction of the calcium that enters may be involved in the release process. That fracton may not have to go all the way through the membrane, only to some critical site within it. Finally, there is the still unsettled matter of what role synaptic vesicles play. Everyone agrees that transmitter release is quantal in the sense that transmitter molecules impinge upon the postsynaptic membrane in groups of perhaps 10,000, not one by one at random; this is observable by physiologic means and has been verified many times. Most neurobiologists, but not all, believe that the physiologically detected quanta are caused by the expelled contents of the vesicles, which can be seen clustered beneath the presynaptic membrane in electron micrographs. The doubters have their reasons (Cooper et al., 1982; Tauc, 1982). The most compelling ones are: (1) the turnover of vesicular acetylcholine is too slow to service release at the rates it is known to occur; (2) quantal release can be detected in embryonic chick cilliary ganglion before vesicles develop; and (3) sampling error and artifact severely compromise the ultastructural data. This is a classic problem in correlation of function with structure. The vesicles are at the site of the action, appear well suited for a function that cannot be simply explained without them, and have no other known function. But final demonstration that they in fact do what so much circumstantial evidence insists they should is a very difficult ultrastructural problem. Something rather close to it has been achieved for the NMJ, but even if the matter is settled there, the same controversy will go on for years over central transmission. The clinician who does not wish to follow the rather intricately technical arguments involved can safely assume for the time being that the vesicle theory is right, while remembering that the neurobiologists are still in contention over it.

The vesicle question is central to understanding the role of calcium in transmitter release. Most synaptic physiologists believe that the calcium that enters the terminal during depolarization somehow facilitates fusion of vesicles with the cell membrane, perhaps by neutralizing fixed negative charges on its inner surface. One is encouraged to visualize calcium ions traversing a specific conductance during depolarization to neutralize such charges, thereby removing an electrostatic barrier to the approximation of vesicle and membrane, which then fuse, expelling the vesicular contents into the synaptic cleft. The subsequent history of the spent vesicle is yet more speculative; too little direct evidence is available to force a choice among several recycling theories. Obviously, the residual uncertainties about vesicles limit the inferences that can be drawn about the role of calcium in transmitter release. There is no uncertainty about the calcium dependency of that process, only about the nature of the step in it for which calcium is critical. Studies of the effect of calcium concentration on release kinetics suggest that three to five calcium ions are associated with release of each (physiologic) quantum. The other cations of extracellular fluid—mainly sodium and magnesium—compete with calcium for access to the conductance mechanism by which it enters the cell; if elevated sufficiently, they can block calcium entry and therefore release. These facts are not in dispute; it is the intracellular part of the process that is incompletely understood.

Once released, transmitter molecules move by simple diffusion to the postsynaptic membrane, where their action on receptors can affect the follower cell in any of several ways. At the NMJ, acetylcholine causes channels in the end-plate (the postsynaptic side of the NMJ) to allow sodium and potassium to flow down their electrochemical gradients. Unlike the conductances responsible for nerve and muscle action potentials, the endplate channels are not sensitive to the transmembrane voltage; they conduct only as long as acetylcholine is present. They differ also in that both ions probably move through the same channels (in opposite directions) simultaneously. The result of the sodium–potassium current is a depolarization in the range of a few millivolts; it is proportional to the number of effective acetylcholine-receptor complexes and persists as long as they do. Acetylcholinesterase molecules located in the end-plate membrane terminate the end-plate current by splitting the transmitter into acetate and choline, both of which are reabsorbed by the pre- and postsynaptic cells and re-entered into various metabolic pathways, including that for transmitter synthesis.

These events at the NMJ are thought to be a typical example of excitatory postsynaptic potentials (EPSPs) are generated by a very similar process at a variety of other synapses in the autonomic and central nervous systems. A few additional principles are sufficient to give a general view of chemical synaptic transmission throughout the nervous system: (1) several substances besides acetylcholine are transmitters: amino acids and biogenic amines are the best established ones; (2) chemical transmission at some synapses opens postsynaptic channels not for sodium and potassium, but for potassium alone, chloride alone, or both together. The result is a hyperpolarization that reduces the likelihood that the postsynaptic cell will fire an action potential; it is called an inhibitory postsynaptic potential (IPSP); (3) rather than briefly opening normally closed channels, transmitters may reduce postsynaptic currents that flow steadily in the resting state; the result can be excitatory or inhibitory, depending on the kind of ionic currents that are affected; (4) transmitters may not affect postsynaptic conductances at all; there is evidence that in some cases they change the rate of metabolic processes in the postsynaptic membrane. The ultimate effect is still to excite or inhibit the postsynaptic cell, that is, to increase or reduce the likelihood that all the influences bearing upon it at a particular instant will bring it to threshold for action potential generation; (5) a single neuron releases the same transmitter at all its terminals (Dale's principle), but the postsynaptic effect is receptor dependent. Acetylcholine released by terminals of the same cell may cause EPSPs on one set of follower cells and IPSPs on another set; the same transmitter may act on conductances in some postsynaptic membranes and on metabolic processes in others.

Though based on a few briefly statable principles, chemical transmission among billions of neurons, many of them with thousands of transmitter-releasing terminals, is prominent among the reasons why the nervous system is the most densely complex tissue in the animal body. It is also a delicate process, susceptible to influence by drugs at concentrations that do not affect action potential mechanisms or energy metabolism. A number of muscle-relaxing agents used by anesthesiologists act by preventing transmission at the NMJ in any of several ways. Diazepam probably produces muscle relaxation by potentiating inhibitory transmission in the spinal cord. Strychnine causes convulsions by blocking glycine-mediated inhibition in the cord. Blockade of transmission mediated by biogenic amines is probably the basis for both the antipsychotic and parkinsonian effects of phenothiazines. Drugs that block transmission in autonomic ganglia are regularly used to control hypertension. Indeed, except for local anesthesia, clinical neuropharmacology is largely the pharmacology of chemical synaptic transmission.

Electrical Synapses

It is well established that some nerve cells communicate with each other by means of an electric current rather than an organic transmitter molecule (Bennett, 1977). The morphologic correlate of such transmission is a region in which the intercellular cleft between adjacent neurons is obliterated by electron-dense material. It is probable that the cells are connected by bridges of cytoplasm in these regions. The view held by most neurobiologists since the time of Ramon y Cajal regarding the discontinuity of neurons must be modified to this extent. When an action potential invades the membrane on one side of such a junction, some of the current it generates flows through the tiny cytoplasmic bridges and changes the membrane potential of the other cell. The change is usually a depolarization and an excitatory influence, but for complex reasons it can sometimes be inhibitory. Electrical syn-

apses are inherently bidirectional; information can pass from either cell to the other, so that either may be "presynaptic" at different times. Some electrical synapses rectify, meaning that they pass current only in one direction. This does not prevent information from flowing in both directions; it merely imposes a restriction on the kind of information that can flow in a particular direction. Thus, if one cell can depolarize another across a rectifying synapse, the second cell can only hyperpolarize the first; the direction of current flow is the same in both cases. At a nonrectifying synapse, either hyperpolarization or depolarization can spread from either cell to the other.

Electrical transmission is faster than the chemical kind, and it is not vulnerable to derangements of transmitter and receptor metabolism, but it is also less flexible. Both kinds exist in the mammalian nervous system; there is some possibility that the synapses between the afferent and efferent neurons of tendon jerk reflexes are electrical ones. In general, however, little is known about the distribution and function of electrical synapses in higher animals.

MUSCLE

The only aspect of muscle biology that will be covered here is excitation–contraction coupling; a comprehensive discussion of muscle appears in another chapter of this volume.

A decision by the central nervous system to contract the fibers of a motor unit invokes a chain of command consisting of a nerve action potential, transmission at the NMJ, spread of an action potential from the end-plate region of the muscle cell along its plasma membrane (known as the sacroplasmic membrane in muscle), and triggering of the contraction process by the muscle action potential (Constantin, 1977; Gergely, 1981). The basis of excitability in vertebrate sarcoplasmic membranes is an action potential mechanism much like that described in the section on nerve. It is started on the electrically excitable membrane surrounding the chemosensitive but electrically excitable membrane surrounding the chemosensitive but electrically inexcitable end-plate by currents flowing through end-plate channels caused to conduct by acetylcholine.

In order to understand the first link in the chain—excitation–contraction coupling—it is necessary to appreciate certain features of the ultrastructural anatomy of the muscle cell. Figure 16–5B depicts these features schematically. The basic functional unit of a muscle cell is the sarcomere, many of which are joined end to end to form a single myofibril. Each muscle cell contains 1000 or so myofibrils lying side by side. Dispersed among the myofibrils in a regular pattern is the sarcoplasmic reticulum, an extensive system of membranes of generally tubular form that is homologous with the endoplasmic reticulum of other cells and is the main site of calcium sequestration within muscle. The anatomic feature most closely related to excitation–contraction coupling is the T tubule system. T tubules are unique to muscle cells; they are tunnels that extend all the way through the cell and are continuous with the extracellular space at both ends. The fluid within them is essentially extracellular fluid, though its composition is probably altered by interaction of its constituents with the walls of the very narrow tubules. Inside the muscle cell, each T tubule is in close association with enlargements of the sarcoplasmic reticulum known as cisterns. The microstructure of the regions where T tubule and cistern membranes come close to each other is still uncertain. Some critical signal is passed from tubule to cistern at this point during excitation–contraction coupling, but neither its nature nor its mechanism is known.

Contraction occurs when the actin and myosin molecules interdigitated in the sarcomere move in relation to each other. The process by which they move involves an intricate series of biochemical events and is not thoroughly understood. The one unequivocally established step in the process is a brief rise in the concentration of sarcoplasmic free calcium from its resting level in the range of 0.1 micromolar to between 10 and 100 micromolar. Some calcium comes in through the sarcoplasmic membrane during the action potential—which is to say that the muscle action potential is in part a calcium spike—but most of the rise is caused by release of calcium sequestered in the sarcoplasmic reticular system. All the steps in the release process are not known; the action potential spreads from the sarcoplasmic membrane into the interior of the muscle cell along the membranes of the T tubule system and somehow triggers calcium release from the closely approximated cisterns. An obvious adaptive advantage of this is that the rise in free calcium concentration is as evenly distributed throughout the muscle as the T tubule–sarcoplasmic reticular system is. If contraction depended on the calcium that enters through the sarcoplasmic membrane, myofibrils near that membrane would contract sooner than the ones in the interior of the cell; the time required for a muscle to develop full power would be considerably prolonged, and animals could not move as fast as they do. In fact, no part of any sarcomere is more than 2 microns from an abundant supply of releasable calcium.

As soon as the large pulse of calcium required for contraction is released, energy-consuming ion pumps in the membranes of the sarcoplasmic reticulum begin to resequester it. The cell may be called on to contract again before the free calcium concentration has been reduced to its resting level. The calcium released in a new pulse is additive with whatever is left from the previous one; if this results in a significantly higher peak concentration of free calcium, the second contraction will develop more power than the first one did. This potentiating mechanism is the principal reason why sustained contractions can be more forceful than brief ones.

COMPOUND PERIPHERAL NERVES

Some communication between the central nervous system and the rest of the body is mediated by hormones and other blood-borne substances, but most of it travels over nerve fibers, as does all communication with the outside world. Peripheral nerves are simply collections of nerve fibers that handle the information flow necessary for normal function of the body part they innervate. Most of what we know about peripheral neurophysiology would not preclude single axons from running separately to their destinations or from being formed into sheets rather than cables. Their cable grouping, however, permits closely approximated fibers to interact in ways we are only beginning to understand; these may figure in the pathophysiology of clinical phenomena such as causalgia, phantom limb sensations, and certain kinds of fasciculations. Cable grouping is also of considerable practical importance in that it confers upon many different kinds of nerve fibers a common vascular supply; common susceptibility to local mechanical, thermal, and metabolic conditions; and an anatomic identity apparent to the naked eye at surgery.

Anatomy

Figure 16–2 is a schematic representation of the principal anatomic features of peripheral nerves (Thomas and Olsson, 1975; Sunderland, 1978; Dyck et al., 1982). The epineurium is fairly loose connective tissue that does not attach itself firmly to adjacent structures; the mobility of nerve is limited only by the tethering effect of its branches and blood vessels. The nerve-fiber population is divided into fascicles bounded by perineurium. There is a great deal of rearrangement of fascicular structure in the longitudinal dimension; cross-sections of nerve only a millimeter or two apart usually have quite different fascicular patterns. Fibers destined to leave the main nerve in the same branch are concentrated in the same fascicle or in adjacent ones well before the branch point. Apart from this, the functional significance of abundant fascicular rearrangement is not known.

The perineurium, which surrounds fascicles, is quite a different kind of structure from epineurium. It is composed of connective tissue elements mixed with concentric lamellae of flattened polygonal cells. It has been demonstrated to be the main barrier to diffusion of many different kinds of substances through nerve. Electron micrographs show "tight junctions" obliterating the extracellular space between some of the polygonal cells, endocytotic vesicles within them suggesting a transport function, and basement membranes on both surfaces of the cellular lamellae. Such morphologic features are characteristic of tissues that separate metabolically distinct compartments. Tracer studies and electron microscopy also indicate that vascular premeability inside the perineurium is sharply limited compared to all other tissues except the central nervous system (Olsson, 1975). A system like the blood–brain barrier unquestionably exists in peripheral nerves, but our understanding of both its normal and its pathologic functions is still primitive.

Intrafascicular connective tissue is called endoneurium. It is composed principally of fibroblasts and collagen that invest axons and their associated Schwann cells and are usually separated from them by basal laminae. Each myelinated fiber occupies a tubule formed of endoneurium; several unmyelinated fibers enveloped by the same chain of Schwann cells may be found in one endoneurial tubule, as shown in Figure 16–2. When nerves are damaged, the endoneurial tubules do not degenerate, as axons and myelin do; filled with proliferated Schwann cells, they remain available for entry by regenerating axons.

The outstanding features of the vascular anatomy of peripheral nerve are the limited permeability already mentioned and the richness of anastamoses in the longitudinal direction. Because of the latter, nerves can be entirely freed from surrounding tissues for lengths up to several centimeters without losing their functional capabilities. What nerves cannot stand is pressure and stretching; these lead rapidly to functional deterioration, which eventually becomes irreversible and ends in physical degeneration if the pathologic condition is not relieved.

Physiology

Erlanger and Gasser (1937) set peripheral neurophysiology on its modern course when they demonstrated the tight and direct correlation between axon diameter and conduction velocity. This relationship gave physiologists a way of determining what part of the fiber population they were dealing with in the actual course of an experiment. Such information, together with degeneration studies, made possible the kind of empirical definition of peripheral nerve function represented by Table 16–2 and Figures 16–6 and 16–7. For fuller treatment of the subject than can be given here, the reader should consult Brinley (1980) and related sections of standard textbooks of neurophysiology. The largest and fastest fibers in most peripheral nerves are those that bring information about skeletal muscle tension and position to the central nervous system. Fibers of motoneurons to skeletal muscle are almost as large. The prominence of these kinds of fibers clearly reflects the adaptive utility of rapid, precise movement. Sensory information from skin and viscera travels centralward less rapidly and generally in less precise form. Motor fibers to

smooth muscle and glands are small and slow compared to motoneuron fibers.

The segmental portions of the skeletal muscle control system are diagrammed in Figure 16–6. A central component is the motoneuron innervating the agonist muscle. The terminals of such a neuron actually innervate from 12 individual muscle fibers in an extraocular muscle to as many as 2000 in a large leg muscle; all the muscle fibers of a motor unit are usually in the same muscle. The motoneuron must fire if a motor unit is to contract, no matter what the source of the request for contraction; hence its designation as the "final common pathway" for movement. The two best appreciated sources are the muscle spindle and higher centers associated with voluntary movement. The latter is outside the scope of this chapter. The operation of the former is illustrated by the monosynaptic tendon reflex (Henneman, 1980). Its afferent limb is the Ia fiber in Figure 16–6. When the tendon of the agonist muscle is tapped, the muscle and the spindle within it are lengthened slightly. This excites the primary spindle receptor (the annulospiral ending of earlier terminology), which is the distal end of the Ia fiber. Volleys of action potentials traveling up many Ia fibers excite many motoneurons and the muscle contracts. The transmitter at the synapse between the Ia terminal and the motoneuron is not known; it is possible that the synapse is an electrical one. At the same time that the Ia volley excites motoneurons controlling its own muscle it inhibits those controlling the antagonists through a disynaptic pathway represented by the other branch of the Ia fiber in Figure 16–6. The mode of transmission to the inhibitory interneuron is unknown, but the interneuron itself almost surely releases glycine, which causes IPSPs on the motoneurons of the antagonist. Of course, the actual connections are very much more complicated than the diagram; for the simplest reflex several muscles, several segments of spinal cord, and many neurons are involved.

Most of the business of the segmental reflex arc in

TABLE 16–2. SUMMARY OF FIBER TYPES FOUND IN MIXED PERIPHERAL NERVES

Types*		Diameter (microns)	Conduction Velocity (m/sec)	Function	
				Motor	Sensory
A	alpha	12–22	72–120	Skeletal muscle	Muscle spindle primaries (annulospiral endings) (1a) Golgi tendon organs (1b)
	beta	5–12	36–72		Muscle spindle secondaries (flower spray endings), touch, pressure, vibration (II)
	gamma	2–8	12–48	Muscle spindles	
	delta	2–5	6–36		"Fast" pain, temperature (III)
B		<3	3–15	Preganglionic autonomic	
C		<1.3	<2	Postganglionic autonomic	"Slow" pain, temperature, crude touch (IV)

*The letter designations are based on electrophysiological measurement of conduction velocity; Roman numerals in parentheses at right show correspondance to a separate sensory fiber classification system based on both size and origin. A and B fibers are myelinated; C fibers are unmyelinated.

(Modified from Brinley FJ: Excitation and conduction in nerve fibers. In Mountcastle VB (ed): Medical Physiology. St. Louis, Mosby, 1980, with permission.)

(Krumbhaar, 1937). Galen exerted great influence during the Middle Ages and Renaissance. During this time, suppuration was considered to be such a natural part of body healing that efforts were made to induce it if it were not already present.

Most of the concepts that are now held on inflammation were the results of work done within the last 150 years. Virchow thought that the primary cause of inflammation was an excessive intake by cells of liquid nutrients filtering through the blood vessel wall. This ultimately resulted in cloudy swelling and degeneration (Rocha e Silva, 1978). Connheim concluded that inflammation was primarily due to lesions of blood vessel walls. This would permit leakage of all the components of blood including cells (Silverstein, 1968). Metchnikoff, in 1892, found that phagocytes could enter areas far from blood vessels. Indeed, by studying primitive intervertebrates without blood vessels, Metchnikoff emphasized the role of phagocytes in inflammation. He further emphasized the defensive role of inflammation and stressed that this was sometimes beneficial to the organism (Silverstein, 1968).

The next advance was made in the 1930s by Menkin, who proposed that many of the clinical and morphologic changes in inflammation were caused by endogenous substances called mediators (Spector and Willoughby, 1968). Menkin, Spector, and Willoughby were responsible for the broad outline of the modern concept of inflammation as a somewhat stereotyped response of the organism to a wide range of foreign irritants. Furthermore, it was realized by the middle of the twentieth century that many of the stereotyped clinical and pathologic features of inflammation were caused by endogenous substances (mediators and cells). The specific aspect of the inflammatory response was realized to be the province of the recognition (immune) system. Certain responses could only be triggered by specific foreign substances (antigens), but once triggered, the response was stereotyped.

PATHOPHYSIOLOGY

Chronic inflammatory joint disease is the clinical manifestation of inflammation that is of most interest to the orthopaedic surgeon. The normal joint has a synovial cavity lined by a synovial membrane. This membrane has a layer of lining cells, one to two cells thick covering a loose meshwork of connective tissue. At the reflection of the synovial membrane, the cartilaginous surface of the bone is found. The cartilage is made up of a ground substance that contains mucopolysaccharides, collagen, and cells known as chondrocytes. In human bone, there are the ground substance, collagen, mineral phase, and the bone cells known as osteocytes.

The acutely inflamed joint at the gross level is red, warm, and swollen, and on x-ray, at this stage, it shows only soft-tissue swelling and perhaps some para-articular osteoporosis. At a microscopic level, one sees an increase in tissue fluid leaking from permeable blood vessels and a variable number of acute inflammatory cells (Movat, 1972; Cotran and Majno, 1964). The chronically inflamed joint is warm, red, and swollen but also shows signs of tissue destruction such as instability and deformity. Radiographically, one sees in addition to soft-tissue changes, the characteristic erosions. At a microscopic level, one sees in the synovial fluid a large number of neutrophils. In the rheumatoid synovium, one sees hypertrophy and proliferation of the lining cells and a large number of chronic inflammatory cells such as macrophages and lymphocytes. In addition, there is destruction and not just disorganization of normal structures; hence, any explanation of inflammation must account for all these changes.

Any explanation of chronic inflammation must account for two things. First, it should define those mechanisms responsible for the persistence of the response. Second, it should explain the mechanisms of tissue destruction. The mechanisms of persistence of inflammation is easy to understand when the initial stimulus persists in the tissue. An example of this is chronic osteomyelitis. Here, a viable bacterium persists in the tissue and stimulates an inflammatory response. Another example is a foreign body reaction that produces a chronic granuloma (Spector, 1974). Less easy to understand is the chronic inflammation seen in diseases of unknown cause such as rheumatoid arthritis. The presence of certain abnormal immunoglobulins in a high percentage of patients with rheumatoid arthritis, and the presence of inflamed tissues and large numbers of lymphocytes, cells known to be involved in the immune response, have led to the strong suspicion that the immune system is involved in the pathogenesis of this disease. If the immune system is involved, it must be activated in response to something. For a long time there was speculation that a microbial antigen persisted in some form in the tissues of patients with rheumatoid arthritis; however, it is now thought that although a microbe could trigger the initial response, an inappropriate response to self-antigen is responsible for the chronicity of the response.

The second task is to explain the mechanism of tissue destruction seen in chronic inflammation. The death of cells, the destruction of the extracellular matrix with the dissolution of the mineral phase, and digestion of collagen, elastin fibers, and ground substance must all be explained. Cell death usually follows loss of integrity of cell membranes, and here endogenous inflammatory body systems, complement, certain enzymes contained in the phagocytes, and substances produced by lymphocytes play their part. The digestion of collagen, elastin, and ground substance is usually accomplished by enzymes produced by phagocytes, synovial cells, and perhaps chondrocytes (Ryan and Majno, 1977).

MEDIATORS

A mediator is an endogenous substance that produces some or all of the manifestations of inflammation. Any substance proposed as a mediator must fulfill several criteria. First, the substance should be demonstrably present when the effect is present and absent when the effect is absent. Second, the substance should be able to produce the effect for which it is held responsible. Third, the administration of specific antagonists to the mediator should lead to a diminution of that aspect of the inflammatory response for which the mediator is deemed responsible. Fourth, depletion of the experimental preparation of the mediator (by specific substances that destroy or deplete it) should likewise lead to a decrease of that aspect of the inflammatory response for which the mediator is deemed responsible (Spector and Willoughby, 1968). Few of the proposed mediators fulfill all of these criteria.

Some of the mediators are normally in the fluid phase, although usually in an inactive or precursor form; however, some of the mediators are produced by and contained in cells either in the circulation or at the site of tissue inflammation.

The cells of the acute and chronic inflammatory response have several important roles. They are ultimately the source of many of the mediators of inflammation. Proliferation of these cells contributes to the swelling and instability of chronically inflamed joints. Interaction among cells modulates the immune response in both a positive and negative way. One of the most exciting developments of research on rheumatoid arthritis has been the elucidation of the interaction among several different cell types in rheumatoid pannus. This interaction is very important in the destruction of joints.

Control of the inflammatory response is of great importance. Although a good deal of the inflammatory response is produced by endogenous substances and cells, inflammation does not occur continuously in normal people. We must explain how substances and cells that are native to the body are held in check until they are needed. The activities of mediators can be controlled in several ways. First, the substances could be preformed and active but enclosed within granules inside of the cells (e.g., histamine, serotonin and lysosomal enzymes). Second, the substance could be circulating in the blood in an inactive form and activated on demand (e.g., the complement system, the kinin-forming system, and the coagulation and plasmin system). Third, the substances could be formed at the time of inflammation (e.g., prostaglandins, lymphokines, and monokines). Fourth, preformed or induced inhibitors could limit the activity of mediators. And finally, the level of certain simple chemicals known as cyclic nucleotides could be important in providing a "set point" against which stimuli of inflammation can act (Goldberg, 1974).

The control of the cellular response of inflammation is equally complex. During the inflammatory response, normal cells are induced to participate. The changes that occur when a normal cell is induced to become a part of the inflammatory response include the expression of new substances on cell membranes that act as receptors and antigens, enhancement of secretion of various substances, and quite fundamental and irreversible functional and morphologic changes in the cell itself.

The following section examines the individual mediators and the contribution of various cells. Some of the cell-derived mediators are discussed under the heading of their respective cells. Next, the discussion focuses on three disease processes in which endogenous inflammatory systems play an important role. These are hives, rheumatoid arthritis, and gout. Finally, the chapter concludes with a discussion of the mechanism of action of various anti-inflammatory drugs.

The mediators histamine, serotonin, the mixture of leukotrienes known as slow-reacting substances of anaphylaxis, and eosinophilic chemotactic factors will be discussed here. These are the products of cells or platelets, but unlike other cell products, these are released into the systemic circulation and have a general effect.

Histamine

Histamine is a substance that has been implicated in playing a direct and contributory role in several forms of the inflammatory response. Histamine in humans is found in the central nervous system, in the oxyntic cells of the stomach, and most important for our purposes, in the granules of circulating basophils and in tissue mast cells (Beaven, 1976). Histamine can be released from the granules of these cells by a number of mechanisms. Probably the most familiar is that circumstance in which antigen reacts with IgE antibody bound to the cell membrane. In addition, histamine can be liberated by a number of nonimmunologic stimuli including trauma, radiation, heat, trypsin (Uvnas, 1969), and anaphylatoxins (C5a and C3a) (Levy, 1974). As will be apparent later, the last mechanism mentioned may be important in the early stages of immune complex–induced inflammation.

Exogenous histamine can reproduce many of the signs of inflammation. In experimental systems, it has been shown to mediate the early increase in vascular permeability caused by separation between the endothelial cells of the postcapillary venules (Majno et al., 1969). In addition, it causes dilatation of small blood vessels, contraction of smooth muscle, and stimulation of secretion from exocrine glands (Levy, 1974).

There is evidence in experimental animals and humans that histamine levels in tissue, fluid, or lymph are increased in association with various forms of inflammation (Lichtenstein and Gillespie, 1972). Furthermore, early portions of some experimental inflammatory reactions are decreased by antihistamines and by substances that deplete the tissue of histamine.

Hence, histamine fulfills all the criteria demanded of a mediator; however, there are important effects, for instance, chemotaxis, that are not produced by histamine. Furthermore, even those effects that are mediated by histamine eventually show tachyphylaxis. In addition, the amount of histamine in granules is limited. It is most likely that histamine has an important role primarily in acute inflammation, such as that of allergic rhinitis and hives. Its pathogenic role in more chronic inflammation is not clear and is probably more complex. In such cases, histamine may be important in causing an early increase in vascular permeability, which may allow deposition of mined. Animal experiments, however, have demonstrated that exposure to an antigen, even in small amounts, during fetal life or the neonatal period may induce a state of immunologic unresponsiveness to that specific foreign antigen. This phenomenon is referred to as *tolerance* (or acquired neonatal immunologic tolerance) and can be maintained throughout adult life by periodic exposure of the individual to small quantities of the same antigen. The failure or inability of an individual to respond to self-antigens is called natural tolerance.

Immunologic Paralysis

A state of tolerance can also be produced in adults under specific circumstances. This usually requires exposure to large quantities of antigen, and the ensuing lack of responsiveness is termed *immunologic paralysis*. It is most easily produced during times of generally reduced immunologic responsiveness (such as during immunosuppressive therapy), and it also may be maintained by repeated exposure to small amounts of the antigen. The ability to induce tolerance depends upon genetic factors of the host, the nature of the antigenic material, and the route of administration. The mechanisms of neonatal tolerance and immunologic paralysis will not be discussed here, but they appear to be similar.

Autoimmunity

Occasionally the system of self-recognition appears to break down, and antibodies are formed against self-antigens. Examples of antibodies to native proteins include those directed at antihemophilic globulin, thyroid tissue (Hashimoto's disease), α-globulin (rheumatoid factor), and antinuclear factor (lupus erythematosus). Although the actual mechanisms by which autoimmunity is induced remain obscure, several possible modes have been suggested. First, exogenous influences (microorganisms, drugs, radiation) may alter native structures sufficiently to make the body recognize them as foreign. If the change is great, the immune reaction is directed at the aberrant structure and is unlikely to result in antibodies that will cross-react with normal tissues. If, on the other hand, the change is subtle, the induced response may result in antibodies that cross-react with normal tissues. Second, autoantibodies may appear if an exogenous foreign material is introduced that is similar enough to a native structure so that antibodies directed against the foreign material will also cross-react with normal tissues. Third, normal antigens may become sequestered during life, and the continuous antigenic stimulus needed to maintain a state of neonatal tolerance is absent. Reappearance of the antigen at a later date may then result in an immune response. Articular chondrocytes are, for example, normally embedded in an avascular matrix and sequestered from both afferent and efferent arms of the immune response. Breakdown of the matrix may, among other things, expose these self-antigens to an immune system no longer tolerant of them. Fourth, unlike the previous mechanisms that are based upon antigenic abnormalities, a defect in the immune system itself may occur that leads to an increased state of responsiveness to native structures with

the production of autoantibodies. Similarly, an imbalance in normal regulation of the immune response may be at fault. Loss of suppressor T-cell function may, for example, result in the development of autoimmune responses.

Enhancement

Enhancement refers to the prolongation of allograft survival mediated by graft-specific host antibodies. It appears that humoral antibodies or antigen–antibody complexes may interfere with the expression of cell-mediated cytotoxicity by influencing the afferent or, more likely, the efferent limb of the immune response. Enhancement is specific in that antibodies mediating the phenomenon react specifically with graft antigens. *Blocking factors* are humoral antibodies capable of abrogating a specific cell-mediated response in vitro, generally described in relationship to tumor models, and may be indistinguishable from enhancement, which is defined by in vivo characteristics.

RELEVANCE OF IMMUNOLOGY TO ORTHOPAEDICS

Infections

The occurence, recognition, and treatment of infection is a practical and common problem for the orthopaedic surgeon. Individuals are constantly confronted by a wide variety of bacteria, fungi, and viruses, some of which are beneficial to the host, some merely innocuous, and others pathogenic. The clinical manifestations of infection are related to both the nature of the offending organism and the host's resistance to the etiologic agent. A knowledge of the immune response can help the physician plan preventative approaches and, where necessary, therapeutic direction aimed at reducing host morbidity.

Microorganism Factors of Significance. The virulence of different types of organisms varies tremendously. Under certain circumstances a single organism of one species may result in a fulminant disease with considerable morbidity and perhaps even mortality (*Pasteurella pestis*). Less virulent strains may fail to produce clinical disease even in high concentrations. In healthy individuals, staphylococcal organisms generally fail to produce a clinically significant infection with less than 10^6 organisms present in the wound. Microorganism characteristics such as the capsule of pneumococcus, the endotoxin of *Escherichia coli*, the powerful exotoxin of clostridial organisms, leukocidins (enzymes capable of impairing leukocyte function) produced by many staphylococcal and streptococcal species, and hyaluronidases of *Streptococcus pyogenes* are factors that favor virulence. Any factor that renders a microorganism less vulnerable to phagocytosis, renders it more resistant to intracellular digestion once ingested by a macrophage, or facilitates dissemination contributes to the noxious nature of the insult.

Host Factors of Significance. As previously mentioned, the nonspecific immune response involves increased vascular permeability, accumulation of a white cell infiltrate containing numerous phagocytic cells, ingestion, and finally digestion or degradation of the foreign material by the phagocytic cells. Interference with this sequence at any level results in diminished defense capabilities of the host. Numerous causes exist for decreased vascular responsiveness including aspirin, steroids (and other anti-inflammatory agents), vasopressors, shock, and occlusive vascular disease. Many factors also exist that can interfere with delivery of the inflammatory cell infiltrate to the site of infection and include the presence of necrotic tissue, foreign bodies, dead space filled with tissue fluid (seroma or hematoma), and anemia. Even in the presence of adequate vascular and cellular responses, abnormalities may exist in the phagocytic cells themselves, either in their ability to ingest or to successfully digest foreign material. In the complicated substructure of cellular metabolism, there exists the possibility of a multitude of genetically determined, developmental, or acquired defects in cell function. Regardless of the deficiency, the impaired response may be inadequate to handle the number of offending organisms that would fail to be pathogenic under more ideal circumstances.

Certain systemic ailments also predispose the individual to diminished immune defenses, especially chronic illnesses such as malnutrition, diabetes mellitus, adrenal insufficiency or hyperfunction, multiple vitamin deficiencies, and extremes of age (young and old).

Nonspecific proteins and enzymes exist that normally increase the effectiveness of the host's nonspecific response. These include natural antibodies, lysozymes, interferon (an antiviral protein), opsonins, and complement. Deficiencies of any of these agents will also result in a less effective response.

The list of primary (genetically determined) and secondary (acquired) immunologic deficiency diseases is extensive. Agammaglobulinemias, hypogammaglobulinemias, and dysgammaglobulinemias are diseases characterized by specific immunologic deficiencies that in turn are manifest clinically by inadequacies of host defense. Knowledge of the immune response and its defects makes the clinical symptoms and problems of patient management associated with these illnesses more understandable. An individual with hypogammaglobulinemia (Bruton's disease) is most deficient in immunoglobulin production but has essentially normal cell-mediated immunity. The clinical course is marked by recurrent pyogenic infections normally handled successfully by specific immunoglobulin responses. There is also a physiologic hypogammaglobulinemia of infancy that occurs when maternal antibodies decrease and before increased production of immunoglobulins by the child. This effect is most apparent in the form of frequent bacterial respiratory tract infections between 3 and 18 months of age. Conversely, a genetically determined deficiency of thymic origin (DiGeorges syndrome) results in frequent viral and fungal ailments.

Secondary immunologic deficiencies include those subsequent to renal disease, malignancies (including multiple myeloma, lymphomas, leukemias, Hodgkin's disease, or underlying malignancies completely unrelated to the reticuloendothelial system), viral infections (rubella, measles), and drug-induced immunosuppression.

Immunity or resistance to infection may be natural (nonspecific inflammatory response) or acquired, either actively (postinfection or immunization) or passively (transfer of humoral factors or cells from an appropriately sensitized host).

Diagnostic and therapeutic directions are of great interest but beyond the scope of this chapter. Needless to say, however, efforts at prevention of infectious disease should be of utmost concern, and the importance of routine immunization procedures must be brought to mind before leaving the subject of infections.

Arthritis and Autoimmune Disease

Autoimmune disease is characterized by an immune reaction directed against native proteins, resulting in injury to host tissues. Put another way, the host is no longer self-tolerant. The growing list of diseases that appear to include autoimmune mechanisms as part of their pathogenesis includes systemic lupus erythematous (SLE), polymyositis, scleroderma, Sjögren's disease, Hashimoto's thyroiditis, glomerulonephritis, and, of greatest significance to the orthopaedic surgeon, rheumatoid arthritis (RA). This discussion will be limited to rheumatoid arthritis, a systemic inflammatory disease of connective tissue manifest clinically by noninfectious inflammatory arthropathies.

Rheumatoid arthritis involves a characteristic synovitis and articular cartilage degradation mediated by nonspecific and specific effector mechanisms. The cellular infiltrate of rheumatoid synovium or pannus contains macrophages, Ia-positive T-cells, and leukocytes, clearly marking the site of an immune reaction. The serum and involved synovial tissues contain rheumatoid factor (IgM) complexed with IgG and IgG complexed with complement components (especially $C\bar{3}$ and $C\bar{4}$). Articular cartilage possesses several groups of potential antigens: chondrocytes, matrix components, and collagen. Active rheumatoid arthritis may be associated with a decreased level of synovial fluid complement, presumably because of local consumption, while serum complement is generally normal or slightly elevated.

The ongoing interaction between rheumatoid synovium and articular cartilage has been well documented clinically and involves some destruction mediated by direct contact but also includes effects by soluble mediators as well. The tissue damage (cartilage breakdown) may be mediated by complement activation subsequent to immune complex (antigen–antibody complexes) deposition in the affected tissues in and around the joint, lysozymal enzymes released by the characteristic inflammatory infiltrate, or both. A mononuclear cell factor (MCF) has been described that causes synoviocytes to release collagenase and prostaglandin E_2, a catabolinlike factor appears to cause local matrix degradation mediated through chondrocytes, and a third soluble factor, osteoclast-activating factor (OAF) may be responsible for the bony erosions characteristic of RA.

IgM and IgA levels are mildly elevated in active rheumatoid arthritis, and an antinuclear antibody (ANA) is found in 10 to 20 percent of patients with more severe forms of RA. The ANA of rheumatoid arthritis is IgM, in contrast to IgG in the case of SLE. The reason why the nuclear material to which this antibody is directed should be antigenic is unknown, but a similar situation is seen in SLE and a variety of other collagen diseases.

The etiology of rheumatoid arthritis is still unknown, but theories include one or more of the following points: (1) autoantibody production to host globulins, (2) an immune response to a microorganism resulting in antibodies that cross-react with native proteins, (3) the direct etiologic role of an exogenous agent such as a virus or other form of microorganism, and (4) a genetic predisposition to the disease combined with the presence of abnormal connective tissue. The most convincing evidence supporting an autoimmune aspect to this disease is the presence of rheumatoid factor, an IgM (or less frequently IgG) antibody to the Fc fragment of IgG. There are problems with this theory, however, including the fact that rheumatoid factor is absent in a small percentage of adults with rheumatoid arthritis as well as in most children with the same or a similar illness. Furthermore, rheumatoid factor alone will not duplicate the pathology in normal individuals, and it is found in a variety of diseases other than rheumatoid arthritis.

Drug Hypersensitivity

Most adverse reactions caused by drugs are not a reflection of an immune response but, rather, related to an exaggerated pharmacologic action of the drug or a metabolic abnormality present in the host. There are, however, many drugs commonly used by orthopaedic surgeons that have demonstrated their ability to evoke morbidity on a basis of a hypersensitivity response, and these include many antibiotics, anti-inflammatory drugs, sedatives, and anesthetic agents. Allergic manifestations in different individuals may vary with the same drug; penicillin, for example, may cause a constellation of signs and symptoms from urticaria to a bleeding diathesis and even anaphylactic shock. The intensity of the drug reaction will usually be dependent upon the dose and route of administration and degree of hypersensitivity of the individual patient. Oral medication generally causes less severe symptoms than intravenously administered ones.

Because most drugs are of relatively low molecular weight, they or their antigenic metabolites probably act as haptens in order to evoke an antibody response. Several metabolites of penicillin, especially benzylpenicilloyl (BPO), are antigenic when combined with larger serum proteins.

A large portion of allergic manifestations of drug hypersensitivity are reagin-mediated (IgE) cutaneous reactions (urticaria). Reagin or IgE specific for antigenic determinants related to the drug or its metabolites fixes to cutaneous tissues where an urticarial reaction follows. Immunoglobulins (usually IgG or IgM) that have a high affinity for specific tissues (or cells) may also be produced, and specific target tissues are subject to injury because antigen–antibody complexes are formed on their surfaces and the complement system is activated. Autoimmune mechanisms have also been implicated in hypersensitivity responses to certain drugs and, along with the other humoral mechanisms mentioned, appear to be responsible for pathology including hemolytic anemia, thrombocytopenia, neutropenia, glomerulonephritis, and hepatitis. Cell-mediated responses are responsible for allergic contact dermatitis and perhaps some forms of systemic drug reactions.

Serum sickness was originally described following injection of foreign serum (usually a horse-derived antitoxin) into a human. The use of human antitetanus immunoglobulin has markedly reduced the incidence of this disease, but the introduction of antilymphocyte serum, an immunosuppressive agent prepared by sensitizing an animal to human thymocytes, caused renewed interest in this problem. Clinically, the syndrome is characterized by varying degrees of urticaria, nephritis, myocarditis, and arthralgias.

There are no uniformly adequate tests for safely predicting drug hypersensitivity. A cutaneous test for penicillin allergy using a synthetic molecule (penicilloyl-polylysine) that is antigenically similar to BPO has an accuracy varying between 30 and 75 percent. The physician is left with a knowledge of the patient's past experience with the drug, a history indicating the individual's hypersensitivity to other agents, and a family history of allergies as a guide to therapy. A high index of suspicion and observation of the recipient for known patterns of hypersensitivity reactions for the particular drug offer a means of ensuring discontinuation of the offending agent at the earliest possible time and institution of appropriate supportive therapy, if necessary.

Transplantation

Transplantation of allografts offers many exciting therapeutic possibilities for a variety of traumatic, degenerative, and neoplastic diseases but is fraught with challenging problems. Attention will first be focused on blood transfusions, the most common and successful type of viable tissue transplant, and then the immunobiology of bone and cartilage allografts will be discussed.

Blood Transfusions. As in the case of drug reactions, adverse responses associated with blood transfusions may have an immunologic basis or may be unrelated to hypersensitivity. Immunologic responses during or following the administration of blood are usually due to plasma proteins or antigens associated with cellular components (such as the membrane-related antigens of erythrocytes, leukocytes, or platelets).

An allergic reaction to blood may be characterized by urticaria, pruritis, angioedema, arthralgia, and bronchospasm if the blood being transfused contains antigens to which the recipient is sensitive. Fever may reflect bacterial contamination (that may lead to septic shock), antibodies to leukocytes or platelets, pyrogens, or a major hemolytic reaction. Antibodies present in the recipient to incompatible transfused antigens or erythrocytes may result in complement activation, hemolysis, capillary plugging because of erythrocyte agglutination, a bleeding diathesis (disseminated intravascular coagulation), or sequestration of red cells with subsequent phagocytosis and cell lysis (in the spleen or liver).

Unlike the case with most other tissue allografts, histocompatibility or transplantation antigens play a relatively minor role in "blood graft" success or failure. HLA antigens, or their equivalent, are not expressed on the surface of erythrocytes that comprise the bulk of the usual blood transfusion, although they are strongly represented on leukocytes. The existence of blood group phenotypes (A, B, AB, and O) and their alloantigens (A, B, and H) has already been discussed, and these antigens, plus a small handful of additional blood group systems, constitute the most important consideration in matching blood for compatibility. One of these major blood group categories is the Rh antigen system, which involves approximately 30 distinct antigens; the most significant antigen is D, and its presence or absence is generally reflected by the statement Rh-positive (D) or Rh-negative (d).

Although prevention of transfusion reactions through careful crossmatching offers the most desirable solution, the need for treatment of adverse immunologic reactions still arises. If the infusion of incompatible blood is in progress when symptoms are first noted, then the transfusion should be terminated immediately. The need for antihistamines, epinephrine, or induced diuresis (for acute renal failure) remains, of course, commensurate with the presence and severity of specific transfusion-related signs and symptoms.

Tissue Transplantation. The field of tissue transplantation is one of the most spectacular and exciting areas of surgery. It brings the skills of the clinical surgeon and the laboratory scientist into a mutual spotlight. Surgical technology, however, appears to have exceeded the expertise of the immunologist in understanding graft rejection and ways to effectively deal with it. This gap has closed, somewhat, with the introduction of the immunosuppressant drug, Cyclosporin-A. It remains beyond the scope of this chapter to discuss the fascinating problems related to viable allografts of complex organs (e.g., kidney, liver, heart and lung) and tissues (including viable skin or marrow). This section will deal briefly with transplantation terminology and then review concepts related to bone and cartilage allograft antigenicity.

General Concepts. The earliest model for studying transplantation immunology in laboratory animals involved skin grafts. Grafts between genetically dissimilar individuals even of the same species (allografts) are routinely rejected within 10 to 14 days. This requires ingrowth of vascular channels followed by an inflammatory infiltrate composed of macrophages, lymphocytes, and plasma cells and eventually vascular occlusion and graft death. This pattern of response is termed a first-set, or primary, rejection and exemplifies a cell-mediated response. If a second skin graft is applied to the same recipient from the same or genetically similar donor, the rejection is accelerated,

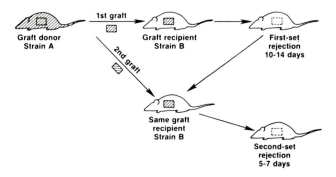

Figure 19-19. First-set and second-set skin-graft rejection.

usually requiring 5 to 7 days. This is called a second-set, or accelerated, rejection (Fig. 19–19). It occurs even if a different donor bed distant from the first site is used, emphasizing the systemic nature of the response. Transfer of viable lymphoid cells from an animal demonstrating a first-set response will result in a second-set reaction in a nonsensitized recipient if that second animal receives a primary graft from the same (or genetically similar) donor used to sensitize the lymphocyte donor (Fig. 19–20).

This again emphasizes the cellular basis of skin graft rejection. Humoral antibodies may also be detected following tissue or organ transplantation (blocking, helper, and cytotoxic antibodies), but their role in graft rejection is less clear and probably varies with the nature and timing of the particular graft and the animal model being used. Although accelerated graft rejection can be transferred by living cells and not serum, there does appear to be a soluble mediator of cell-mediated immunity. This substance, called transfer factor, is produced by immunocompetent cells, which, in certain animals and under certain circumstances, can transfer properties of cell-mediated immunity from one host to another.

It is apparent that privileged sites exist within the body where allograft acceptance is routine, most notably the anterior chamber or cornea of the eye. The lack of vascularity and lymphatic drainage to these areas may explain the unusual property. Certain tissues, such as collagen, appear to be immunologically privileged in that rejection is markedly delayed or nonexistent. The low order of collagen antigenicity is related to its relatively con-

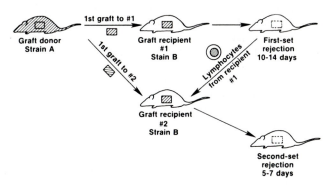

Figure 19-20. Passive transfer of cellular immunity.